— Dr. Jonathan V. Wright's —

TREASURY
OF
NATURAL
CURES

NUTRITION & HEALING

Additional orders and inquiries can be directed to *Nutrition & Healing*, Subscriber Services, P.O. Box 925, Frederick, MD 21705; tel. (443)353-4231, fax (410)558-6359.

All material in this publication is provided for information only and may not be construed as medical advice or instruction. No action should be taken based solely on the contents of this publication; instead, readers should consult appropriate health professionals on any matter relating to their health and well-being. The information and opinions provided in this publication are believed to be accurate and sound, based on the best judgment available to the authors, but readers who fail to consult with appropriate health authorities assume the risk of any injuries. The publisher is not responsible for errors or omissions. The material in this report has not been approved by the Food and Drug Administration. The products discussed are not intended to diagnose, treat, cure, or prevent any disease.

Cover image property of Jupiterimages Corporation.

600R011583

Table of Contents

Part X: Essential Health Secrets

Part I
Cancer

Chapter 1:

Toss your sunscreen and step out of the shadows! You can prevent skin cancer and still enjoy time in the sun this summer

As the days are getting longer, the weather is getting warmer, and the dermatologists and sunscreen salesmen are getting down to business with their annual chorus. Like the best of self-proclaimed "saviors," they threaten us with Skin Cancer Hell if we "sin" by exposing our bodies to the Great Sun Satan.

If some dermatologists had their way, we'd all dress like people in the Victorian era, covering up in ankle-length dresses and long pants whenever we're outdoors, carrying parasols and wearing gloves whenever sunshine threatens to come too close, and having just the smallest bit of skin peeking out whenever we go swimming.

And sunscreen salesmen would like nothing more than for us to believe the only way to avoid skin cancer is by slathering every inch of exposed skin with SPF 10,000 (or thereabouts).

Sometimes I wonder if they think that humans were originally an underground species, with skins not adapted to the rays of the sun. Or perhaps we're all originally from some planet further from the sun—Mars or Jupiter maybe—where the sun's rays are weaker?

For some reason that continues to perplex me, they seem to forget that the sun has been around for billions of years (probably more), and human beings date back quite a ways as well—existing in times where the only clothing came from scraps of animal skin and there was no such thing as sunscreen.

Anthropology vs. dermatology: Are we on the wrong planet?

Before attending medical school, I received my undergraduate "A.B." degree (in 1965, Harvard liked "A.B." instead of "B.A.") in anthropology. I still like to keep track of this field of research today. Knowing the history of the human race has given me a different (and sometimes unique) perspective on health care, including skin cancer prevention.

Anthropologists have determined that the earliest humans lived in Africa. The sun's intensity is much greater there, and people spent nearly all of their time outdoors wearing very little clothing. While it's likely that "early man" and "early woman" sought shade whenever the sun's heat was just too much, it's also likely that our remote ancestors got enormously more direct-skin sun exposure than we do now.

For hundreds of thousands of years, humans lived mostly outdoors, and, odds are, our skin is quite adapted to sun exposure—as long as we pay attention to the early twinges of sunburn.

And just to drive the point home, no anthropologist has ever reported finding anything even remotely resembling sunscreen along with the remains of prehistoric man, so let's move on and dispose of…

The sunscreen myth

You've probably seen pictures from the 1920s depicting women on the beach reveling in their newfound liberation by shedding inhibitions and what was, at the time, a shocking amount of clothing. Of course, we men joined in the fun, too—and bathing suit manufacturers saved a lot on cloth. Sunscreen use was rare in the '20s compared to the present, but the skin cancer rate was notably very low.

Sunscreen use has risen every decade since then, and the rate of skin cancer has risen right along with it! No, I'm not claiming that sunscreen *causes* skin cancer, but the data shows that sunscreen doesn't do a terribly good job of *preventing* skin cancer, either. So, if you want to prevent skin cancer, what do you do?

Could your diet lead to skin cancer?

Before we became "civilized," humans relied completely on whole foods. There were no processed or junk foods, no one added sugar to anything, and, of course, there were no food chemicals, herbicides, pesticides… you get the picture. As long as there was enough food to eat, nutrient deficiencies didn't exist except in areas of the world with specific soil mineral deficiencies. That's certainly not the case today! Nutritional deficiencies and "insufficiencies" (not an outright deficiency you could die from, but not enough to "get the job done" for all your body's needs, either) are absolutely rampant. Many of the most common deficiencies involve nutrients that can protect your skin from sun damage and cancer.

To sharply reduce your risk of skin cancer, what foods and specific nutrients are most important? The food list won't come as a surprise: Vegetables, nuts, beans, fish, eggs, and whole grains are first in line. Specific nutritional supplements include folic acid, vitamin A, vitamin B12, zinc, and vitamin C.

What do folic acid and your tax refund have in common?

Folic acid is destroyed rapidly by heat, cold, and exposure to light, including sunlight. So it's sunlight's destructive effect on folic acid in the skin, not the actual sun exposure itself, that accounts for a significant part of the skin cancer problem. Folic acid (along with vitamin B12 and zinc) is absolutely key to DNA reproduction and repair. When skin cell DNA is damaged by errant or excess sunshine, intracellular enzymes dependent on folic acid, vitamin B12, and zinc get right to work repairing the damage, and the skin cell is much less likely to become cancerous.

For decades, folic acid has been the No. 1 dietary vitamin deficiency. If folic acid levels are low to begin with, sunshine can make the situation even worse. It's no wonder skin cancer rates have risen in response. By supplementing with the right amount of folic acid, you can ensure that your body has enough to offset the amount destroyed by the sun.

Just a few years ago, after considerable arm twisting, criticism from other government agencies, and congressional pressure, the FDA reluctantly mandated folic acid "enrichment" of certain foods. Unfortunately, food "enrichment" is much like your tax refund—a few dollars given back each year to make you feel better about forking over a big chunk of every paycheck to the government: It's enough to quiet most complaints, but not enough to do much good. So folic acid still competes with essential fatty acids for the No. 1 spot on the vitamin deficiency list. And folic acid deficiency and insufficiency is a major contributor to skin cancer risk.

At the risk of sounding like your mother, I'll tell you once again: Eat your vegetables! It really is the best way to ensure that you get adequate folic acid to reduce your risk of skin cancer. Spinach and other deep green vegetables are particularly good sources. Other good food sources of folic acid include brewer's yeast (it's actually the best source), beans (especially lima beans), cantaloupe, watermelon, and wheat germ. Liver is a good source, too, but it *must* be from entirely organically raised animals.

Even if you already eat the foods listed above, it's a good idea to take a folic acid supplement too. Use at least 1 milligram (1,000 micrograms) daily, more if you like to be out in the sun or have a family history of skin cancer. Unfortunately, you won't find folic acid supplements in

1,000 microgram quantities because our "guardians" at the FDA limit the amount that can be put into one tablet to 800 micrograms. But there have been no recorded folic acid overdoses, so you can go ahead and take two or more 800-mcg tablets without worrying about taking too much—you can't!

Bringing vitamin A out of the shadows and into the light—literally!

Aside from seeing it listed on the label of your daily multivitamin/mineral combination, you probably don't spend a whole lot of time thinking or worrying about vitamin A. But vitamin A is a crucial element in the war against skin cancer.

Vitamin A is very similar to folic acid in its connection to skin cancer. Like folic acid, vitamin A assists with cellular repair and lack of this nutrient can result in the cellular damage dermatologists blame only on the sun's rays.

The protective metabolite of vitamin A is called retinoic acid. (When we take vitamin A, our body naturally metabolizes some of it into retinoic acid.) Researchers have reported that ultraviolet irradiation from the sun causes a major loss of retinoic acid receptors in skin cells.[1] But if levels of vitamin A are sufficient, more retinoic acid can be formed, which appears to protect retinoic acid receptors, and much of the "sun damage" is prevented. The bottom line: Skin cells can repair themselves better with sufficient retinoic acid, which is only possible with sufficient vitamin A. (Using retinoic acid itself is the very best way to use vitamin A to protect against sun damage, but it must be done carefully.

While vitamin A may not always catch your attention, I'm sure you've heard of carotenoids, especially beta-carotene. Carotenoids are vitamin A precursors: Your body must break them down to get vitamin A, and, unfortunately, like many other things, the older we get, the more this process slows down. So it's best to make sure you get some actual vitamin A, not just beta-carotene.

There are relatively few dietary sources of vitamin A as vitamin A itself (and not carotenoids). Eggs, liver (from organically raised animals only), and fish liver oils are the most widely available and healthful sources. Carotenoids are present in all yellow-orange and green vegetables, but don't rely on them for your entire vitamin A intake.

It's important to keep in mind that while it's nearly impossible to truly overdose on beta-carotene (although you can turn a very interesting carrot color if you take very large amounts), you can overdose on vitamin A itself, so you should be very careful about quantities. Symptoms of vitamin A overdose include headache, very dry skin, loss of hair at the outer edges of the eyebrows, and pain in the "long bones," just to note a few. Quantities up to 75,000 IU are generally safe, but you don't need to take quite that much for skin cancer prevention. To lower your risk of skin cancer, take 40,000 IU of vitamin A daily. (Don't be afraid of taking or eating extra carotenoids such as beta-carotene along with a vitamin A supplement. Even if your body already has enough vitamin A, extra carotene *will not* cause a vitamin A overdose.)

Do you have this risk factor for skin cancer? The answer might be written on your fingernails

Although zinc is a well-known supplement for a variety of skin conditions (eczema and acne are among the best known) its potential to reduce skin cancer risk is a well-kept secret, even among many skin cancer researchers. But if you remember zinc's critical role (along with folic acid and vitamin B12) in helping repair damaged DNA, it makes sense that zinc will help damaged skin cells restore themselves to health before the damage leads to cancer. And it also makes sense that if your body has a deficiency of this mineral, it won't have all the tools necessary to get the repair job done.

In the early 1960s, the USDA (the federal "agriculture department") published a map showing that 31 states had insufficient levels of zinc in their agricultural soils for optimal crop growth. The situation has only worsened in the 40 years or so since! You don't need me to tell you (but

I'll remind you anyway) that if there's not enough zinc in the soil for optimal crop growth, then there certainly won't be enough zinc in those crops to ensure optimal health in the people eating them.

My patients are usually surprised to learn that zinc deficiency is sometimes literally written on their bodies in what might seem like an unlikely place: The fingernails. Go ahead and take a look at your own fingernails right now. Do you see any little white spots? These are "zinc deficiency spots," first identified and publicized by Dr. Carl Pfeiffer. Zinc is most "used up" when a large mass of cells are rapidly growing and dividing, which happens to the greatest extent during puberty, so teenagers are particularly at risk for zinc deficiency and insufficiency. But unlike many of the other aspects of puberty, this isn't one that you can simply thank your lucky stars to be finished with. Zinc deficiency can happen at any age. And it's important to keep in mind that zinc deficiency or insufficiency more often occurs *without* the telltale "zinc spots," so even if you don't see any on your fingernails, you should still consider taking extra zinc as extra insurance against skin cancer.

The best food sources of zinc—by far—are oysters. I don't know about you, but I just haven't been able to develop a taste for these slithery mollusks, so I usually rely on herring and other seafood, eggs, liver (yes, organic only), and beef, which are all good zinc sources. The best vegetable sources of zinc include sunflower seeds, nuts, mushrooms, and whole grains.

Regardless of how many of the foods above you decide to incorporate into your diet, you should also take 25 to 30 milligrams of zinc (picolinate or citrate) in supplement form each day for the best chance of lowering your risk of skin cancer. To prevent zinc-induced copper deficiency, take 2 milligrams of copper along with the zinc. Many good multiple vitamin/mineral combinations already contain these amounts, and I recommend that all my patients take such a formula, so there may be no need to buy additional supplements. But check the quantities on the label of your multi to be sure.

Eating meat may reduce your skin cancer risk

The final member of the "DNA repair group" that can help you reduce the risk of skin cancer is vitamin B12. But do you get enough? I worry that many of my patients put themselves at significant risk for B12 deficiency by listening to the nutrition "experts" who advise eliminating most animal protein from the diet.

My concern lies in the fact that the vitamin B12 in our diets is almost exclusively from animal sources. Liver (organic) is far and away the best source, but other organ meats, regular cuts of meat in general, and seafood are good sources too. There are very, very few plant sources of B12 other than algae, chlorella, and spirulina. Don't get me wrong, I'm not arguing against vegetarian diets (they're actually best for some people), but if you follow such a diet, be very careful to take adequate amounts of vitamin B12 and iron.

While the possible lack of this nutrient in the diet is an important aspect to consider, it isn't the major problem with vitamin B12 nutrition. The biggest problem is with the digestion and absorption of the vitamin.

I know you've read this from me over and over, but hypochlorhydria, poor stomach function with inadequate production of hydrochloric acid and pepsin, (which happens increasingly with age) is such a common—and often ignored—problem that I feel it's necessary to remind you about it as often as I can. In this case, you need to know that hypochlorhydria is the major cause of vitamin B12 deficiency and insufficiency.

I could go on and on about this problem (and I have—in the September 2001 issue of *Nutrition & Healing*, as well as in the book *Why Stomach Acid Is Good For You*, which I co-authored along with Lane Lenard, Ph.D.). So, I won't write any more about it here but recommend that if you're over 40, have your stomach acid levels tested and take the necessary steps to correct any imbalances.

In the meantime, take at least 500 micrograms of vitamin B12 daily. You can do so worry-free, since, as with folic acid, it's nearly impossible to overdose.

Vitamin C: Stress relief for your skin

Even though our ancestors have genetically prepared us to handle exposure to sunlight, intense or prolonged exposure does impose a certain amount of extra stress on your skin. For most creatures, this isn't a problem because their bodies produce extra vitamin C naturally in response to any stress. So when they remain in the sun for long periods of time, the *internal* production of vitamin C is stepped up and it is then "rushed" to the skin to help prevent damage and repair any that may have already occurred. But humans are among the "select" few species to have a unique genetic defect that prevents our bodies from making vitamin C internally under any circumstances, stress or otherwise—so we must make sure we get adequate amounts from supplements and food sources like fruits and vegetables.

(Just a quick bit of trivia: We share our vitamin C defect with gorillas, monkeys, chimps, and other primates, which you may have guessed, since their internal makeup is very similar to ours. But I'll bet you never thought you shared a genetic link with guinea pigs! They're among the very few other species that have this internal shortcoming.)

If you know you're going to stress your skin with sunshine, make sure to take at least an extra gram of vitamin C twice daily—and more if you're on the beach in a tropical environment. (It's the least you can do for being lucky enough to go on such a getaway!)

Damage control and antioxidants

The word "antioxidant" is relatively new on the medical scene, but it describes nutrients that have been around forever. For example, all of the specific nutrients you've read about so far are antioxidants to one degree or another. I've always suspected that the "powers that be" in academic medicine coined the term and popularized it as the "latest breakthrough" in order to cover up their possible embarrassment at finally being forced to agree with all us "health food nuts" that vitamins, minerals, and other nutrients can prevent and treat disease.

But "antioxidant" has some actual meaning when describing a specific function these nutrients share: Slowing or preventing oxidative damage. One example of oxidative damage is the kind caused to your skin cells by excess or prolonged exposure to sunlight.

For this reason, other antioxidant nutrients have great potential for lowering your risk of skin cancer. First among these is vitamin E, but the list of potential skin-protective antioxidant nutrients is incredibly long. In addition to the specific recommendations made in this chapter look for a well-rounded antioxidant formula at your local natural food store or compounding pharmacy to lower your risk of skin cancer even further.

Giving the blessing to bask

Ignore the chorus of dermatologists who are undoubtedly good at many things they do but have forgotten that we belong on Earth, descended from tens of thousands of generations who never used sunscreen but rarely got skin cancer. Being in the sun is good for you! It's one of the places you, your children, and grandchildren belong! So, as long as you take the right dietary precautions and heed your skin's warning twinges of sunburn, go ahead and soak up some rays.

Chapter 2:

The cancer-fighting mineral you can't afford to ignore

If someone had predicted 30 years ago that iodine would become one of the most important breast cancer treatments, I doubt many people would have believed it. And they would have been right—it *isn't*. In fact, it's hardly used at all.

But it should be.

Iodine kills breast cancer cells without killing off normal cells in the process. In other words, it's ideal for both the treatment *and* prevention of breast cancer.

Chances are your doctor hasn't heard of this. (I'll tell you why in just a minute.) So if you want the treatment—and believe me, you should—it's up to you to share this information with your doctor.

Solid research conveniently ignored

In the 1960s and 70s, pioneering iodine researcher Benjamin Eskin, M.D., reported time and again that iodine is a key element in breast health. (At one time, I counted over 80 of his research papers on the topic.)

In one of his studies, Dr. Eskin demonstrated that deliberately block-ing breast cells from access to iodine resulted in precancerous changes—changes that were aggravated when those same cells were exposed to ei-ther estrogens or thyroid hormone. Surprisingly, in the absence of iodine, thyroid hormone appeared to be more likely than estrogen to produce abnormalities in breast cells.[1]

In another report, he noted that when breast tissue cells are lacking in iodine, the cells are more likely to be abnormal, precancerous, or cancer-ous. He said, "Iodine-deficient breast tissues are also more susceptible to carcinogen action and promote lesions earlier and in greater profusion. Metabolically, iodine-deficient breasts show changes in RNA/DNA ra-tios, estrogen receptor proteins." He concluded that: "[Iodine] presents great potential for its use in research directed toward the prevention, diagnosis, and treatment of breast cancer."

Despite its obvious potential, not much has been done with this treat-ment over the past 30 to 40 years—at least not in these United States. Since iodine isn't patentable (and is therefore unlikely to be "approved" for use to prevent or treat breast cancer), Dr. Eskin's work has been ig-nored. Patent medicine companies simply looked elsewhere for profits. Sadly, since most mainstream doctors are dependent on patent medicine company reps, the doctors have been kept in the dark regarding this po-tential use for iodine.

Over the past two years, though, researchers in Mexico and India (where low-cost, unpatented medicine is a necessity) have begun further investigations into iodine's potential as a breast cancer treatment. So far, all of their results confirm Dr. Eskin's original research: Iodine directly kills many types of human breast cancer cells, and it doesn't kill healthy cells in the process.

Traveling beyond the border for natural cancer cures

In 2005, researchers from the Autonomous National University in Juriquilla, Mexico, reviewed evidence showing that iodine supports breast health by slowing or preventing the spread of cancerous cells. They said, "In animal and human studies, molecular iodine [I(2)] supplementation exerts a suppressive effect on the development and size of both benign and cancer neoplasias…Iodine, in addition to its incorporation into thyroid hormones, is bound into antiproliferative iodolipids [iodinated lipids with anti-cancer activity] in the thyroid called iodolactones, which may also play a role in the proliferative control of the mammary gland." They concluded that breast cancer patients should consider supplementing with I2 in addition to their traditional breast cancer therapy.[2]

In June 2006, a group from the Sanjay Ghandi Institute of Medical Sciences in Lucknow, India, found that iodine is cytotoxic (deadly) to several human breast cancer cell lines, including (for the technically inclined) MCF-7, MDA-MB-231, MDA-MB-453, ZR-75-1, and T-47D. When iodine was applied to human blood cells (monocytes), it inhibited growth and proliferation, but it didn't kill the cells.[3]

Then, in December 2006, the group in Mexico tested the effect of iodine on the MCF-7 form of human breast cancer cells. They found that iodine (but not iodide), along with an iodinated fatty acid, inhibited the MCF-7 cancer cells. At the same time, the iodine neither harmed nor inhibited fibroblasts—normal human connective tissue cells that help to support breast tissue and other tissues throughout the body. Other technical details led the researchers to suggest that iodine may become active against cancer cells when it is bound to certain lipids or proteins that are normally present in the breasts.[4]

A safe adjunct treatment to conventional cancer therapies

These recent research reports give new hope and an added tool for breast cancer patients. It's true that the research isn't conclusive at this point, but you don't need to wait for academic and scientific certainty—which will likely take many more years—to try out the benefits for yourself.

If you have breast cancer and are undergoing regular treatment, adding iodine to your treatment plan will only increase your odds of a favorable outcome—and it's perfectly safe. Numerous studies have proven that iodine (and its iodide form) are among the safest of all the elements.

In one case, a 54-year-old man mistakenly drank 600 ccs (over 20 ounces) of a saturated solution of potassium iodide—100,000 times the recommended daily allowance. The initial reaction was a bit scary: He developed swelling in his neck, mouth, and face, and he experienced transient heart rhythm abnormalities—but he recovered uneventfully.[5]

In another instance, a researcher had 2,400 patients with asthma take 5,000 milligrams of potassium iodide daily on a cycle of four days on followed by three days off. Only 12 of the individuals (1/2 percent) became hypothyroid as a result, and four developed swollen thyroid glands. There was no report of any adverse reaction among the rest.

Even though it's generally safe, some individuals are sensitive to iodine and/or iodide. There have been anecdotal reports of iodide's causing auto-immune thyroiditis, hyperthyroidism, and hypothyroidism. Too much iodine in a few individuals has caused iodism—an acne-like rash, a runny nose, and a bad taste in the mouth, all of which went away when the dosage was reduced or eliminated.

But the possible consequences of unchecked breast cancer are considerably more likely—and, of course, much worse—than experiencing a negative reaction to iodine. So if I were you, I'd give it a try.

Rub away your breast cancer?

A suggestion for you and your doctor to consider: Put the treatment right onto the problem! Mix a solution of 50 percent iodine/50 percent DMSO and rub it directly onto your breast as near as possible to where the cancer is (or used to be). The DMSO will ensure penetration deep into the tissue. A 70-percent DMSO solution is widely available, and iodine is available by prescription as Lugol's Iodine and in natural food stores and the Tahoma Clinic Dispensary as Triodide (from Scientific

Botanicals). If you're worried about the breast cancer spreading, you can also rub the mixture into the area under the arms that is rich in lymph glands (nodes) where breast cancer spreads first.

But please don't do any of the above without consulting a physician skilled and knowledgeable in the use of high-dose iodine!

You should also be sure that your physician monitors your thyroid function and gives you other nutrient suggestions while you use iodine as an adjunct to your regular breast cancer treatment. (To find a physician, see the Alternative Health Resources section on page 485 or check with the International College of Integrative Medicine, www.icimed.com, (866)464-5226.)

You can get more information on the many uses of iodine, including its effectiveness in breast cancer prevention, in the August 2005 issue of *Nutrition & Healing*. I also recommend reading two excellent books: Dr. David Derry's *Breast Cancer and Iodine: How to Prevent and How to Survive Breast Cancer* and Dr. David Brownstein's *Iodine: Why You Need It, Why You Can't Live Without It.*

Chapter 3:

The "unimportant" molecule curing cancer: Do-it-yourself tips for boosting your levels—without Big Pharma's help

You may have read about Panzem®, one of "Big Pharma's" aggressive moves into bio-identical hormones. But for decades before the pharmaceutical industry changed its name and spent hundreds of millions of dollars trying for FDA "approval" Panzem was actually known by its _real_ name, 2-methoxyestradiol.

For much of that time, no one really knew the function of 2-methoxyestradiol, and since there are such tiny quantities of it in our bodies, it was dismissed as "unimportant" (as scientists so often do when they don't yet know what one of Nature's "minor" molecules is for).

But now the gold rush of research is on for 2-methoxyestradiol, because it appears that it may be able to actually cure—or at least significantly slow—many types of cancer, including some of the most commonly feared forms, including prostate, breast, and ovarian.

An "inactive" hormone shows its true cancer-fighting potential

As usual with patent medicine research, the emphasis (and the rush) is on the "gold" that can be produced by selling an "approved" form of this entirely natural molecule (at an unnaturally high price), rather than learning how to work with Nature as closely as possible, which would offer the most benefit at the least possible cost to patients everywhere. But that's just one of many "fatal flaws" of the current "health care" system here in these United States. And even though that's unlikely to change anytime soon, we still may be able to salvage something from this situation.

Before turning the spotlight on 2-methoxyestradiol itself, it's always important to have a little bit of general background on how these things work in the body. Estrogens and androgens are steroid hormones (Nature's own original steroids, not the "extraterrestrial-molecule," pumped-up-to-be-patentable, pseudo-steroids currently scandalizing professional athletics). These natural steroids are produced by the ovaries or testes, adrenal cortices, and other body tissues of both men and women.

But, too much estrogen, especially too much of the "wrong kind" of estrogen increases the risk of new cancers and promotes the development of any tumors that are already present. This occurs primarily when two of the major forms of estrogen, estradiol and estrone, follow a pathway that metabolizes them into estrogen compounds that promote tumor formation. Other pathways produce estrogen metabolites that protect against tumors.

As it turns out, 2-methoxyestradiol isn't inactive, as the "experts" once assumed.[1] In fact, it's one of the most potent anti-carcinogenic estrogen metabolites. This metabolite is formed from the hydroxylation of 17β-estradiol followed by O-methylation in the liver.[2,3] (I know that's highly technical, but remember the word "methylation" for later.)

Some recent studies have shown that 2-methoxyestradiol inhibits the growth of prostate cancer cells by inducing apoptosis (cell "suicide") and preventing tumor growth in rapidly growing cells.[4] It showed similar benefits for both breast[5] and prostate cancer[6] when it was used in combination with other chemotherapeutic therapies.

And speaking of its role among chemotherapy drugs, not only does 2-methoxyestradiol have potent effects against pancreatic and gastric cancers that have become resistant to other chemotherapeutic drugs,[7] but it also reduced the amount of other chemotherapeutic drugs needed in cases of ovarian cancer by enhancing their anti-tumor effects.[8] Researchers have seen similar results using 2-methoxyestradiol in many other kinds of cancer, including osteosarcoma,[9,10] leukemia,[11] and chondrosarcoma, a type of cancer affecting the cartilage.[12]

In addition to promoting apoptosis in cancer cells and working with chemotherapy drugs to boost their effects with lower doses (which, hopefully, will help minimize the harsh effects of these drugs), 2-methoxyestradiol also works against cancers by inhibiting angiogenesis, the formation of new blood vessels, which is how many cancers nourish themselves.[13,14] To top off this roster of benefits, 2-methoxyestradiol has also shown the ability to inhibit the spread of cancer through metastasis.

All of these various approaches to fighting cancer (and likely some that haven't even been discovered yet), make 2-methoxyestradiol an extremely promising tool for treating the disease at many different stages.[15,16]

Giving Nature the cancer-curing credit it's due

The study results I listed above are really just the tip of the proverbial iceberg when it comes to the clinical trials being done on 2-methoxyestradiol. As a matter of fact, just as I was sitting down to write this chapter, yet another "2-methoxyestradiol might cure cancer" study was released—and made quite a splash in the media (probably because it was done at one of the most mainstream of mainstream institutions, the Mayo Clinic). The press report started:

"A new study of an estrogen-derived drug shows promise as a

treatment for breast cancer and breast cancer metastases to bone. A drug that has shown promise in treating sarcoma, lung and brain cancers, demonstrates that the drug may also be effective in treating breast cancer, in particular the spread of breast cancer."[17]

I'm sure you've noticed the typical patent medicine company language "spin" right away. 2-methoxyestradiol is a natural estrogen, not a "drug," but the word "drug" is used three times in the first two sentences. And the spin didn't stop there.

> "[Mayo Clinic researchers] studied the effect of 2-methoxyestradiol on the bone...In breast cancer, the cancer commonly lodges in the bone, destroying it in a debilitating painful process called osteolysis. Osteolysis can lead to bone fractures and causes patients to feel tired, or even to lose consciousness."

According to one of the researchers, 2-methoxyestradiol is potentially very important in the treatment of breast cancer metastatic to bone because it has few of the unpleasant side effects of most chemotherapy drugs and targets both bone resorption and the cancerous tumor cells. According to another researcher, "We were expecting the 'drug' (quotation marks added) to have an effect, but we were not expecting to have as big of an effect as it did."

I suppose getting the mainstream to credit Nature instead of "drugs" is too much to hope for. But at least they haven't tried twisting all-natural 2-methoxyestradiol into a patentable, space-alien version—yet.

And these researchers did make one other bit of progress: They appear to be among the first to notice that swallowing steroids is not Nature's preferred route of administration. Of course, that should have been obvious from the start to any M.D., Ph.D., or intelligent student of the human body. But, obvious or not, nearly all other researchers have had their volunteers swallow 2-methoxyestradiol, which may be one of the reasons such enormous doses have been required in the research to-date. According to the news report on the Mayo Clinic study:

"Clinical trials of 2ME2 for breast cancer patients are in progress. These trials are based on an oral version of 2ME2 to treat primary tumors, but this method has limitations as the oral version of 2ME2 is poorly suited to getting into the blood system and reaching tumors. Researchers resolved this problem by delivering 2ME2 by injection and found it was much more effective."

To put it simply, the Mayo Clinic study found that 2-methoxyestradiol:

- Effectively targets breast cancer cells

- Prevents the spread of breast cancer cells to bone

- Protects bone from osteolysis, which is a type of bone metastasis in which the bone is eaten away by cancer cells.

- Is much more effective in smaller quantities when not swallowed, but (in this case) injected.[18]

Safety in numbers— and larger-than-normal doses

The Mayo Clinic study may be the most recent—and accurately conducted—research on 2-methoxy-estradiol so far, but there are lots of other studies on this estrogen metabolite as well that show just as much promise, even with some wrinkles in the methodology.

In a phase I clinical trial of 2-methoxyestradiol in 15 women with metastatic breast cancer, 10 patients stabilized in their disease progression and two reported reductions in bone pain and the use of painkillers. And there were no adverse effects from daily oral doses of 200, 400, 600, or 800 milligrams, although at 1,000 mg per day all 15 patients in the study reported hot flashes.[19]

Another phase I study of 2-methoxyestradiol examined its effects when combined with the cancer drug docetaxel in 15 patients with metastatic breast cancer. This time, no adverse effects were observed when oral 2-methoxyestradiol was administered in concentrations between 200-

1,000 mg per day for 28 days following 4-6 weeks of docetaxel therapy.[20]

The next clinical trial on 2-methoxyestradiol's resume involved 11 men and nine women who were given oral doses of the metabolite to find the maximum-tolerated dose and determine any level of toxicity. To be enrolled in the study, patients had to have malignant, metastatic, inoperable solid tumors and to have exhausted standard treatment options. Prostate and ovarian cancers were the most commonly represented tumors in the study group. Patients were initially given a specific oral dose of 2-methoxyestradiol over the course of 28 days. When a treatment cycle was completed without adverse effects or progression of disease, doses were escalated to the next highest dose. Results of the study determined that 2-methoxyestradiol was well tolerated orally at dose levels ranging from 400 mg to 3,000 mg, though side effects, such as hot flashes and thrombosis, did occur in some participants.[21]

As the previous study indicated, 2-methyoxyestradiol may be as beneficial for men as it is for women. In one randomized, placebo-controlled study specifically on PSA levels and prostate cancer, 33 patients were given either 400 or 1,200 milligrams per day of oral 2-methoxyestradiol over the course of 16 weeks. PSA numbers either stabilized or declined by as much as 40 percent in many of the patients receiving the 1,200-milligram dose. Several patients did developed abnormalities in liver function that resolved when 2-methoxyestradiol was discontinued, but other than those few instances, the 2-methoxyestradiol was well tolerated in the study participants.[22]

Once again, no matter how the media—or the patent medicine industry—tries to spin it, 2-methoxy- estradiol is a naturally occurring estrogen metabolite, not a "drug." And this natural substance has enormous potential as an anticancer agent for a wide variety of cancers, particularly when it's administered properly (into the bloodstream first, before the liver gets a chance to change it and destroy it, which is actually the liver's job with steroid hormones). But even the studies that used the wrong method of administration demonstrated that 2-methoxyestradiol has few adverse effects and little toxicity.

The good news and bad news about this revolutionary cancer therapy

The good news we can take away from the 2-methoxyestradiol research to date is that a much safer and effective form of cancer treatment is coming. Now for the bad news: Given the "approval" process, it's still years away. And, unfortunately, like all other newly introduced "approved drugs" it will be enormously expensive (although more likely to be covered by insurance than non-"approved" natural treatments).

But by now you might be wondering why you need to wait around for approval at all. Since 2-methoxyestradiol is a naturally occurring estrogen, doctors—especially ones skilled and knowledgeable in the safe and effective use of bio-identical hormones—should be able to order it through their compounding pharmacies, and prescribe it for you just like the other estrogens used in an overall bio-identical hormone replacement therapy (BHRT) program. Not to mention the fact that even though they've been proven safe, it's also very likely that you wouldn't need doses as large as the ones used in the research studies: There's every reason to believe that much lower doses of 2-methoxyestradiol will be just as effective if they're used as part of an overall, natural anti-cancer approach, in combination with excellent diet, detoxification, immune support and stimulation, and many other safe and natural anti-cancer compounds.

So why not just talk to your doctor about adding this safe and all-natural hormone to your current BHRT regimen now?

Well, unfortunately, it's not that easy—and, believe me, I've tried. One compounding pharmacist told me that chemical supply sources advertising 2-methoxyestradiol for sale on-line refused to sell to compounding pharmacies, giving various excuses. Another compounding pharmacist actually was able to purchase a very small amount, which arrived in a package emblazoned with a skull and crossbones, accompanied by a safety sheet that cautioned about potentially toxic effects of 2-methoxyestradiol! Either these sources don't have a clue what they're selling, or the fix is in (but most likely it's a mixture of both).

Since 2-methoxyestradiol is in fact a relatively harmless natural metabolite with great potential for good, I'm hoping it becomes available through the same sources as other bio-identical hormones at a reasonable price sometime in the near future. Otherwise, it'll be the same ol' story: If you develop cancer, don't call your doctor, call your travel agent!

In the meantime, though, there are some things you can do to increase your body's own 2-methoxyestradiol levels.

Stockpiling your own internal reserves

2-methoxyestradiol is one of the metabolites monitored in the 24-hour urine evaluation (more information can be found in the December 2007 issue). Even though it's present in very tiny quantities, don't be fooled by the research studies using huge doses by unnatural means (oral administration). As I mentioned above, even tiny quantities can be pivotal as "signaling molecules" when they occur naturally in your body.

For example, one research study found that an exceptionally tiny quantity—1 micromole—has "antiproliferative, antiangiogenic, and apoptotic effects" on uterine fibroid cells.[23] Although there's no concrete proof, it's very likely that one function of the very tiny quantities of 2-methoxyestradiol in our bodies is to prevent both benign hormone-related tumors such as fibroids as well as hormone-related cancers before they get started.

So how can you increase your own level of 2-methoxyestradiol? Remember the term "methylation" from the beginning of this chapter? It's the process that produces 2-methoxyestrdiol from other forms of estrogen. Methylation relies on certain enzymes and molecules called "methyl donors" to function properly. Making sure you're supplying your body with enough of these methyl donor molecules is key to raising your 2-methyoxyestradiol levels.

The list of foods that contain the most of the necessary methyl donor molecules will probably look familiar: Green leafy vegetables, legumes, citrus, berries, and nuts. Although in this particular case, it's very important that the foods have been processed as little as possible before you eat them—and that includes heating and freezing. Keeping these foods as fresh and "raw" as possible helps preserve the methyl donor molecules they contain.

There are also a few supplements that supply methyl groups, including S-adenosylmethionine (SAMe), followed by methylsulfonylmethane (MSM), betaine (including the betaine from betaine hydrochloride), 5-methyltetrahyrofolate (a "new-in-the-stores" and more natural form of folic acid), and methylcobalamin (a form of vitamin B12).

If your 24-hour urine test reveals that your levels of 2-methoxyestradiol are low, increase your consumption of the foods listed above, and check with your physician skilled and knowledgeable in bio-identical hormone replacement therapy about which and how much of these supplements to take.

And on a non-supplemental note: Stress, especially prolonged stress, reduces methylation of estrogens since the required "methyl groups" get used by the body to make adrenaline instead. Meditation, biofeedback, and other stress and "adrenaline reducing" techniques can make more methyl groups available to make 2-methoxyestradiol, and reduce your risk of cancer at the same time.

Thanks to Lauren Russel N.D. for her organization and summary of the data I collected for this chapter.

Chapter 4:

The astonishing eggplant cure for cancer

Would you believe that studies have shown that an extract from eggplant can cure—that's cure, not just improve—the majority of skin cancers, usually in two to three months or less? This may seem like groundbreaking information, but researchers have known about it for nearly 20 years.

Actually, extracts from plants of the Solanaceae family, (which includes eggplant, tomato, potato, "Bell" peppers, and tobacco) were reported effective for treating cancer as long ago as 1825. But scientific investigation of these anti-cancer effects didn't happen until the second half of the 20th century, and the first few years of the 21st.

Results in no-time flat

The first reported study compared the effects of a topical eggplant extract called BEC with a placebo on two different types of skin cancer—basal cell and squamous cell—and actinic keratosis, a condition characterized by small, rough, yellow or brownish patches of skin that almost always occur on sun-exposed skin of individuals over 50.

Thirty individuals had basal cell cancers, usually a form that spreads locally if untreated. All 28 of the patients using BEC had complete regression of all of their basal cell cancers (some had more than one) in three to 13 weeks. None of the patients using placebo had improvement after 14 weeks.

Twenty of the volunteers had squamous cell cancers, a form which starts and spreads locally but can metastasize. Again, all of the patients using BEC (20 this time) had complete regression of their squamous cell cancers in three to 11 weeks. There were no placebo treatments in this group.

The actinic keratosis group experienced the same effects: Of the 24 in the BEC-treated group, 100 percent had complete regression, this time in just one week to a month. None of the 12 patients using placebo had any improvement at all in 14 weeks.

In another small study, which used a slightly different version of BEC called BEC2, 13 individuals with 24 basal cancers had 83 percent of those cancers completely regress in less than two months. Five people with squamous cell cancers also had 83 percent of their cancers completely regress within one to three months. And eight individuals with actinic keratoses had 100 percent regression in just two to six weeks.

Cost-effective and non-invasive

In a letter dated April 23, 2002, Drs. Rino Cerio and Sangeeta Punjabi of the Dermatology Department of the Royal London Hospital describe their experience participating in trials using a form of the extract called BEC5 to treat both invasive and non-invasive forms of basal cell carcinoma. The first was a placebo-controlled, double-blind, multi-centered study of 94 patients. The second trial with 41 individuals was done only at Royal London Hospital, and was mostly to assess safety, so no placebo was used. The doctors reported that in both trials, approximately 78 percent experienced complete regression within eight weeks.

The doctors noted that with twice daily use, only a few patients reported skin irritation and redness. They pointed out that the cosmetic outcome is "comparable to that resulting from surgical excision."

The doctors concluded: "In our view and experience BEC5 is a topical preparation which is safe and effective, ideal therapy for outpatient treatment… It is a cost-effective treatment for both primary and secondary skin cancer care."

And follow-up research on patients who have used BEC shows that once their cancer or actinic keratosis goes away, it doesn't recur.

The "backdoor approach" to cancer treatment

BEC5 is a name for a mixture of 1/3 solasonine and 1/3 solamargine in the "triglycoside" form, and 1/3 "diglycosides and monoglycosides" of these two basic molecules.

Solasonine and solamargine themselves are actually very similar (but not identical to) human cholesterol and steroid molecules.

By themselves, solasonine and solamargine don't have anti-cancer activity because they can't penetrate into cells, cancerous or normal. That's why just eating the foods that contain these compounds won't eliminate your skin cancer or even reduce your risk of getting it.

In order for them to be effective, they need to be able to get into the cells. That's where the glycosides come in.

Glycoside is a term used to describe molecules with various simple sugars attached to them. One of these simple sugars, called rhamnose, selectively latches on to receptors present only in skin cancer cell membranes and in actinic keratosis. When you combine the solasonine and solamargine with rhamnose, they can get into the cells where they cause cancer cell death by destroying cell components called lysosomes.

Normal cells escape any harm, since the BEC5 can't get into them.

80,000 success stories

According to Dr. Bill Cham, who has developed BEC since the 1980s, BEC5 is effective at extremely low doses and is safe to use even very frequently.

Dr. Cham writes: "BEC5 is applied at least twice daily to the skin and may be applied much more frequently if rapid regression of the tumor is required. Some patients apply [it] up to 10 times daily. The cosmetic results after using BEC5 are very impressive and over 80,000 patients have now used BEC5 successfully."

Also, please note that BEC5 does not contain the part of the eggplant that can cause "nightshade sensitivity" in arthritis sufferers.

You can get BEC5 from the Tahoma Clinic Dispensary (888-893-6878, www.tahomadispensary.com), or on-line from International Anti-aging Systems (www.antiaging-systems.com).

Remember: What's reported here are preliminary research results concerning BEC5 and squamous cell cancer, basal cell cancer, and actinic keratosis. Even though these results are very good, they may not apply to you.

As always, consult with a physician skilled and knowledgeable in nutritional and natural medicine if you'd like to try BEC5. And since skin cancer (especially squamous cell cancer) can be very dangerous if neglected, it's always wisest to consult a dermatologist, too.

Chapter 5:

The mustard miracle that can wipe out deadly cancers

We all know Grandma was right when she told us to eat our vegetables. Over the last decade or so, researchers have added their findings to Grandma's advice, concluding in one study or another that more vegetables in your diet helps reduce your risk of heart disease, stroke, cancer, and other ailments. So what's new about eating your vegetables? Now it looks like certain kinds might actually be able to cure illnesses, even ones as deadly as cervical and prostate cancer.

Preventing and curing cancer of the cervix

In May 2000, Maria Bell, M.D., revealed study results that pointed to the reversal and apparent cure of a certain type of cervical cancer with a natural substance found in vegetables belonging to the mustard family, including cabbage, broccoli, Brussels sprouts, and bok choy (these are also known as Brasicca vegetables).

The natural cancer-fighting substances in these vegetables—isothiocyanates and indoles—help regulate and improve the 2/16 hydroxyestrogen ratio, which is a proven predictor of all hormone-related cancers (like breast and prostate). In essence, a normal 2/16 ratio means less cancer risk.

In this study, Dr. Bell's group used a specific type of indole, called indole-3-carbinol (I3C), to reverse a significant proportion of cervical cancers.

Results that speak for themselves

Dr. Bell explained that 95 percent or more of all cervical cancer is directly related to infection with the human papilloma virus (HPV). She noted that HPV infection lowers the 2/16 ratio.

So in her 12-week study, Dr. Bell researched 30 women with moderate or severe cervical dysplasia (HPV is thought to play a role in causing cervical dysplasia).

Ten of the women took 200 milligrams of I3C daily, 10 took 400 milligrams of I3C daily, and the remaining 10 took placebos. At the end of the 12 weeks, both I3C groups' 2/16 ratios had gone up, while the placebo group's had gone down. And as for the women's cancer, 50 percent of those who had been taking 200 milligrams of I3C showed complete regression, as did 44 percent of the group taking 400 milligrams a day. (None of the patients in the placebo group experienced a regression.)

Research also shows dramatic prostate health benefits. In one study, men who ate as few as three servings of Brassica vegetables a week experienced a 41 percent reduction in prostate cancer risk.

Eating your vegetables can help you *remain* cancer-free

Although the study lasted only 12 weeks, I'd say it's a reasonable prediction that if the women whose cancers regressed continued their I3C and ate Brassica vegetables, their cancers wouldn't return. I think it's also a reasonable prediction eating these vegetables and/or taking I3C regularly may very well prevent a significant proportion of cervical and prostate cancer.

It's also apparent that the 2/16 ratio is a worthwhile risk factor screening tool. Testing your 2/16 ratio is simple and relatively inexpensive.

And, best of all, you can do it from home. All that's required is a small urine specimen that you send to the lab by regular mail. In Washington State, where I'm located, you don't even need a doctor's order for the test.

So as Grandma said, "Eat your vegetables!" And she's right. To help prevent cervical, breast, and prostate cancer, eat cabbage, broccoli, Brussels sprouts, cauliflower, or bok choy three to four times a week. Occasionally, Brassica vegetables can inhibit thyroid function, though, so don't eat more than three or four servings a week for an extended period of time without having your doctor do a thyroid test to make sure everything is running smoothly.

If you do eat right, exercise, take your vitamins, minerals, and botanicals…you may reduce your risk of ever needing cancer treatment at all, nontoxic or otherwise.

Part II

Heart

Chapter 1:

Could a stroke steal your future? Know your risk and prevent it from happening!

You probably know someone who's had a stroke—wheelchair bound or walking difficulty, unable to use an arm or a leg (or both). In seconds, a stroke can render you physically helpless, without the ability to speak or even to smile. It always makes me sad to see a patient who was active, funny, and independent suddenly turn info a shell of their former self after a stroke. It can literally steal your quality of life—with absolutely no warning.

But while stokes sneak up on us, we are certainly not defenseless against them. By following some simple guidelines, you can significantly reduce your risk of suffering a stroke.

Not all strokes are created equal, but they are preventable

First, let me clear up a common misconception that allows far too many of us to assume we're "stoke-proof." It's not true that you're only at risk if you have high blood pressure or high cholesterol levels. While high blood pressure is a major risk factor, men and women with perfectly normal blood pressure have strokes, too. Other stroke risk factors include tobacco smoking, heavy alcohol consumption, and physical inactivity.

To understand how to avoid a stroke, you need to understand how it happens.

There are at least two "basic" types of stroke: Hemorrhagic (bleeding) and ischemic/thrombotic (lack of blood flow associated with a clot).

So, either a blood vessel in the brain breaks, spewing blood into brain tissue where it doesn't belong, or the blood vessel gets blocked with a clot, depriving an area of the brain of blood. Or, just maybe, the blood vessel goes into an intense spasm with the same result. In any of these cases, the affected area of the brain can't function, and often dies.

Common sense tells us that strengthening blood vessels will reduce their risk of breaking and causing hemorrhagic stroke. Common sense also says that reducing the tendency of blood to clot abnormally, and increasing blood's clot-busting potential will reduce the risk of thrombotic/ischemic strokes. Reducing the tendency of blood vessels to spasm will likely reduce your risk of stroke, too. But how can you possibly do all of that when you can't even see the area needing improvement, you might wonder?

I'll admit, the results aren't very easy to measure—in a visual sense. You can't stand in front of a mirror and see if your blood's ability to clot has been regulated. These results are ones you're more likely to feel in the form of more energy and an overall sense of wellbeing. And even better: You don't need a gym membership to get your blood vessels "pumped up" and strong. This is where Mother Nature steps in and gives us all the tools we need to protect ourselves from strokes.

Forget pumping iron… strengthen your blood vessels with vitamins, minerals, and herbs

There are many, many nutrients and herbs that help to strengthen blood vessels; I'll just mention a few of the basics and particularly important ones here. Let's start with vitamin C.

Without enough vitamin C blood vessels simply break down. Although only a few milligrams of vitamin C daily are enough to prevent blood vessels from breaking easily, it takes much more to maximize blood vessel strength—though research has yet to determine precisely how much more. Since there's no definitive conclusion on this point yet, and since vitamin C is so important for so many reasons, I have *two* recommendations. Choose the one that works best for you.

If you want to optimize health and even fight the aging process, take "bowel tolerance" levels of vitamin C. ("Bowel tolerance" is as much vitamin C as your intestines will tolerate without provoking excess gas and loose stools.) For most people this is between three and nine grams a day. You should take the amount you need in divided—between two and four—doses daily.

However, I understand that the "bowel tolerance" amount can be quite large and involve taking quite a few pills every day, which some people are hesitant to do. So it isn't absolutely essential to take that much (though it will make a considerable improvement in your health, I guarantee it). But the bare minimum you do need to take is 1 gram of vitamin C, twice daily.

Just like thunder and lightning, vitamin C and flavonoids go together for a reason

Where there's vitamin C, there's flavonoids…at least in nature. Vitamin C and flavonoids are always found together, probably because when they're together they work better to keep you healthy. In the 1930s, flavonoids were found to correct the fragility of the smallest blood vessels (capillaries) in cases of scurvy. Over the decades, they have been found to strengthen all sizes of blood vessels, as well as ligaments, tendons, connective tissue, and many other body tissues.

So where do you find flavonoids? Check the bowl of fruit on your table, or the "crisper" in your refrigerator. Flavonoids (along with carotenoids) give fruits and vegetables most of their colors. The best way to ensure you're getting enough flavonoids to reduce your stroke risk is to eat as many differently colored fruits and vegetables as possible.[1]

You've read this from me many times before, but here it is again: Diets high in vegetables and fruits and lower in animal protein are associated with fewer diseases of all kinds, including stroke.[2] In a 12-year study of 859 men and women, *only one additional* serving of vegetables or fruits daily lowered the risk of stroke by 40 percent![3] (And just as a side note while I'm talking about your diet, consider that eating whole grain products lowers the risk of ischemic stroke, but refined flour products give no protection.[4])

Herbs and minerals: More blood-vessel-strengthening tricks up Mother Nature's sleeve

Sometimes even I'm amazed at just how many options nature has for us (and I've been doing this for 29 years now!). In addition to vitamin C and flavonoids, there are a number of herbs—and at least one mineral—you can take to help strengthen your blood vessels. You've heard of most of these before, so instead of spending a lot of time giving you their history, I'll just outline what they do and how much you'll need for maximum stroke protection.

Hawthorn has been is the No.1 traditional European botanical for blood vessel strengthening for centuries. "Modern" scientific research confirms hawthorn's effect on the heart and blood vessels.[5] Although there are many hawthorn supplements available, I usually recommend Hawthorn Solid Extract by Scientific Botanicals, a local Seattle firm (with which I have no connection), one teaspoonful daily.

Ginkgo has been most heavily advertised for preservation and improvement of memory, but it's been demonstrated beyond a doubt that it also strengthens blood vessels and improves blood flow all over the body. Take 80 milligrams of a standardized ginkgo preparation, twice daily.

Ginkgo helps prevent strokes in other ways, too, by helping to prevent clots and blood vessel spasms. It's even helpful *after* a stroke has occurred, by reducing brain swelling, promoting better ATP (energy) production and blood sugar use following ischemia (lack of blood flow.)[6] A word of caution here: If you are taking a blood-thinning medication,

---

Stroke prevention in one easy-to-follow outline

Here's what you need to do:

- eat more vegetables and fruits
- eat whole grains (not refined flour products)
- eat more fish (and reduce animal protein)
- quit smoking
- cut alcohol consumption to no more than one drink daily
- exercise!

And here's what you need to take:

- vitamin C: 1,000 milligrams twice daily (more for optimal health)
- cod liver oil: 1 tablespoonsful daily always with
- vitamin E: 600 IU daily
- ginkgo (standardized extract): 80 milligrams twice daily
- hawthorne solid extract: one teaspoonful daily
- centella asiatica (standardized extract): 60 to 120 milligrams daily
- turmeric: 20 (or more) milligrams daily (or put turmeric into your cooking regularly)
- magnesium: 250-400 milligrams daily
- copper: 2 milligrams daily
- nattokinase: 138 milligrams three times daily

consult your physician before adding gingko to your routine.

While flavonoids strengthen the blood vessels themselves, centella asiatica (also known as gotu kola) strengthens the connective tissue sheath that surrounds blood vessels, thus providing an additional layer of protection against blood vessel rupture.[7] Centella also reduces hardening of the blood vessels and improves blood flow. Take 60 to 120 milligrams of a standardized preparation daily.

It's also important for larger blood vessels to maintain their elasticity, and not become hardened or stiffened. Copper is absolutely essential to the formation and repair of elastic tissue throughout the body, including blood vessels. Make sure you're taking at least 2 milligrams daily. But you may not need to take a separate copper supplement. Most multiple vitamin-mineral supplements have at least 2 milligrams, so check the label on yours before buying more.

Keeping clots out of your strengthened blood vessels

Strong blood vessels are the first part of the stroke prevention equation. Next on the list is eliminating blood clots and keeping things flowing smoothly in your body.

The essential fatty acids contained in fish oil lessen the risk of abnormal blood clotting. Fish oil makes platelets (the tiny blood elements that clump together into clots) more "slippery," so they can't stick together as easily. Fish oil literally does a "lube job" on platelets.

Eating fish two or three times weekly is the best way to get a start on fish oil consumption. However, if you're really concerned about stroke prevention, take 1 to 1 1/2 tablespoonful of cod liver oil daily. (Of course, cod liver oil helps prevent osteoporosis, reduce your risk of heart attack and heart rhythm disorders, and many other things, too!) And remember, additional vitamin E should always accompany essential fatty acid supplementation. Take at least 600 IU of vitamin E for the amount of cod liver oil noted above.

"Fibrinogen" is a precursor of "fibrin," a key element in clot formation. Elevated levels of fibrinogen are an "independent risk factor" for easy blood clotting. Turmeric helps reduce abnormally high levels of fibrinogen.[8] Using turmeric in cooking is the easiest way to use a turmeric supplement. You only need 20 milligrams daily—which is about 1/14,000 of an ounce—to do the job. If you'd rather take a supplement, that's fine. Most turmeric capsules contain much more than the "necessary" amount, but, fortunately, there are no known turmeric overdoses.

The Japanese soy-cheese clot buster

Until very recently, there have been no known substances (except for incredibly expensive, intravenously administered ones) actually effective in *breaking up* clots once they start to form in our blood vessels. But thanks to the persistent research of Professor Hiroyuki Sumi of Miyozaki Medical College, Japan, a safe, effective, orally administered enzyme that breaks down the fibrin component of clots has very recently become available.

Professor Sumi discovered a potent fibrinolytic (clot-busting) enzyme naturally present in the soy cheese, natto, a food consumed in Japan for at least two thousand years.[9] In one study, volunteers ate either natto (200 grams, approximately 7 ounces) or took 1,300 milligrams of nattokinase, the active enzyme in natto. Both groups demonstrated significantly improved "clot-busting" activity that lasted for approximately eight to twelve hours.[10]

As I said above, natto has been eaten by millions of people for centuries. So even though it's "new" to nearly all of us in the United States, we can safely add this soy cheese to our list of stroke-preventing foods. I recommend several ounces three to four times weekly along with regular consumption of fish and other stroke preventing foods. Of course, as a traditional Japanese food (and one that's referred to even there, with its sour flavor and stringy texture, as an "acquired taste"), you may have a hard time finding it in your local health food store or ethnic-food grocer.

If you can't find natto, or prefer to forego acquiring a taste for it, you can now get it in supplement form. Nattokinase supplements are being marketed by Allergy Research Group in 138 milligram capsules, with a suggested use of four capsules daily. While this quantity is significantly lower than the amount used in Professor Sumi's research, when you add it to the other supplemental items I've outlined for you so far, it should still be of significant help. Nattokinase is available through Tahoma Clinic Dispensary (with which I'm of course affiliated) and other outlets carrying Allergy Research Group products.

Stroke risk: More than just a plumbing problem!

So far, I've been using common-sense "plumbing principles": Stronger "pipes" with smooth flowing blood will cut the risk of stroke. But blood vessels aren't just pipes, they're alive, and can do at least two things a regular pipe can't. Blood vessels can spasm, and they can become inflamed.

Magnesium is by far the most important essential nutrient needed to prevent spasm in your blood vessels. And even though deep green vegetables are excellent sources of magnesium, most of us should be taking and additional 250-400 milligrams daily, not only to help prevent blood vessel spasm and potential stroke, but also to reduce the risk of nearly every cardiovascular problem known. (But please don't exceed this amount of magnesium…see Clinical Tip #80, *Magnesium: Are you getting too much of a good thing?*, December 2000.)

Cardiovascular research has increasingly focused on blood vessel inflammation as a triggering event for blood vessel damage. It appears that much of the plaque in blood vessels (which was previously thought to be caused solely by excess cholesterol and other blood lipids) is actually formed as the body's response to inflammation.

If you're eating fish and taking cod liver oil or other omega-3 fatty acid containing oils (along with vitamin E) you've got this one covered already—these all help prevent blood vessel inflammation from occurring in the first place.

But just to make sure, tests for cardiovascular inflammation such as "C-reactive protein" are (or should be) part of your routine check-ups. Ask your doctor if he's ever given you this test. If he hasn't, tell him you'd like to have it done on a regular basis.

The sum of the stroke prevention equation

I know the items mentioned throughout this chapter add up to a hefty, and probably overwhelming, list. So, I tried to boil it down for you at least somewhat in the box on page 43. Read through it and take the advice to heart. Taking action now to prevent a future stroke, and all of the heartache it can bring with it, is well worth the effort!

Chapter 2:

The egg risk you need to know about before you order your next omelet

Poached, hard boiled, over easy—just about any way you cook them, eggs are good sources of nutrition. Except scrambled, that is.

You've probably heard numerous reports claiming that eggs are too high in cholesterol. But if you're eating your eggs cooked in one of the ways listed above, that cholesterol isn't likely to cause any damage to your heart or arteries.

To get a better understanding of why scrambled eggs are the only variety taking the blame, let's back up and go over how the whole "cholesterol is bad for you" myth originated in the first place.

Almost 100 years ago, now-famous Russian researcher Nikolai Anitschkov fed cholesterol to rabbits. When the rabbits developed atherosclerotic vascular disease, it was said to "prove" that cholesterol "causes" atherosclerosis.

Objections were raised, including the obvious: As born vegetarians, rabbits in Nature have never eaten cholesterol, and even lab rabbits show no inclination to eat cholesterol if there are tastier (to a rabbit) alternatives. Despite this, the myth that cholesterol itself causes atherosclerosis has persisted, fueled largely by manufacturers of cholesterol-lowering patent medications and their friends, ex-colleagues, and future colleagues working for *los Federales.*

But in a much-less-publicized experiment approximately half a century later, another researcher tried to duplicate Anitschkov's research. He too fed rabbits cholesterol, but, unlike Anitschkov, he was very careful not to allow the cholesterol to lie around the rabbit cages exposed to air, which causes it to oxidize quite rapidly. Surprisingly (except perhaps to this researcher) the rabbits *did not* develop coronary atherosclerosis. Their arteries remained clear.

What this follow-up study proved is that *oxidized* cholesterol— not cholesterol itself—can cause atherosclerosis in rabbits. However, as there's no money to be made publicizing this detail, many people have never heard or read of it.

So where do scrambled eggs fit in? Well, when you cook scrambled eggs, you break the yolks. Since the yolks contain most of the egg's cholesterol, breaking and scrambling them allows that cholesterol to be exposed to much more air and heat than other cooking techniques that leave the yolk intact. That air and heat can cause the cholesterol in the scrambled egg yolks to oxidize before you even have a chance to eat them, potentially contributing to atherosclerosis.

This information isn't meant to terrorize you into fearing the very sight of scrambled eggs. If you're otherwise eating quite well and taking your daily supplements (including anti-oxidants), the occasional scrambled egg while you're traveling or visiting friends or relatives certainly won't kill you, and likely will be offset by the rest of what you're doing. But if you're a "scrambled egg lover" and eat your eggs cooked this way frequently, you might want to consider giving poached or sunny-side-up a try.

Chapter 3:

How to drop your cholesterol level by as much as 134 points without drugs or deprivation

"The doctor I saw for my check-up wants me to take a cholesterol-lowering drug," David MacElroy began, "and his wife won't let him!" Wendy MacElroy finished. "He finally took a step to check on and protect his health, and I won't let him take that...that poison as a result."

That's what brought the MacElroys to my office at the Tahoma Clinic.

David admitted that he'd been a junk food eater all his life. His father and grandfather died from heart attacks at ages 56 and 61. With David's cholesterol level at 322 and his HDL or "good" cholesterol at 34, he was definitely at high risk.

Determining the proper diet

I asked David to follow a low-fat diet (although not everyone benefits from low fat) and also explained the idea of "good fat" and "bad fat" to him. Until recently, the general consensus among mainstream health "authorities" was that saturated fats are bad and unsaturated fats are good. But as some research supporting high-fat, high-protein diets (like the Atkins diet) suggests, it's not quite that simple.

There's only one general type of fat that you should always avoid, and that's the artificial, man-made type of fats—especially hydrogenated and partially hydrogenated vegetable oils.

You've probably noticed that these oils have been inserted into a myriad of products in the supermarket. Snack foods are the worst offenders: Try to find a potato or corn chip without it and you'll see what I mean. Even natural food stores carry a lot of products that contain partially hydrogenated oils. Make sure to read the labels of the packaged foods you buy. If it contains hydrogenated or partially hydrogenated oil, don't buy it.

So these man-made fats are definitely the ones you should stay away from. But you can't go without any fat at all. Essential fatty acids are definitely a must. The best way to make sure you are getting enough essential fatty acids is to eat whole foods containing them. The best food sources are fish and unroasted nuts and seeds.

Other naturally occurring fats (polyunsaturated, monounsaturated, and even saturated) are also safe as long as you eat them as part of a whole, unprocessed, unrefined diet.

Even though milk, ice cream, and cheese aren't on that list of man-made fats to avoid at all costs, it's still a good idea to eliminate as much dairy from your diet as possible. Dairy is one of the most common food allergens and just generally does more harm than good. It's like I always say: Milk is for baby cows—not people!

On the other hand, you <u>should</u> eat eggs. They've gotten a bad reputation because of their cholesterol content. But they contain phospholipids, which offset any possible adverse effects of egg cholesterol. Plus, phospholipids have a unique function in keeping brain cell membranes healthy. Eggs and soy are the only dietary sources of phospholipids. Soy is still rather controversial, and while I don't think it's necessary to give it up entirely, I do think it's a good idea to limit how much you eat to just a couple of servings a week at the most. So eggs are your only other food option for getting those nutrients that are crucial to brain cells.

Also try to include plenty of the following in your diet as good cholesterol-lowering foods: Garlic, onions, oat bran, carrots, and alfalfa sprouts.

Supplement, supplement, supplement!

There are so many vitamins, minerals, and botanicals known to lower serum cholesterol that drugs are almost never necessary. There's inositol hexaniacinate, lecithin, pantethine, L-carnatine, beta-sitosterol, fish oil and fish-oil concentrates, phosphatidyl choline, choline itself (usually with inositol and methionone), vitamin C, calcium, vanadium, magnesium, chromium, and vitamin E, which have all been found to raise levels of HDL cholesterol, the "good" cholesterol. Then there are the botanicals, including guggulipid, garlic oil, "red yeast rice," ginger, pectin, curcumin, fenugreek powder, reishi mushrooms, silymarin, turmeric, garcinia, and artichokes.

But perhaps the most effective way to lower cholesterol naturally is with something called policosanol, a natural supplement derived from sugar cane. In numerous studies comparing it directly with patent cholesterol-lowering medicines, policosanol was more effective at lowering levels of LDL (bad) cholesterol. But that's not all.

Unlike the patent medicine products, policosanol also lowered triglyceride levels and elevated HDL (good) cholesterol levels. In two studies, it also significantly lowered blood pressure as well. The good news is that it does not require a prescription and is available at most natural food stores, compounding pharmacies, and even online. And it doesn't come with the negative side effects associated with statin drugs.

You don't need to take ALL of these different supplements, of course; the point is, there are so many to try that chances are good you won't ever need to take cholesterol-lowering drugs.

David MacElvoy's program:

David began taking vitamin E, the "mixed tocopherol" type, 400 IU daily; inositol hexaniacinate, 600 milligrams twice daily; vitamin C, 2 grams twice daily; and a high-potency multiple vitamin-mineral with at least 200 micrograms of chromium and 300 to 400 milligrams of magnesium. (You may need to get a separate multiple mineral if you can't find a vitamin-mineral combination.) And last, lecithin. Remember those phospholipids for brain cells? Besides eggs, soy lecithin is the only other diet source, and as a "bonus," lecithin lowers serum cholesterol. Take two 19-grain capsules daily.

After six months, David's total cholesterol level was down to 237 and his HDL cholesterol level had risen to 41. At the end of one year, his numbers were 188 and 46—that means his total cholesterol dropped an impressive 134 points!

But even better than just improving his "numbers," David had substantially reduced his risk of following his father and grandfather to an early cardiac death.

This exact combination of supplements and this diet plan may not work for you. But there are many different combinations you can try. It's best to check with a doctor skilled in natural and nutritional medicine who can help you tailor a supplement program suited exactly for your needs. For a list of such doctors in your area, contact the American College for Advancement in Medicine at (800)532-3688 or www.acam.org.

Cholesterol: How low should you go?

Let's face it: Much more attention is given to high cholesterol than low cholesterol. But like any other biologic marker, there's always a range that's "too high," "too low," or "just right."

I'm not denying that having high serum cholesterol carries a risk for heart disease. I'm just saying that many people probably don't know that low serum cholesterol may also carry risks—namely cancer, stroke, and depression.

All naturally occurring steroid hormones such as DHEA, estrogens, progesterone, testosterone, and pregnenolone are made in our bodies from a single starting material: Cholesterol. And cholesterol is a key component in every cell membrane in our bodies. That's why it's important not just to make sure cholesterol isn't too high or too low, but that it's just right.

High serum cholesterol is usually considered at or above 200 mg/dl (milligrams per 100 cc's of blood). Low cholesterol is defined by many researchers as being at or below 160 mg/dl.

I pay particular attention to my patients' low cholesterol levels when they get to be around 140 mg/dl and advise them to take manganese. Manganese is a key co-factor in the transformation of cholesterol to steroid hormones. Although manganese doesn't raise serum cholesterol to the normal range 100 percent of the time, it is partially or completely effective in more than 50 percent of the cases. I usually recommend 50 milligrams of manganese citrate, once or twice daily. Once your level returns to normal, you can cut your dose to 10 to 15 milligrams a day.

There is one caution in regards to manganese supplementation: Very high levels of manganese intake have been found to cause Parkinson's disease in manganese miners and other industrial workers. However, case reports of manganese poisoning from oral intake are extremely rare (only one case report exists of toxicity from supplementation; others have been from well water with excess manganese).

But in my 30 years of practice, I've never observed problems from the doses necessary to raise low serum cholesterol.

The high-fat/low-fat debate:
Choosing which diet is best for you

There are two basic approaches to a cholesterol-lowering diet: The first is the politically correct, low-fat, high-complex-carbohydrate plan, which was the mainstay of nutritional "experts" for years. And there's also the high-protein, low-carbohydrate approach. It seems strange that such opposite plans can both work, but remember that no one diet is best for every person. Before choosing what's best for you, you will need to find out a bit more about your insulin response to sugar and carbohydrates (yes, sugar and carbohydrates, even though the subject is cholesterol regulation).

High-protein diets work well for many people struggling with cholesterol problems because these individuals' bodies generally manufacture much more insulin than others in response to sugar, refined carbohydrates, and excess carbs in general. This overproduction of insulin causes the liver to produce too much total cholesterol and triglycerides, and not enough HDL cholesterol.

Insulin is one of the hormones that regulates blood sugar. Some people (especially if they have type 2 diabetes or even have a genetic family tendency toward type 2 diabetes) have high insulin levels that go up much more rapidly in response to sugar and carbohydrate intake. In this case, the insulin is not used properly by the cell membranes, so the insulin can't take the sugar from the blood into the cells as it's supposed to. Then, their bodies keep making more and more insulin to try to force the sugar from the blood into the cells. The excess insulin causes other problems, including high blood pressure and cholesterol abnormalities.

Just recently, more and more evidence has been coming out in favor of the high-protein, low-carb approach to lowering cholesterol and triglyceride levels. In fact, according to a study published in the May 22, 2003 edition of the *New England Journal of Medicine*, people following a high-protein diet for six months had higher levels of HDL (good) cholesterol and bigger decreases in triglyceride levels than those people following a low-fat diet. There was no difference between the groups' LDL (bad) cholesterol levels, which shows that restricting protein and fat intake doesn't do as much to help cholesterol levels as the "experts" once thought.

It's possible that many people with weight problems have them due to this excess insulin response to sugar and carbohydrates. If your cholesterol levels are high, ask your doctor to administer a glucose-insulin tolerance test, which can tell you how much insulin your body makes in response to a standard amount of sugar. Then you can make an informed choice about your diet.

The hidden high cholesterol culprit you might not be looking for

Saturated fat gets a lot of blame when it comes to high cholesterol. Carbohydrates come in a close second. While they're both important factors, they aren't the only ones to consider. Diets high in saturated fat are responsible for approximately one in five cases of high serum cholesterol, and high carbohydrate intake is responsible for approximately one in three. That still leaves a little less than half of all high serum cholesterol cases unaccounted for.

The fact is, if you have high cholesterol, you may need to look further than your diet to find the real culprit.

Researchers from the Japanese National Institute of Agrobiological Sciences think they may have found a missing piece of the cholesterol puzzle. They discovered that small quantities of lead caused elevated serum cholesterol in experimental animals. In their experiments they found that lead induces the genes responsible for creating the liver enzymes that produce cholesterol.

To compound the problem, lead also suppresses a gene responsible for the production of a liver enzyme that breaks down and destroys cholesterol. With cholesterol production "turned on" and cholesterol breakdown "turned off" by lead, the animals' serum cholesterol increased significantly.

Although the lead/cholesterol connection hasn't been proven by research on humans yet, it still helps to explain some observations that holistic doctors have made over the years. Holistic doctors who do chelation therapy (a process that removes lead and other toxic metals from the body) have noted that cholesterol levels often drop after chelation.

If you've tried following a strict diet and your serum cholesterol is still high, have a physician skilled and knowledgeable in nutritional and natural medicine check your lead levels. The most accurate way to test for lead is to get an intravenous drip of a chelating agent (EDTA is typically used for lead chelation) followed by a six- to eight-hour urine collection, which is then tested for lead and other toxic metals.

If a chelation test shows you have too much lead (or other toxic heavy metal) in your system, work with your physician to get the lead out. Not only will it help your serum cholesterol levels, but it will also help lots of other natural biochemical processes in your body operate better.

Chapter 4:

How to drop your blood pressure by 20, 30, or even 40 points—naturally

The mainstream medical industry certainly seems determined to get us all on patent hypertension (blood pressure) medications. With the new guidelines issued by the National Heart, Lung and Blood Institute, people whose blood pressure levels were once considered well below normal (a 120 over 80 reading) suddenly became "pre-hypertensive"— essentially overnight. And, of course, one of the first recommendations out of all the so-called "experts'" mouths was more widespread use of patent hypertension medications.

But you can beat high blood pressure—most of the time without drugs. And even if you can't completely avoid patent medicines, taking the right natural measures may be able to help you use substantially less.

What works for someone else may not work for you

In many cases, the old saying "you are what you eat" holds true. It might do some good in some cases to cut out a few of the cream sauces and slices of pizza. In some cases, a diet containing more fruits, vegetables, and whole, natural starches rather than a lot of protein could be your best bet. However, the key words here are "in some cases" and "could."

Decades ago, public health researchers observed that women and men who had been strictly vegetarian all their lives had lower blood pressure readings in their 60s and 70s than did men and women who ate considerable animal protein. A vegetarian diet provides a better potassium-to-sodium ratio. Having more potassium and less sodium helps regulate blood pressure. But a vegetarian diet isn't the best choice for everyone and, in fact, could cause more harm than good for some.

People with high blood pressure who have personal or family histories of type 2 (adult onset) diabetes usually have insulin resistance/hyperinsulinemia. The term insulin resistance refers to the impaired use of insulin by cell membranes. Hyperinsulinemia occurs when the pancreas overproduces insulin in an attempt to overcome insulin resistance. (Insulin resistance/hyperinsulinemia is easily diagnosed via a glucose-insulin tolerance test.)

Hyperinsulinemia is a known cause of high blood pressure. To bring insulin overproduction under control, the most necessary dietary changes are total elimination of sugar and refined carbohydrates and a sharp reduction in overall carbohydrate intake. It's especially important to eliminate such starches as potatoes, beans, pasta, and grains. Obviously, this diet pattern is not vegetarian, but, as it helps bring hyperinsulinism under control, blood pressure is also better regulated.

You can also take natural supplements to help regulate your insulin. There are so many nutrients shown to be helpful in type 2 diabetes that taking them all individually would be a real chore. You'll find several "multiple" formulas designed specifically to aid in blood sugar control in natural food stores. The one I helped formulate is called Glucobalance. (If you can't find it in your local natural food store, it's available from the Tahoma Clinic Dispensary.) One of Glucobalance's most important blood sugar controlling ingredients is chromium. Chromium helps to restore the cell membrane response to insulin.

There are also two more ingredients you should take in addition to Glucobalance or any other blood sugar controlling multiple supplement.

The first is niacin. With chromium, niacin forms part of a molecule called the glucose-tolerance factor, which helps insulin do its job. Both chromium and niacin will get your cells to pay attention to the insulin again, so your insulin and blood sugar levels should go down. It's important to do initial and follow-up testing with your doctor to monitor your progress. Finally, you should also consider taking flaxseed or flaxseed oil capsules. Flaxseed also helps your cells use insulin.

However, there has been a shadow cast over it recently because it contains the essential fatty acid alpha-linolenic acid (ALA), which several studies have linked to a higher risk of prostate cancer and cataracts. While not all the research agreed, there's definitely enough to be cause for concern.

However, these studies definitely aren't the "last word" on ALA. It's important to remember that ALA is an essential-to-life fatty acid, and it's highly unlikely that Nature would require us to have it in order to survive if there was no way around these potential negative effects. It's very possible that another nutrient or several nutrients are involved in the ALA-prostate cancer and ALA-cataract connection, and that using more (or less) of these would "erase" any possible harm from higher levels of ALA. Unfortunately, researchers rarely consider nutrients in more complex interactions. So it'll likely be a long time until this aspect of the "ALA question" is considered.

In the meantime, this does not mean that you need to eliminate flaxseed and flaxseed oil from your diet! In addition to ALA there are many other healthful nutrients present, especially in whole flaxseed. However, it's probably wisest to consult your nutritionally knowledgeable physician about what quantity of flaxseed or flaxseed oil might be best for you. And since too much ALA can suppress "5-alpha-reductase," if you're a man, you might want to have your "5-alpha reductase" enzyme activity measured. This is easily done from a 24-hour urinary steroid test. Some physicians may also recommend a red blood cell membrane essential fatty acid test to make sure your ALA levels aren't out of balance with other fatty acids.

Food allergy may be the culprit

For some people with hypertension, food allergies can play a big part in the problem. Eliminating the allergens or desensitizing to them can help lower blood pressure levels, though no one has been able to successfully explain the connection. If you have a personal or family history of allergies, it's worth investigating. Contact a member of the American Academy of Environmental Medicine (316-684-5500; www.aaem.com) for a list of doctors near you who can help with thorough allergy screening.

The most notable individual case of allergy aggravated hypertension I've worked with involved a gentleman who was undergoing maximum antihypertensive drug therapy but still had blood pressure readings ranging from a minimum 180/120 to a maximum 220/150. Once he discovered and eliminated all food allergies, his blood pressure dropped to a level ranging from 160/100 minimum to 180/120 maximum.

Biofeedback and exercise—old news, but underrated and underused

Biofeedback is another valuable and frequently effective "non-drug" tool for lowering blood pressure. It's not so much a "treatment" as it is a training program. Using external instruments, a reading is obtained of your body's reactions to stress. Through practice, you learn to recognize the physiological responses you have that might be causing unhealthy reactions and teach yourself how to control those responses. Biofeedback centers are found in all major and most midsize cities. Check your local Yellow Pages for listings.

Exercise also can significantly lower high blood pressure. Even light exercise can make a big difference. The amount that's healthy varies from person to person. Of course, it's best to check with a doctor or other knowledgeable individual before starting a strenuous exercise program.

If you're concerned about blood pressure and wonder what your level might be, there are many places to have it measured for free, including drugstores, fire stations (when the firemen aren't fighting fires), health fairs, and "senior centers." Home blood pressure monitoring equipment is quite accurate, and most places that sell it will teach you how to use it as well.

Nutrients: Which to cut back on and which to increase

Sodium. You've probably heard that cutting WAY back on salt intake is an important step in lowering high blood pressure. However, researchers are finding more and more evidence that sodium restriction might not be best for everyone after all. If you have high blood pressure you might want to determine through trial and error whether or not salt restriction makes a difference for you.

Potassium. Sometimes it reduces blood pressure, sometimes it doesn't. Since a higher potassium level does reduce the risk of stroke, it's always wisest to take extra potassium if you have high blood pressure, even if it doesn't lower your actual blood pressure numbers.

Calcium and magnesium. For some individuals, about 1 gram (1,000 milligrams) of calcium daily can greatly reduce blood pressure by five to 10 points. For others, calcium makes very little difference. It appears to work more often for those with insulin resistance/hyperinsulinemia. If you do supplement with calcium, it's important to balance it with magnesium. Magnesium by itself can lower your blood pressure level, since it helps relax muscles, including those of the smaller blood vessels, thus helping to dilate them and improve blood flow. Supplementing with 300 to 400 milligrams daily is usually sufficient.

Vitamin C. A recent research letter sent to the medical journal *Lancet* reconfirmed that vitamin C lowers elevated blood pressure. Although this study used less, you should take a minimum of 1 gram twice daily.

Vitamin D. During the last few years, I've observed significant reductions in blood pressure in people I've worked with when they take vitamin D supplements. Vitamin D achieves its blood pressure lowering effect by addressing one of the major causes of high blood pressure—a substance called angiotensin II.

Without adequate vitamin D, one of your genes (a tiny part of your DNA) initiates the formation of excess quantities of a molecule called renin. Renin breaks down another molecule, called angiotensinogen, into angiotensin I. Angiotensin I is converted into angiotensin II by a substance known as angiotensin converting enzyme (ACE). That's why most popular patented "space alien" antihypertensives are ACE inhibitors and angiotensin II receptor blockers (ARBs).

But vitamin D helps prevent high blood pressure by targeting the very first step in the process: It persuades the gene that controls the production of renin to become less active. When less renin is produced, less angiotensin is produced.

While vitamin D is very effective at lowering blood pressure, don't expect overnight miracles: It frequently takes two to three months for significant changes to start taking place and six to eight months for the vitamin D to take full effect.

How much do you need? Well, recent research has reevaluated the safe upper limit for this vitamin, and many experts now agree that it's 10,000 IU daily (though some say it's as low as 4,000 IU daily). But my target for optimal vitamin D intake is whatever it takes to achieve a serum level of approximately 60 ng/ml. Since achieving this level will mean a different dose for everyone, it's always best to work with your doctor to monitor your blood level of vitamin D.

The building blocks of healthy blood pressure

Amino acids are the "building blocks" from which all proteins are made. In certain cases, supplementing with them has led to lower blood pressure.

At least one study devoted to each demonstrated that L-tryptophan and taurine can lower blood pressure in essential hypertension (high blood pressure with no known cause). The amount of L-tryptophan used was 3 grams daily. L-tryptophan has been available by prescription for two to three years now, but it also very recently became available over the counter once again (as it used to be until about 1989). At present, over-the-counter L-tryptophan can be found in a few natural food stores, compounding pharmacies, and the Tahoma Clinic Dispensary.

Quantities of taurine used in the study were relatively large (but safe)—6 grams daily. However, when taurine is used in combination with other nutrients and botanicals, you need only 1 to 2 grams daily.

L-arginine has gained considerable "notoriety" lately as the precursor to nitric oxide (NO), the blood vessel-dilating metabolite essential to male sexual function. However, that same blood vessel-dilating ability has been found to improve heart function in cases of congestive heart failure, and I've observed cases in which this same blood vessel-dilating effect has lowered blood pressure.

The benefits of metabolites: Coenzyme Q10 and DHA

Metabolites are molecules made in our bodies from other (precursor) materials. Sometimes, directly supplying the body with extra quantities of certain metabolites can be much more effective than supplying the precursor materials. This is definitely the case with coenzyme Q10, as our bodies make less and less of this metabolite as we grow older.

Coenzyme Q10 aids in metabolism in every cell in the body. It's found in greatest concentration in the mitochondria, the "energy engines" of the cells. It's such an important metabolite that, even though it can be fairly expensive, I recommend a small amount (30 milligrams) for everyone over 60 and more (50 to 150 milligrams daily) for everyone with high blood pressure.

Another important metabolite that helps lower blood pressure levels is docosahexaenoic acid, or DHA (not to be confused with DHEA). This is an omega-3 fatty acid, a metabolite of the essential fatty acid called alpha-linolenic acid. A recent study reported that 4 grams daily of DHA lowered blood pressure in hypertensive patients by a small but significant degree.

The garlic and herb recipe for blood pressure success

Although you'll encounter a few foods that your doctor will tell you to stay away from if you have high blood pressure, there are certain foods and herbs that can help. Garlic may not make for the freshest breath, but it does usually help to lower blood pressure readings.

A lesser-known (but still important) blood pressure-lowering botanical is olive leaf. Only powdered olive leaf in capsule form is presently available in the United States, and you should take 500 milligrams four times daily. Like many of the items noted above, olive leaf can take three to four months to show an effect.

Sarpaganda (better known in Western medicine as rouwolfia) has been used in India for centuries to treat ailments like fevers and snakebites. Early 20th century pharmaceutical chemists searching for a "magic bullet," single-ingredient, patentable, FDA-"approvable" drug treatment managed to isolate one of the active ingredients in sarpaganda—reserpine.

Herbalists have been telling us for most of the 20th century that it's really better to use the whole herb containing the active ingredient(s), for at least two reasons. First, a smaller quantity of an active ingredient is usually effective because of synergistic effects of other parts of the herb—and the whole herb usually holds less potential danger than the isolated active ingredients. Second, herbalists have told us that combining the whole herb with other selected herbs can further lessen the quantity of each active ingredient necessary to achieve significant results and further lessen potential danger.

But western physicians still went ahead using reserpine instead of whole natural sarpaganda to combat high blood pressure. Unfortunately, many of them prescribed excess dosages of reserpine. These excess dosages caused various ailments, including depression and occasional suicide, so reserpine fell out of common use.

Unfortunately, since there's not as much money to be made with the whole, natural herb itself, the medical world basically forgot about sarpaganda after the problems with reserpine: Only a few practitioners outside of Ayurvedic medicine are even aware of its existence. Most of the sarpaganda products available these days combine this herb with others also useful for the heart. Although side effects are rare and sarpaganda is definitely a very effective "big gun" in hypertension treatment, products containing sarpaganda are usually only available through health care practitioners.

I usually recommend sarpaganda as a part of the Ayurvedic combination, Cardiotone, which contains 50 milligrams of sarpaganda per capsule; take one capsule three to four times daily. Cardiotone is available from the Tahoma Clinic Dispensary (425)264-0059; www.tahomadispensary.com.

An underactive thyroid: An often overlooked culprit

Incidence of hypothyroidism (an underactive thyroid) is higher in individuals with high blood pressure than in those with normal blood pressure. Even the most up-to-date thyroid blood tests can miss instances of "subclinical" hypothyroidism. Some signs of an underactive thyroid are low body temperature, dry skin, and a slow ankle reflex. It's best to talk to your doctor if you think there's a problem.

Make sure you know how much metal you're really carrying around

Heavy metal toxicity is another often-overlooked cause of high blood pressure. But even if your doctor does test you for heavy metal toxicity, chances are the results won't be accurate. That's because blood tests for heavy metals are virtually useless.

Since these toxic substances are damaging to so many different cell structures, your body clears them from your bloodstream as rapidly as possible. If there's too much toxic metal to be immediately excreted through your liver and kidneys (and there usually is), it gets tucked away in your bones or other less metabolically active tissue where it causes less immediate damage. So a blood test won't necessarily pick up any toxicity—even if there's a ton of it stored in your body (well, not literally a ton, but you get the idea).

Unfortunately, wherever the unexcreted toxic metal is stored, it still does some damage, and if and when it's finally released from storage, it can do further damage.

Hair testing for toxic minerals isn't much better than blood tests. If one or more metals are found to be high based on a hair test, there's definitely a toxic mineral problem. But if the hair test comes back negative, it doesn't necessarily mean that you're free from heavy metal toxicity.

The best test for the presence of heavy metals is a chelation test. In my experience, more than 50 percent of individuals with blood pressure higher than 140/90 have significant excretion of toxic metals found by a chelation test.

And if you do have heavy metal toxicity, chelation therapy will usually help lower your blood pressure. Chelation therapy is an intravenous process that binds to the heavy metals and removes them from the body. Oral chelation can also be effective, but it takes considerably longer and doesn't necessarily remove as much toxic metal.

For more information or advice about both chelation testing and treatment for toxic metals, consult a physician from any of the groups listed below:

- The American College of Advancement in Medicine: (800)532-3688; www.acam.org

- The International College of Integrative Medicine: (866) 464-5226; www.icimed.com

- The American Academy of Environmental Medicine: (316)684-5500; www.aaem.com

• The American Association of Naturopathic Physicians:
  (866)538-2267; www.naturopathic.org

If you have high blood pressure, nearly all the diet and supplementation ideas discussed are safe to try. If you don't have high blood pressure but it runs in your family, it can't hurt and may help in prevention to follow a few of the basic suggestions outlined in this section.

Chapter 5:

Beyond cholesterol and blood pressure—two more heart risk factors you need to know about

The next cardiovascular risk factor on the list has been "generally accepted" as such for over a decade but is just now starting to make some noise in the health world. It's called C-reactive protein and some sources are saying it's even more important than homocysteine and other risk factors. For instance, one recently published study of 27,939 women found women with elevated C-reactive protein levels were more likely to have a heart attack, stroke, and death from cardiovascular disease than those with elevated levels of LDL ("bad") cholesterol.

Regardless of whether it's a more important risk factor than homocysteine or cholesterol, the point is that C-reactive protein is a risk factor and you should have your levels tested.

If your levels are elevated, the best way to tackle the problem is by reducing the inflammation the C-reactive protein is, well, reacting to. And in my experience, the best way to reduce inflammation is to concentrate on your omega-3/omega-6 fatty acid ratio. Omega-3 fatty acids are considered anti-inflammatory; omega-6s are pro-inflammatory. So, to put it simply, you want more omega-3s than omega-6s.

Minimize (or even better, eliminate—at least temporarily) sources of omega-6 fatty acids, especially hydrogenated vegetable oils, which are present in many processed and packaged foods, like crackers, cookies, potato and corn chips. Read the labels of the foods you pick up off the supermarket shelves. If it lists hydrogenated or partially hydrogenated vegetable oil as an ingredient, don't buy it.

Next, if you aren't already using it, switch to olive oil for cooking and flavoring your food. Nearly all other vegetable oils contain 100 percent omega-6 fatty acids.

Also, even though nuts and seeds are generally very good foods, the essential fatty acids in almonds, peanuts, and nearly every other nut or seed are mostly omega-6. So if your C-reactive protein levels are high, stick to walnuts and flaxseed (and its oil), which contain more omega-3 than omega-6 fatty acids.

But the absolute best sources of omega-3 fatty acids are fish and fish oils. I recommend taking at least one tablespoonful of cod liver oil and 1,500 milligrams of DHA each daily. (Remember to take at least 400 IU vitamin E as mixed tocopherols whenever you take any extra essential fatty acids.)

Blood clots: Not just a stroke risk

Fibrinogen is a protein involved in blood clotting. If it sounds familiar, you may have heard of it in terms of its more well-known role as a stroke risk factor. But elevated fibrinogen levels are also a well-established, though very little known, independent risk factor for cardiovascular disease. (Where's that "National Fibrinogen Education Program" when you need it?) Like many other less than desirable changes, fibrinogen levels tend to increase with age—though researchers aren't sure why.

However, one group of researchers has found that the spice turmeric (best known as an ingredient in the traditional Indian flavoring curry) and one of its components, curcumin, can lower elevated fibrinogen levels to normal. If testing shows your fibrinogen levels are elevated, take either 500 milligrams of turmeric twice daily or 200-500 milligrams of curcumin daily.

Researchers have also found that eating fish two to three times a week or taking fish oil lowers fibrinogen levels by as much as 20 percent. Take 1 1/2 tablespoons of cod liver oil daily, along with 400 IU of vitamin E. Or if you simply can't stand the oil, take a DHA/EPA supplement providing 2 to 3 grams of DHA daily.

Chapter 6:

Two signs on your body that may point to heart trouble

There are some physical signs to look for on your body that can be used as a basis for further investigation or treatment. Of course, this method isn't 100 percent accurate—and you must keep in mind that self-diagnosis can be tricky and deceptive. Any serious symptoms deserve medical attention. With that said, these physical signs can be a great starting point on your way to good health.

A message to your heart written on your earlobes

If you have diagonal creases across your earlobes, it may be a sign of increased susceptibility to cardiovascular disease. If you're eating right, getting regular exercise, and taking vitamin E, it's probably not anything to worry about. But just to be on the safe side, you may want to have your cholesterol, triglyceride, homocysteine, and C-reactive protein levels checked.

Beware of a pink nose and rosy cheeks

If you have dilated capillaries in your cheeks and nose (a red nose or rosy cheeks), it could be a sign of low stomach acidity. (See Chapter 7 on page 77.) This means that you may not be properly digesting and absorbing important nutrients, supplements, or medications.

Also, low production of hydrochloric acid and pepsin in the stomach is associated with hardened arteries, high cholesterol, high triglycerides, high blood pressure, and even obesity—all of which can spell trouble for your heart.

Chapter 7:

The natural artery-cleaning program that starts in your stomach

Hernando wasn't an old man, but his diseased arteries made it so difficult for him to get around that he could barely hobble into my office. As he put it, "I'm just waiting around for things to get bad enough so I can have my legs amputated."

Is your body starving itself of essential nutrients?

It turned out that one of Hernando's problems was a condition called hypochlorhydria, in which his stomach wasn't digesting his food and nutrients efficiently. This is by far the most common digestive problem we see at the Tahoma Clinic. It happens when the stomach doesn't produce enough acid for digestion to proceed normally. In fact, according to one medical text book, *The Pharmacological Basis of Therapeutics*, 10 to 15 percent of the general population have this problem. And if inefficient digestion isn't corrected, then even the best of diets and supplementation won't help.

Having seen firsthand how many problems this condition can cause, I always recommend having stomach function tested.

One way to test this is by radio telemetry using the Heidelberg capsule. To take this test, you'll swallow a small, plastic capsule that contains electronic monitoring equipment. As it moves through the stomach and intestines, the capsule can measure the pH of the stomach, small intestine, and large intestine and transmit a signal, which you'll receive through antennae that you wear outside your body. This information can help your doctor determine whether or not your stomach is producing adequate amounts of gastric acid. (This test can be obtained by contacting a doctor-member of the American College for Advancement in Medicine, or ACAM, at (800)532-3688, www.acam.org or the American Academy of Environmental Medicine AAEM at (316)684-5500, www.aaem.com.) Other laboratory clues can also help to diagnose this condition. One is a mineral analysis of a hair specimen. If six or more minerals are low, excluding sodium and potassium, have your stomach acid checked.

Although the mainstream medicine deals with the problem of low stomach acid by ignoring it or treating it with a bland diet, there is a much better solution. But it must be monitored by a doctor. If your test results indicate low levels of stomach acid, it's a good idea to supplement with either betaine hydrochloride-pepsin (or glutamic-acid hydrochloride-pepsin) before meals. To start, I usually recommend taking one capsule (5, 7 1/2, or 10 grains) before each meal. After two or three days, if there are no problems, use two capsules in the early part of the meal, then increase your dose to three capsules per meal several days later. The dose is gradually increased in this step-like fashion until it equals 40 to 70 grains per meal.

This method should only be used when testing indicates a need for it. Although problems rarely occur, they can be bad ones. Hydrochloric acid should never be used with aspirin, Butazolidin, Inodicin, Motrin, or any other anti-inflammatory medications. Also, hydrochloric acid is usually taken in combination with pepsin. Stomachs that don't produce adequate hydrochloric acid are presumed not to produce enough pepsin either.

If during treatment you feel bad in any way—for example, if you experience pain, burning, or additional gas—STOP. In certain cases, I've treated patients with small, gradually increased quantities of lemon juice or vinegar and found the effects to be similar to (but slightly less than) treatment with hydrochloric acid.

There's a long list of diseases frequently associated with low stomach acidity: Diabetes mellitus, both underactive and overactive thyroid problems, childhood asthma, eczema, gallbladder disease, osteoporosis, rheumatoid arthritis, chronic hives, lupus, weak adrenal glands, chronic hepatitis, vitiligo, and rosacea, for example. Unfortunately, simply getting older is also associated with an increasing frequency of low stomach acidity. In fact, some investigations have found it in more than 50 percent of those over 60.

Hernando's natural artery-cleaning program

Hernando began the following natural "artery-cleaning" program that put him on the road to recovery:

- Vitamin C, 1 gram three times daily.

- Vitamin E, 800 units of the mixed tocopherol type daily.

- Inositol hexanicotinate, 1 gram three times daily. (Vitamin E and inositol hexanicotinate can improve walking distance for individuals with blood-flow impairment in the legs.)

- L-carnitine, 250 milligrams three times daily. This has also been shown to increase walking distance.

- Cod liver oil, 1 tablespoon daily or the equivalent in capsules. Fish oil makes platelets more slippery, reducing the risk of clotting, and as an omega-3 fatty acid source reduces inflammation.

- A high-potency multiple vitamin-mineral. It's always wisest to add a multiple to back up individual nutrients in high amounts.

- Chelation (IV treatment) with EDTA (a synthetic amino acid shown to improve circulation remarkably in some individuals with atherosclerosis) and magnesium. Taken intravenously, these absorb more efficiently.

Hernando's results

Hernando decided to take chelation therapy. He changed his diet, found he needed digestive aids, took all his supplements, and even took a small quantity of testosterone. Soon he was back walking at least two miles, three times every week, without sitting down once.

Chapter 8:

Putting an end to agonizing chest pain

John had been having angina chest pains for three years when he came to the Tahoma Clinic for the first time. He had been to a cardiologist who gave him a "treadmill electrocardiogram" test and an angiogram. He was told that several of his arteries had some blockage but that it wasn't too severe. He was taking two prescriptions, nitroglycerin (he was currently taking six to eight pills every week) and calcium channel blockers. And his doctor had recommended that he take vitamin E, although he couldn't assure him of its efficacy.

John's wife had already changed their diet at home to whole grains, no chemicals, less meat, more fish, and more vegetables. John underwent a physical exam and was checked for key minerals, blood levels of homocysteine, and "C-reactive protein." He also underwent routine testing for cholesterol and HDL cholesterol levels, triglycerides, kidney functioning, and allergies. In addition to diet changes and supplements, chelation therapy is usually very helpful for relieving angina and improving circulation. To make sure chelation therapy is safe, kidney functioning must be monitored.

I recommended that John take the following supplements:

• Vitamin E, 800 IU daily to start.

• L-carnitine, 500 milligrams.

• Coenzyme Q10, 100 milligrams.

• Magnesium (aspartate), 125 milligrams.

All of these should be taken three times daily. In addition, I advised John to take a high-potency vitamin-mineral supplement with at least 50 milligrams of vitamin B6, 800 milligrams of folate, and 500 micrograms of vitamin B12.

In addition to taking the recommended magnesium supplement by mouth, John must also come to the Tahoma Clinic for a short series of intravenous magnesium injections. And, along with the suggested chelation therapy, he also used mineral replacement IVs to replace any beneficial minerals that may have been lost during the therapy.

Testosterone can be extremely valuable in strengthening the heart muscle, so I also recommended that John have his serum levels tested.

Like many individuals, John had inefficient stomach function, with low production of hydrochloric acid and pepsin. I advised him to take supplemental hydrochloric acid and pepsin with his meals. Without these, his body wouldn't have been able to make optimal use of his food and dietary supplements.

Two weeks to dramatic angina pain reduction

John's cholesterol and triglyceride tests were both slightly abnormal; his testosterone was OK. Since his kidney function tests were normal, he went ahead with chelation therapy. He made sure to stick to his healthy diet, took the vitamin E, L-carnitine, coenzyme Q10, magnesium (both orally and injected), as well as a "back-up" high-potency vitamin-mineral.

John's angina started to diminish just two weeks after his program started. By six weeks, he was down to only two "nitros" per week, and after six months, he was off all medications and free of chest pain unless he exerted himself maximally. John undertook a gradually increasing exercise program after four months, and after one year could run two miles without angina. Five years later, he remains free of any chest pain.

Chapter 9:

A contaminant in your water may be clogging your arteries

There are a few, if any, communities around the world that have both chlorinated drinking water and a low incidence of atherosclerosis. Chlorine is a powerful oxidizing agent (that's why it is used for bleaching) that is capable of causing severe damage to blood vessels. American servicemen fighting in Korea and Vietnam who were killed in battle were found to have atherosclerosis in more than 75 percent of all cases. The water given to these men was so heavily chlorinated that it was virtually undrinkable. In animal studies, chlorine has been found to promote the development of atherosclerosis. The good news is that it's fairly simple to remove the chlorine from your drinking water. Just boil the water for five to 10 minutes or add a pinch of vitamin C crystals to the water.

It can also be removed by charcoal filtration, as well as through "reverse osmosis." Check with the filter manufacturer of whatever brand you choose to be certain.

Chapter 10:

Testosterone testing: Important for heart health in men **and** women

Congestive heart failure patients should always undergo a testosterone test. Why? Remember, our hearts are muscles—specialized muscles. And testosterone is the body's major muscle builder. There's a small amount of testosterone in women's bodies naturally, just as there's a small amount of estrogen in men's. People with congestive heart failure often have testosterone levels that are much lower than usual for their respective sex. Supplementing identical-to-natural testosterone, when done carefully, is often a major help in relieving heart failure. And the form that I work with is a balanced group of identical-to-natural hormones, not just testosterone (though testosterone is the most important of these hormones for strengthening the heart muscle).

In one placebo-controlled study, Drs. S.Z. Wu and X.Z. Wan reported on 62 men, 60 of whom had suffered a heart attack in the five years prior to the study and two of whom had experienced complete occlusion of at least one coronary artery. Prior to the study, the 62 men had significantly lower testosterone levels than did members of a "control group."

Angina pain plummets in 77 percent of patients

The men were given either the testosterone or a placebo for 10 weeks and then were switched to the opposite treatment. The testosterone groups reported 77 percent reduction in angina symptoms as compared to 7 percent in the placebo groups. EKG measurements reflected the symptomatic improvement, showing 69 percent improvement with testosterone vs. 8 percent with the placebo. Improvement shown by portable monitors was even better, showing 75 percent improvement (testosterone) vs. 8 percent (placebo).

Unfortunately, heart patients of both sexes are almost never offered testosterone to prevent or treat heart disease. Testosterone patches are widely available these days, but they're marketed by patent medicine companies primarily for men with low libido or impotence as a result of testosterone deficiency—not to treat or prevent heart disease. While physicians are free to prescribe testosterone to any patient for any reason, most are locked into the conventional treatment of cardiovascular disease, and few are aware how beneficial testosterone might be for prevention or treatment.

If your doctor won't test your testosterone level or consider testosterone therapy for heart disease, find a nutritionally oriented doctor who will. Contact the American College for Advancement in Medicine (ACAM) at (800)532-3688 or www.acam.org for a list of such physicians near you.

Chapter 11:

Coenzyme Q10—a treatment for cardiomyopathy

O ne of the greatest tragedies of modern medicine is that doctors continue to ignore coenzyme Q10 (coQ10), a nutrient that, if used appropriately, would relieve the suffering of millions of Americans (especially heart patients) and save billions of health care dollars. Of course, the "medical establishment" has a reputation for being oblivious to the most nutritional treatments. However, with the volumes of scientific research on coQ10, that ignorance is inexcusable.

One study, published in the *American Journal of Cardiology*, showed that patients with "terminal" cardiomyopathy had a dramatically increased survival rate when they took coQ10. The typical mortality rate is usually 75 percent within two years, but in this case, 60 percent of the coQ10 patients were still alive after 5 years. Shortness of breath and blood flow from the heart also improved when the patients took coQ10.

All chemical processes in the body that require energy (including the workings of the heart) also require an adequate supply of coenzyme Q10—of course they require an adequate supply of other things too, but it seems that coQ10 is one of the most important.

Coenzyme Q10 is available at most natural food stores, pharmacies, and grocery stores. It can be on the expensive side, but it's one of those things that really is worth the additional cost. The usual dosage of coQ10 for preventative purposes is 30 milligrams per day. Larger amounts are used to treat certain medical conditions. Please check with your doctor.

Chapter 12:

OPCs—what are they and how do they help your heart?

Scientists are still baffled by the French paradox: Although the French have a similar intake of saturated fat to the British, their incidence of heart disease is substantially lower. Various causes have been attributed to this phenomenon, but much attention has focused on the high French intake of red wine. Red wine is rich in OPCs. OPC stands for oligomeric procyanidins, compounds that have been found to be useful in the prevention and treatment of a wide variety of heart problems. OPCs are also a key chemical component in hawthorn, a popular herbal cardiac treatment.

Some people will obviously prefer to take their OPCs in the form of wine. The quality of the wine does make a difference to its potential health benefits. If the wine contains any sort of preservative, like sulfites, it's just as likely—if not more so—to do harm as it is to do any good. Vineyards are required to state the presence of sulfite on the label of any wine containing it, so this is another instance where it's important to read labels.

The key word in terms of wine's health benefits is moderation. Of course, there's no final word about how much wine is "optimum" for your health. But it's pretty safe to say that the negatives associated from drinking too much would undoubtedly outweigh any positives. Stick with a glass or two a day, at the most.

If you prefer not to drink wine, there are various OPC herbal products, including hawthorn, available in natural food stores. The clinical support for hawthorn is strong, so regular intake might be an important contributor to the prevention of heart disease.

Chapter 13:

The No.1 heart-protecting mineral

Among its many other heart health functions, magnesium reduces the risk of abnormal heart rhythm, helps blood vessels to relax and dilate, and raises levels of HDL ("good") cholesterol. So it makes sense that low levels of magnesium can contribute to heart problems.

The most accurate way to measure your magnesium level is by having a white blood cell magnesium (WBC-Mg) test.

The remedy for low levels of magnesium is simple: Eat more magnesium-containing food and take magnesium supplements. A general rule of thumb for finding magnesium-rich foods: Anything that's green—naturally green, that is (lime Jell-O doesn't count!)—contains magnesium. And one word of caution about supplements: Don't take more than 400 milligrams of supplemental magnesium without measuring your own "intestinal transit time." Intestinal transit time describes the length of time food takes to transit from the entrance to the exit of the gastrointestinal tract. Higher doses of magnesium can sometimes "speed things up," which means you may not be absorbing it or the other nutrients your body needs.

Although estimates vary, a reasonable range for "normal" transit time appears to vary from 12-24 hours. You can measure your own transit time by eating beets or corn or swallowing charcoal tablets and observing how long it takes them to emerge. If magnesium appears to speed up your own normal transit time, cut back on your dosage until you reach the amount that brings things back to normal.

Chapter 14:

Sweat your way to a healthier heart in 4 weeks or less

Saunas have been around in Europe, especially Northern Europe, for hundreds (probably thousands) of years. In America, some of the earliest inhabitants developed and passed down the tradition of "sweat lodges" for both health and spiritual benefits. Saunas are still great for their traditional uses: Meditation and detoxification. But believe it or not, there are actually a surprising number of controlled studies on the physical health benefits of saunas.

And some of the recent research shows that they may improve heart function in patients with clogged arteries, high blood pressure, and even congestive heart failure.

Big benefits after just one week

Most of the recent research has been done on a specific type of sauna known as a far infrared sauna. Far infrared saunas are sort of the "new kid on the (sauna) block," having become very popular in Japan over the past century. Far infrared saunas are a bit different than the traditional steam versions. Far infrared waves warm things without actually heating up the air in between the heat source and the object. So in a far infrared sauna, the air is warm and dry, as opposed to the humid heat in traditional saunas.

The first study on the health effects of far infrared saunas took place in Japan and involved golden hamsters. (If you want a quick laugh, try picturing a hamster in a sauna.) One group of hamsters received actual sauna temperatures—usually between 105 and 140 degrees (Fahrenheit)—daily for four weeks. The control group was placed in a room-temperature sauna (it wasn't turned on) for equal lengths of time.

Chemical analysis showed greater amounts of a substance called nitric oxide synthase in the endothelial (lining) cells of the aorta, as well as the coronary, carotid, and femoral arteries of the hamsters that got the real sauna treatments. The reason this finding is so important is that increased levels of nitric oxide synthase will produce more nitric oxide. Nitric oxide dilates coronary arteries, helping to improve heart function. That's good news on its own, but it gets even better.

More detailed analysis showed a 40-fold increase in nitric oxide synthase in the endothelial cells of the aorta after just one week. After four weeks of treatment, the increase leveled off but steadied at 50 percent.

Saunas tackle congestive heart failure, atherosclerosis, and hypertension

With such encouraging results from the hamster study, the researchers decided to test this approach in individuals with congestive heart failure.

The researchers treated 20 congestive heart failure patients with far infrared sauna daily for two weeks. They were compared with 10 "control-group" individuals, matched for age, sex, and degree of heart failure (according to the widely accepted New York Heart Association, or "NYHA," classification system).

After just two weeks of far infrared treatment, 17 of 20 sauna-treated individuals had significant improvement in clinical symptoms. Their ultrasound evaluations and blood tests were also significantly better. None of the 10 control group individuals had any change.

Previously, the same researchers had studied 25 younger men (ages 31-45) with one or more "coronary risk factors," including diabetes, hypertension, high cholesterol, and smoking. They were compared with 10 healthy younger men (ages 27-43) who had none of these risk factors. Compared with the "normal" men, the men with risk factors had impaired blood vessel dilation. But after just two weeks of daily far infrared sauna treatments, the risk-factor group had very significant improvements in blood vessel dilation. The researchers wrote that these results "suggest a therapeutic role for [far infrared] sauna therapy in patients with risk factors for atherosclerosis."

Given the hamster-in-the-sauna results, it's very likely that the improved blood vessel dilation in the men with cardiovascular risk factors resulted from higher levels of nitric oxide synthase.

Although none of the studies have measured it specifically, far infrared sauna therapy will very likely lower blood pressure for many individuals too. This theory makes sense, since the mechanism of action is the same as in congestive heart failure: An increase in nitric oxide dilates blood vessels and lowers blood pressure. If the studies I mentioned above are any indicator, it shouldn't take long to find out, either, since the effects in both hamsters and humans occurred in just two to four weeks.

And even though there's no clinical proof yet, I also think it's very likely that combining the amino acid L-arginine (another precursor of nitric oxide) with far infrared sauna therapy would produce even better results than either therapy alone—whether you're using it for hypertension or congestive heart failure.

Get all the benefits of saunas without even leaving home

The most economical way to use sauna therapy is probably to buy one for your own home. I did a quick search of the Internet and found literally dozens of companies selling far infrared saunas. They range in price, so shop around. Keep in mind that I'm not connected with any of these vendors, and I don't have any information on them, but I have a bit more faith in any company that provides complete copies of articles (or at least citations to studies) concerning their products or technology.

So far, the one that has far and away the best citation list is High Tech Health, Inc., (800-794-5355, www.hightechhealth.com). If you want to start investigating far infrared saunas (which are usually easy to assemble, and simply need to be plugged in to use), you might want to start there.

Part III
Pain

Chapter 1:

Two weeks to bursitis relief— minus the aspirin, NSAIDs, and cortisone shots

You'd be amazed at how many different symptoms can be related to a single underlying cause. And I think you'd be even more amazed at how ineffective conventional medicine is in treating something that alternative medicine can nip in the bud in as little as two weeks. Although this applies to a host of conditions, one of the most fitting examples that comes to mind is bursitis.

I see it frequently at the Tahoma Clinic. Take Bill, for instance. Bill was 63 years old when his wife Rose, who had been a Tahoma Clinic client for several years, was finally able to drag him in to see me. Bill had suffered on and off from shoulder pain for two to three years. When the pain flared up, he typically took aspirin for a few weeks until it went away. But the last time the pain flared up, aspirin hadn't worked—neither had stronger over-the-counter pain relievers. When it got to the point where he couldn't work, he went to his primary care physician, who predictably injected a dose of cortisone into his shoulder.

The pain promptly went away, but three months later it was back again. Bill was geared up to get another cortisone shot when his wife finally put her foot down. She had called the doctor's office and found out that Bill hadn't been given real cortisone after all. Instead, his doctor had given him a formerly patented and much more powerful "space alien" version of naturally occurring cortisone called Kenalog. Once Rose read about the potential long-term adverse effects of repeated Kenalog injections, she convinced Bill to see if I had any alternative treatments.

At his appointment with me, Bill demonstrated trying to lift his arm away from his body. As he raised it, he grimaced with pain and stopped before his hand even became level with his shoulder. I checked his shoulder by putting a little pressure at the point just past the bone where it sloped down into his arm. He jumped a little, squirmed, and promptly said, "Enough! That's it!"

That was all I needed to know that he had bursitis.

In another case, a 56-year-old woman named Ellen came to the Tahoma Clinic because she was always tired and low on energy. She also had some general aches and pains. The most bothersome pain was in her right hip, but it usually only hurt her when she lay in bed. If she unconsciously rolled onto her right side during the night, the pain often woke her up.

I asked her to stand up and applied pressure to the area of her upper right hip where the bone came closest to the surface. She had a similar reaction to Bill's—jumping and saying, "That's it! And I hope that's enough pushing!"

Although it was in a different spot than Bill's, Ellen also had bursitis.

Sixty-seven-year-old Jay's bursitis was a bit more obvious than Bill's or Ellen's. His left arm looked as if he'd had a golf ball inserted under the skin at the point of his elbow. The swollen area was red and tender, and it felt as if it were filled with fluid (which, in fact, it was). He kept his arm bent, since it hurt too much to straighten it out.

What is bursitis?

Bursitis is the name given to a painful, tender, sometimes swollen bursa. A bursa is a very slender, usually unnoticeable structure located at body angles where bone lies almost immediately under the skin, as it does in shoulders, elbows, hips, knees, and heels. A bursa contains a very small sack of fluid, which allows it to function as a shock absorber, protecting bony prominences from damage when you occasionally whack them into walls, doors, and other solid objects. Once the pain and any swelling from acute injury is gone, an injured bursa usually returns to its usual unnoticed shock-absorbing role until the next inadvertent whack.

But that's not always the case, especially once you reach 50. Whether it's due to years of recurrent injury or other reasons, some bursae don't recover normally from a whacking. Sometimes the pain continues for an extended period of time. At other times the bursa will seem to recover but then become painful again, often repeating the on-off pain cycle for months or even years. I've also worked with many people who were absolutely certain they hadn't recently whacked or even lightly bumped their shoulders, knees, or elbows, yet they still developed bursitis.

"I know it's bursitis" Jay said. "I've had it right at the point of my elbow before, but it never swelled up like this. I'm told it might need to be drained, but my chiropractor said you might be able to help it without that, so here I am."

His chiropractor was right: Jay had come to the right place. But before I tell you how I treated him, Bill, and Ellen, let me tell you about Sharon.

When Sharon was only 45, she'd been diagnosed with depression. She didn't want to take any of the synthetic antidepressants because she suspected such drugs could have contributed to her mother's suicide. She had also read a lot about them in books and on the Internet (on sites like www.drugawareness.org) and was disturbed by the high proportion of high school shooters who'd been taking synthetic antidepressants at the time they shot up their schools.

But aside from her depression, Sharon mentioned a few other problems, including pain in her right knee. Although she could feel it hurting when she stood up, her knee bothered her the most when she tried to kneel down in her garden or at church. Sometimes she couldn't kneel down at all on her right knee for days at a time.

I asked her to stand up, and I applied gentle pressure to the skin over the bone an inch or two below her right knee. I knew it was the right area when she flinched and leaned away from the pressure.

"It's likely bursitis," I said. "And I think I may know why you've been experiencing depression."

The vitamin that beats bursitis

Routine treatments for bursitis include everything from aspirin and other NSAIDs to more dangerous and recently notorious COX-2 inhibitor drugs like Vioxx and Celebrex, and onward to injections of the "space alien" varieties of cortisone (such as the Kenalog shots Bill had received). But these are just temporary treatments that don't get at the root of the problem—not to mention the fact that they all come with a long list of potential side effects.

But over the past 33 years, I have recommended an entirely different treatment for bursitis sufferers—one that's completely natural, with no side effects.

And even though Bill, Ellen, Jay, and Sharon all had different complaints and varying degrees of pain, I gave them all the same advice for treatment.

Nearly 50 years ago, Dr. Irving S. Klemes discovered that the best treatment for bursitis pain is vitamin B12. Nothing has come close to it since then. When Dr. Klemes treated 40 individuals with acute subdeltoid bursitis with vitamin B12 shots, he found that they almost all experienced rapid pain relief—in some cases starting in just a few hours—and that complete relief was often achieved within a few days.[1] All but three individuals were completely pain free within two to three weeks.

Dr. Klemes recommended that vitamin B12 (1cc, 1,000 micrograms) be given by injection every day for a week, then tapered to three times weekly, then to twice weekly, and then to once weekly until the pain was completely gone. Early on, I asked bursitis sufferers to follow these instructions exactly. Later, I discovered that taking 2 ccs of vitamin B12 every day until the pain went away—with no tapering—worked even better.

That's exactly what I recommended to Bill, Ellen, Jay, and Sharon. And like hundreds of others before them, they all made complete recoveries within two weeks with no other treatment. In 33 years, I've seen vitamin B12 fail to relieve bursitis pain only once. In all other cases—even with the worst pain and swelling—vitamin B12 injections have always taken care of the problem.

Digging deeper: Rooting out the cause of bursitis pain

But as I explained to Bill, Ellen, Jay, and Sharon, even though their bursitis pain was gone, they'd just started on the road back toward good health. Unlike conventional medicine, which so often appears to be satisfied with symptom relief (particularly if it involves continuing everyday use of a patent medication), a basic goal of the natural approach to medicine is to find the cause and eliminate it safely. (See http://www.bastyr.edu/academic/naturopath/principles.asp for a great explanation of the principles of naturopathic and natural medicine.) In some cases the cause can't be found, but with bursitis it's usually clear.

I asked each one of them to have a gastric analysis done. As I suspected, they all had varying degrees of low stomach acid secretion—just like everyone else I've tested who has bursitis.

Bill wanted to know what his stomach acid—or lack of it—had to do with his shoulder. I explained that certain cells (called parietal cells) that line the stomach normally secrete hydrochloric acid. They're also supposed to secrete intrinsic factor, a poorly named molecule responsible for vitamin B12 absorption. When the parietal cells are impaired, they don't make either hydrochloric acid or intrinsic factor very well, and sometimes they don't make them at all.

So to review: If vitamin B12 by injection (which bypasses the digestive system and goes straight into the bloodstream) solves a health problem (like bursitis) but vitamin B12 from food or supplements doesn't, then vitamin B12 absorption must be poor or absent. The most likely cause for this is that the parietal cells aren't making intrinsic factor. And if that's the case, it just makes sense to expect that they can't do their other job—making hydrochloric acid—very well either.

What a stomach acid test could tell you about your energy levels

When Ellen heard this explanation, she caught on right away but asked why it was necessary to find out about her stomach if the vitamin B12 injections were the remedy for her bursitis. I explained that although the vitamin B12 improved her symptoms, we were just scratching the surface of a deeper problem.

To understand why that's the case, we need to follow the rabbit trail even further. Hydrochloric acid activates pepsin, which is responsible for digesting and breaking down nearly all protein into amino acids and peptides (which are linked amino acids) in the stomach. Hydrochloric acid also frees many minerals from the organic matrix that binds them in food—iron in meat and spinach, for example. Restoring low levels of amino acids and minerals is an important part of recovering energy—Ellen's primary concern when she first came to the Tahoma Clinic.

In Ellen's case, she had virtually no hydrochloric acid, which resulted in low levels of six of the eight essential amino acids. (These amino acids are dietary essentials because our bodies cannot make them at all, but must get them from food in order to build and repair tissue.) Most of her mineral levels were also below normal. I told Ellen that fixing her digestion and, in turn, normalizing her essential amino acid and mineral levels would be an important part of recovering her energy.

Connecting the dots between bursitis and depression

To take this another step further, essential amino acids are responsible for making most neurotransmitters. Most individuals I know of who suffer from mental health conditions are low in some or all of their essential amino acids.

Sharon was one of the few with low levels of all eight essential amino acids. By the time her test returned, she had done her own research and knew all about the connection between amino acids and depression.

"No wonder I'm depressed, and no wonder you knew why right away," she exclaimed. What Sharon had learned was right—nearly every important neurotransmitter is made from an essential amino acid. Brain cells can make plenty of neurotransmitters on their own if they just get enough essential amino acids. But because Sharon's stomach wasn't working well enough, it was depriving her of essential amino acids and vitamin B12. Taking a patented antidepressant just sidesteps the main issue: Instead of giving your body more essential amino acids and vitamin B12, it just artificially raises and alters the level of neurotransmitters.

Sharon and I then looked at two other tests I'd asked her to have done: A mineral analysis and a folic acid test called a neutrophilic hypersegmentation index. Not only did she need additional folic acid, but most of her essential minerals were considerably below normal. I explained that, like vitamin B12, folic acid doesn't absorb as well when stomach acid is low and that most minerals require larger quantities of hydrochloric acid to be adequately separated from their organic "matrix" in foods so that they can be optimally absorbed.

I told her that in the long run, she'd likely need to take hydrochloric acid/pepsin capsules along with injections of vitamin B12 and folic acid.

But if she did that alone, her recovery would take months or maybe even years. The surest and most rapid way for her to recover, I explained, would be through a series of infusions of essential amino acids and essential minerals. (For more information, see the July 2004 issue of *Nutrition & Healing*.) She took the series of infusions, and her depression and insomnia cleared up completely. Her bursitis stayed away too.

Beyond bursitis relief

Even though their bursitis had gone away with the vitamin B12 treatments, Ellen, Bill, and Jay all decided to take the hydrochloric acid/pepsin capsules and the infusions of essential amino acids and essential minerals. It wasn't long before Ellen's energy returned to normal. Both men admitted that they gained back some energy, too. Jay said he'd been a little depressed but hadn't noticed it until it was gone. And Rose joked that Bill "wasn't quite as much of an old grouch anymore."

Chapter 2:

Catch the culprit behind
your arthritis pain

The first thing to determine is which type of arthritis you have. There are two major forms of arthritis: Degenerative arthritis (also known as osteoarthritis) and rheumatoid arthritis.

Osteoarthritis is the most common form of the disease and occurs when the cartilage between the joints begins to break down and wear away, causing pain and stiffness. This cartilage damage is one of the hallmarks of osteoarthritis, but oddly enough, heavy use of the joints isn't necessarily what causes this problem. In fact, many former long-distance runners have perfectly normal hips and knees, while their more sedentary friends become plagued with degenerating joints. No one knows for sure exactly why the cartilage wears away, but those of us who practice natural medicine do know that there are plenty of ways to alleviate the pain it causes. More on that in a minute.

Rheumatoid arthritis involves inflammation, pain, and stiffness of the lining of joints in your body and also causes redness and swelling in most cases. If you aren't sure which form of arthritis you have, your doctor can help determine that. Although both types have very different causes, some of the natural treatments for each type overlap.

And no matter which type of arthritis pain you're battling, you'll need a good starting point for all of the nutrients that can help. So the first thing I recommend is a basic, healthy diet. This includes whole, unprocessed foods, with no added sugar, no so-called "soft drinks," no chemical additives, and no flavorings, coloring, or preservatives. I suggest only whole grains (if you're not allergic or sensitive to them), no artificial sweeteners, and only small amounts of alcohol. And I know it's easier said than done, but it really is best to eliminate caffeine altogether.

Now, let's start with osteoarthritis.

The arthritis triggers that could be growing in your garden

The first thing I recommend for osteoarthritis is changing certain aspects of your diet. In the 1950s, Norman Childers, Ph.D., found that eliminating certain vegetables (known as nightshade vegetables) from the diet could completely eliminate arthritis symptoms in many cases. Nightshade vegetables include tomatoes, potatoes, peppers (including paprika, but not black pepper), eggplants, and tobacco. According to Dr. Childers, nightshade sensitivity isn't an allergy but actually a progressive loss of the ability to metabolize substances known as "solanine alkaloids," which are found in all nightshade vegetables. Unfortunately, there's no test that can tell you if your arthritis will respond to a nightshade-free diet. It's strictly a "try it and see" situation.

It's harder than it might seem to completely eliminate nightshades. Tomato and potato make their way into a wide variety of food products, and pepper gets around a lot too. Check your local library or contact the Arthritis Nightshades Research Foundation (888-501-8822; www.noarthritis.com) for a copy of Dr. Childers' book, variously titled (depending on the edition) *Childers' Diet; Arthritis—Childers' Diet to Stop It*; and similar titles. The information he includes can be a big help in searching out all sources of nightshades. But even eliminating the

Add some oil to those rusty joints

Fish oil is one of my favorite recommendations. There's a good reason: Omega-3 fatty acids may have replaced folic acid as America's No.1 dietary deficiency/ insufficiency. And fish oil is the best source for your body to get the omega-3s it needs.

Make sure the brand you use is "certified heavy metal free," but aside from that, fish oil— always taken with vitamin E—has practically no hazards. (That infamous "cod liver oil burp" can almost always be eliminated by "burying" the oil in the middle of a meal, by blending the oil with rice, almond, or soy milk, and a banana, or by taking it with a "high-lipase" digestive enzyme.)

For osteoarthritis, take 1 tablespoon of cod liver oil (with 400 I.U. vitamin E) once daily— twice daily if you have a particularly bad case. You can take it right along with glucosamine and niacinamide, as they all work in different ways for different aspects of the problem.

most common nightshades (the ones listed above) is definitely worth trying. Eliminate them for at least three to four months and see if it makes a difference in your symptoms. If you're not sure after three or four months, you can do a "nightshade challenge" by eating lots of tomato, potato, and peppers. If the pain comes back after the challenge, you'll know that you are nightshade-sensitive and you should eliminate those foods from your diet permanently.

Sometimes, osteoarthritis is aggravated by "regular" food allergies. If you have a personal or family history of allergies, it's worth having this possibility checked out. For a list of physicians in your area who can help you with allergy screening, contact the American Academy of Environmental Medicine at (316)684-5500 or www.aaem.com. There are various ways to determine specific food allergies, but skin testing is not usually an accurate tool in this case.

The $10 osteoarthritis cure

Once you've determined whether or not allergies or sensitivities play a role in your arthritis, you can move on to other natural therapies, starting with glucosamine. By now, even mainstream medical doctors have heard of glucosamine. Research shows that it works by helping to stimulate the growth of new joint cartilage. This is probably why there's usually a three to four week delay after starting treatment for pain relief to begin. I recommend 500 milligrams of glucosamine sulfate three times a day.

There have been some warnings in mainstream medical publications that glucosamine might affect blood sugar control. If you have significant osteoarthritis and don't have diabetes, this theoretical possibility shouldn't be a problem. If you do have diabetes, checking your blood sugar will tell you whether the glucosamine has enough of an effect to warrant not taking it. In most cases, the improvement you'll likely feel will far outweigh the possibility of any slight effect on blood sugar.

Glucosamine is often combined with chondroitin in natural arthritis formulas. But there's enough question about chondroitin and risk of prostate cancer for me to advise all men to avoid chondroitin at this time. Besides, I've observed that glucosamine usually works just as well by itself. So just use "plain" glucosamine until this question is settled for good.

Complete arthritis relief in less than one month

The next natural osteoarthritis remedy on the list is niacinamide. Even many natural medicine doctors have forgotten, or never learned, just how useful niacinamide (not niacin) can be for controlling the pain and swelling of osteoarthritis.

In 1949, William Kaufman, M.D., Ph.D., published his exceptionally careful and comprehensive research about niacinamide and osteoarthritis titled "The Common Form of Joint Dysfunction: Its Incidence and Treatment." Unfortunately, Dr. Kaufman's research came out around the same time that patented cortisone formulas were being heavily promoted, so niacinamide treatment was hardly noticed. But even though it never made much of a stir, niacinamide treatment works very well. I recommend using 1,000 milligrams of niacinamide three times a day (it doesn't work as well if you only take it once or twice daily). You'll probably start feeling results in three to four weeks. Many osteoarthritis sufferers achieve complete relief of pain and swelling as long as they continue on with niacinamide.

Niacinamide doesn't appear to re-grow cartilage, so it's best to use glucosamine along with it. If you have diabetes and are concerned about glucosamine's effects on blood sugar, niacinamide is a good companion for it. Niacinamide also has many benefits for blood sugar problems, and using it with glucosamine is even more likely to relieve your osteoarthritis symptoms.

And a caution: On rare occasion, people who take this amount of niacinamide get low-grade nausea, queasiness, and sometimes vomiting. Although this only happens in less than 1 percent of people who take niacinamide, if you experience any of these problems, stop taking it immediately. The nausea should go away promptly, but check with your doctor before any further niacinamide use.

Three more great remedies to try

Since glucosamine is on the well-known end of the arthritis-relief spectrum, the final two items on the osteoarthritis-fighting list usually slip below the radar of most physicians. But boron and S-adenosylmethionine (SAMe) can both be quite effective.

Epidemiologic evidence shows a greater incidence of arthritis in areas of the world low in boron. A small amount of research shows that boron can relieve many symptoms of osteoarthritis. Since boron is quite inexpensive, is safe in small doses, and is useful in treating osteoporosis and preventing cancer in addition to osteoarthritis, it certainly can't hurt to take 3 milligrams twice daily.

SAMe is quite effective for some cases of osteoarthritis but not so helpful for others. While it's not a surefire cure, it's quite safe and worth trying if the diet changes and supplements noted above aren't helpful. The only drawback is that it's a bit pricey compared with many other supplements. If you decide to give it a try, take 400 milligrams once or twice daily.

Willow bark is actually the all-natural forerunner to aspirin. It's been

Osteoarthritis relief in one easy-to-use outline

Here's what you need to do:

- Eliminate all nightshade vegetables and other items (tomatoes, potatoes, peppers, eggplants, tobacco, etc.) from your diet for three to four months to see if it helps alleviate your pain

- Have thorough allergy screening done to test for non-night-shade food sensitivities

And here's what you need to take:

- Glucosamine sulfate—500 milligrams, three times a day

- Cod liver oil—1 tablespoon, once or twice daily

- Vitamin E—400 I.U., once or twice daily (along with the cod liver oil)

- Niacinamide—1,000 milligrams, three times a day

- Boron—3 milligrams twice daily

- SAMe—400 milligrams, once or twice daily

- Willow bark—two to four doses per day (of tablets containing 400 milligrams of willow bark extract and 60 milligrams of salicin)

- Myristin—six capsules per day for 80 days

proven to relieve pain equally as well as prescription pain medications.

The most recent study was published in the journal *Rheumatology* in December 2001. Researchers tested two groups of 114 participants each, treating one group with two to four 240-milligram doses of salicin (one of the main pain-relieving ingredients in willow bark extract) per day and the other with the same number of 12.5-milligram doses of rofecoxib (the generic name of Vioxx). After four weeks there was no difference between the results for the two products in terms of pain, requirement for additional analgesics, or side effects. The only difference in the two treatments is that willow bark extract is much less expensive than Vioxx.

In all the trials done so far, researchers administered two to four high potency willow bark extract tablets per day to each patient. The tablets contained 400 milligrams of actual extract and 60 milligrams of salicin. The 400 milligrams of extract corresponds to 6 to 8 grams of willow bark, depending on the type used. Your local compounding pharmacist can help you make sure you're getting the right amounts. To locate a compounding pharmacist near you, contact the International Academy of Compounding Pharmacists (800-927-4227; www.iacprx.org).

Breast-feeding mothers should use willow bark extract with caution, since the remnants excreted in breast milk may cause rashes in babies. If you are currently taking blood-thinning medications or NSAIDs, be sure to consult your physician before taking willow bark extract. It is much less likely to cause problems with bleeding than prescription medications or even aspirin, but a bit of caution can go a long way in keeping you safe, healthy, and pain-free.

One-time treatment can cure arthritis for good

Back in the 1990s, former National Institutes of Health researcher Harry Diehl became intrigued by the observation that mice don't get osteoarthritis. Working in his home lab, he analyzed literally thousands of mice, finally isolating a type of fatty acid called cetyl-myristoleate (CMO) not found in rats (which <u>do</u> get arthritis) or humans.

He invented and patented the first process to create bio-identical CMO. When he tried the bio-identical CMO on arthritic rats, they were cured. But he couldn't interest any patent-medicine companies in CMO. So he "let it go" until he developed arthritis himself at age 80.

Over the course of 10 days he applied small amounts of CMO (which he combined with DMSO) topically to his hands. Not only did it completely eliminate his arthritis pain, but Harry also reported that it cured a long-standing headache he'd been suffering and prevented any more recurrences of bronchitis which he's suffered on a regular basis.

Harry used CMO only that one time, and never need to take it again. He also made it for friends, who had the same experience.

While Harry's original topical CMO formula isn't available anymore, he developed a capsulized formulation, called Myristin, that appears to be just as effective. You can find Myristin in natural food stores, compounding pharmacies, and through the Tahoma Clinic Dispensary.

I usually recommend taking six capsules of Myristin daily for 80 days. (If it hasn't worked by then, it probably isn't going to.) Although it doesn't work for everyone, the majority of the Tahoma Clinic patients who've tried it have had substantial or complete relief.

Chapter 3:

The 100 percent solution for rheumatoid arthritis

Now let's move on to rheumatoid arthritis (RA). RA is a chronic disease of unknown cause, usually manifesting itself as inflammation of multiple joints. The severity of the disease varies from person to person—I've seen cases ranging from minor pain and discomfort to severe pain and inflammation, with joint damage and deformity.

RA can also attack other parts of the body, resulting in heart disease, anemia, nerve damage, lung disease, and general debility. This condition is considered an autoimmune disease, since the immune system appears to go awry and attack the body's own tissues.

As I mentioned earlier, some of the following recommendations are the same as those for osteoarthritis, but there are a couple of distinct differences. First, attention to diet is very important to rheumatoid arthritis control—even more so than in cases of osteoarthritis. I've observed improvement in every case of rheumatoid arthritis with elimination and desensitization of food allergy, and not just elimination of nightshade vegetables. I learned about the link between allergy and sensitivity and all sorts of health problems—including arthritis—back in 1979 when I read

Dr. James C. Breneman's book *Basics of Food Allergy*.

Since then, I've found that at least 40 to 50 percent of the people who come to see me at the Tahoma Clinic have partial to complete relief of all their symptoms—not just arthritis pain—when they uncover their allergies and sensitivities and avoid the offending foods.

Dr. Breneman's technique involves following an elimination diet. During the first week, you'll eat only foods that are less likely to cause allergies (Dr. Breneman had his patients eat things like rice, spinach, and beef). Then you add back the foods you normally eat, one at a time to see if they cause your symptoms to return.

Milk and dairy are almost always major allergens in people with this form of arthritis and have even been the subject of mainstream medical research into RA (which showed that eliminating milk and dairy worked to alleviate symptoms). But even though dairy is usually a primary culprit, there are always multiple allergens aggravating rheumatoid arthritis. The ones that do cause a recurrence should either be completely eliminated from your diet, or you may choose to work with a physician who may be able to help you desensitize to your allergens (you may not be able to desensitize to all trigger foods though). A good place to start is with a member of the American Academy of Environmental Medicine (316-684-5500; www.aaem.com).

But while food allergy elimination and desensitization improve rheumatoid arthritis, sometimes dramatically and always noticeably, it doesn't cure the problem.

A common culprit contributes to rheumatoid arthritis

Over the years, multiple studies have reported a high incidence of stomach malfunction (specifically, low levels of hydrochloric acid and pepsin) in individuals with rheumatoid arthritis. These reports also revealed that just replacing the "missing" hydrochloric acid and pepsin—without making any other changes—can significantly improve many cases of rheumatoid arthritis. Telltale symptoms of hypochlorhydria include bloating, belching or burning immediately after meals, a feeling that food just sits in the stomach undigested, and an inability to eat more than a small amount of food without feeling full. Many people with hypochlorhydria are constipated, some suffer from diarrhea, yet others have normal bowel function.

So with this in mind, I always ask individuals suffering from rheumatoid arthritis to have a gastric analysis done. At the Tahoma Clinic, we test this by radio telemetry using the Heidelberg capsule. To take this test, you'll swallow a small, plastic capsule that contains electronic monitoring equipment. As it moves through the stomach and intestines, the capsule can measure the pH of the stomach, small intestine, and large intestine and transmit a signal, which you'll receive through an antenna that you wear outside your body. This information can help your doctor determine whether or not your stomach is producing adequate amounts of gastric acid. (This test can be obtained by contacting a doctor-member of ACAM at 800-532-3688, www.acam.org.)

In the majority of instances, the test discloses low stomach function (low acid). If this is the case for you, consider supplementing with either betaine hydrochloride-pepsin or glutamic-acid hydrochloride-pepsin before meals.

I usually recommend starting out by taking one capsule (5, 7 1/2, or 10 grains). After two or three days, if there are no problems, use two capsules in the early part of the meal; then, several days later, increase the amount to three capsules. The dose is gradually increased in this step-like fashion until it equals 40 to 70 grains per meal.

You'll probably need to work with a doctor on this aspect of rheumatoid arthritis, too. On rare occasion, treatment with hydrochloric acid can be dangerous, so it should only be used when testing indicates a need.

Hydrochloric acid should never be used at the same time as aspirin, Butazolidin, Inodicin, Motrin, or any other anti-inflammatory medication. These medications themselves can cause stomach bleeding and ulcers, so using hydrochloric acid with them increases the risk.

Low levels of DHEA could be a culprit

People who suffer from rheumatoid arthritis should also be tested for low levels of DHEA. (The DHEA test is a blood or urine test, and requires a lab request signed by your doctor.) DHEA is an adrenal hormone and an important regulator of the immune system that is useful in autoimmune diseases, including rheumatoid arthritis. It normally reaches its highest levels in both sexes between the ages of 25 and 30 and gradually tapers off from there. At this point, it's not known how to reliably restore normal levels of DHEA secretion, so it's best to use a DHEA supplement. (Since lab results will vary, you should work with a physician to determine how much you need to take.) You can find DHEA supplements at most natural food stores or vitamin shops.

Fish oil and its cousins— an arthritis-relieving family reunion

Fish oil: Here it is again, and it's even more important in rheumatoid arthritis than osteoarthritis. Many research studies have shown that the anti-inflammatory omega-3 fatty acids contained in fish oil significantly reduce the inflammation and pain of rheumatoid arthritis. Generally, I recommend taking 1 tablespoonful of cod liver oil with 400 I.U. of vitamin E (as mixed tocopherols) twice daily.

Plain fish oil, such as cod liver oil, on its own is often very helpful, but some individuals have found that particular fish oil "fractions" such as DHA (docosahexaenoic acid) and EPA (eicosapentaenoic acid) can be even more helpful. If you want to try these, I still recommend backing them up with that "plain" fish oil; for example, take 2,000 to 3,000 milligrams of DHA (DHA capsules always contain EPA as well) along with 1 tablespoonful of cod liver oil and 400 I.U. of vitamin E each day.

Another closely related option is eicosatetraenoic acid (ETA). ETA was originally derived from mussels and is a close relative of DHA and EPA. It's

The warning that's not on the back of your Advil bottle

If you have arthritis and have taken aspirin, Motrin, Advil, or another non-steroidal anti-inflammatory medication (NSAID) for several months or more to relieve your pain, you probably need supplemental copper.

Before they can become effective and offer any sort of pain relief, NSAIDs must first form a "complex" with molecules of copper already present in your body. So it's important to replace the copper that's literally been "used up" by these medications.

But, it's also important to balance supplemental copper with zinc. You should consider having your levels of each tested to determine what balance of zinc and copper is right for you. The February 10, 2003 edition of Health e-Tips from *Nutrition & Healing* (subject line: "Your pipes can't help you after all") gave some good tips on testing and finding a general copper/zinc balance. To read it (or to sign up to receive this free e-letter service), visit the *Nutrition & Healing* website at www.wrightnewsletter.com.

And, of course, before you begin taking any new supplement, it's always best to discuss your plans with a physician skilled and knowledgeable in nutritional medicine.

an anti-inflammatory fatty acid and has been very well studied in Australia. You might have heard it called by the brand names Lyprinol and Lyprinex. Some rheumatoid arthritis sufferers have found that 50 milligrams of ETA three times daily noticeably lessens their inflammation. ETA can be a bit hard to find; try your local natural food store first, and if you can't find it there, you can get it online or through the Tahoma Clinic Dispensary by calling (425)264-0059 or visiting www.tahomadispensary.com. (Although I am affiliated with the Clinic Dispensary, I am not associated with the manufacturers of ETA.)

The final ingredients in the
rheumatoid arthritis relief recipe

Rounding out the list of natural rheumatoid arthritis relievers are the following:

Ginger. You can use this tasty spice in your cooking and take it as a supplement as well. It helps stomach function along even more—and it helps relieve the symptoms of RA too. If you have rheumatoid arthritis, use as much ginger in your cooking as you can and also take 1,000 milligrams of ginger in supplement form three times daily. One study showed that after three months of taking ginger root, patients with rheumatoid arthritis reported pain relief, better joint movement, and less swelling and morning stiffness.

Unless you're allergic to it, there's no downside to ginger, and my patients tell me it's usually a significant help.

Zinc and copper. These minerals are helpful individually for rheumatoid arthritis, but since prolonged use of one can lead to insufficiency or deficiency in the other, it's best to use them together (although not necessarily in the same instant). Take 30 milligrams of zinc (from picolinate or citrate) two to three times daily and 2 milligrams of copper (from sebacate) two or three times daily. (Take the three doses a day if your arthritis is more severe.)

Selenium. Garlic and onions are the only common foods high in selenium, so if you're not allergic to them, include plenty in your diet—along with the ginger. And I also recommend supplementing the onions and garlic with 200 to 500 micrograms of selenium daily. But don't over do it; it is possible to overdose at quantities of 1,500 to 2,000 micrograms daily.

Niacinamide. Although it's not a primary treatment for rheumatoid arthritis as it is for osteoarthritis, niacinamide can be particularly useful for "ankylosed" joints—meaning ones that have been partially or completely stiffened and immobilized by long-time rheumatoid arthritis.

Rheumatoid arthritis relief in one, easy-to-use outline

Here's what you need to do:

• Undergo thorough screening for an elimination of food allergies and sensitivities (which may include following an elimination diet)

• Undergo stomach function testing and treatment (if needed) using hydrochloric acid/pepsin therapy

• Have your DHEA levels tested, and work with a physician to determine how much (if any) you need to supplement to return them to the "normal" range

And here's what you need to take:

• Cod liver oil—1 tablespoon, twice a day

• Vitamin E—400 I.U. (as mixed tocopherols), twice daily (along with the cod liver oil)

• DHA—2,000 to 3,000 milligrams, once a day (if you decide to try DHA, you can reduce your dosages of cod liver oil and vitamin E to once daily)

• Ginger—1,000 milligrams, three times daily

• Zinc (picolinate or citrate)—30 milligrams, two to three times daily

• Copper—2 milligrams, two or three times daily

• Selenium—200 to 500 micrograms daily

• Niacinaminde—1,000 milligrams, three times a day

After several months of regular niacinamide use, most cases of ankylosed joints gradually regain mobility. I've seen a few ankylosed joints become more mobile again after a year or more of continuous niacinamide treatment, and many more regain at least partial mobility.

Natural arthritis relief: No news can still be good news

Regardless of which type of arthritis you're battling, you don't have to wait around for the next patent medicine news flash to find relief. All of the items discussed in the preceding pages work safely and naturally to relieve arthritis pain. I've been recommending them for years and have witnessed far more successes than anything the patented formulas have achieved!

Chapter 4:

The simplest solution for gallbladder pain—without surgery

Sometime in the 1980s, the folks who keep track of such statistics noted that approximately 800,000 people per year have their gall-bladders removed. But over 99 percent of all gallbladder removals are totally unnecessary. The only time surgery is absolutely crucial is when a gallstone "stuck" in the duct that travels from the gallbladder and lower through the pancreas to the small intestine. But that only happens in less than 1 percent of all cases.

The other 99 percent of gallbladder surgeries have nothing to do with a "stuck" gallstone. Instead, they're done to relieve recurrent "attacks" of gallbladder pain brought on by food allergies. (Eggs, pork, and onion are the most common offenders, but any food is a possible culprit.) Eliminating the food allergens eliminates the attacks of gallbladder pain, also eliminating the need for surgery.

If you have recurring gallbladder pain, you should see a physician who knows how to work with food allergy as soon as possible. A visit to a member of the American Academy of Environmental Medicine, (316)684-5500, the American College for Advancement in Medicine,

(800)532-3688, or the American Association of Naturopathic Physicians, (866)538-2267, would be a good start.

Chapter 5:

The nutrient "cocktail" that can wipe out chronic pain and more

Mainstream medicine is finally becoming aware of the need to relieve chronic pain. Hospitals now have pain-management teams, and palliative care—a relatively new medical specialty—was developed specifically to address pain relief. Whole centers devoted to pain relief are also cropping up all across the country. But they all concentrate on mainstream "cures"—drugs and surgery, which are rife with uncomfortable and even life-threatening side effects. But I've been using an all-natural nutrient combination to relieve my patients' pain for years, and they tell me it works better than any of the mainstream treatments they'd tried.

The nutrient combination I use is based on the work of Dr. John Myers, M.D., who found this therapy effective for all sorts of conditions—from fibromyalgia to chronic fatigue. It involves intravenous injections of a vitamin and mineral "cocktail" made up of vitamin C, the entire vitamin B complex (including vitamin B5, also known as dexpanthenol), magnesium, and calcium.

You'll need to work with a physician who can determine the exact quantities right for you and help you with the injections themselves. For a list of skilled nutritional doctors in your area, please contact the American College for Advancement in Medicine at (800)532-3688.

Part IV
Diabetes

Chapter 1:

Five steps to curing the common condition your doctor may be overlooking

At least three to four times a month, I see patients with a condition that their primary care doctors have completely missed. In fact, I saw this easy diagnosis completely ignored again—twice—in just one week. And along with the missed diagnosis goes the wrong type of treatment for some of its symptoms. This doesn't help the real problem at all but actually allows it to progress and lead to a whole new set of symptoms and health concerns. I'm talking about the ever-increasing instances of a condition known as insulin resistance.

When Mrs. Williams came to the Tahoma Clinic with this problem, she had a pretty typical case. Her doctor had given her a statin drug for high cholesterol and an ACE inhibitor for high blood pressure. He told her that these problems were caused by her obesity, and that she should go onto a low-fat, calorie-controlled diet to lose weight. She'd tried very conscientiously, and brought in the diet records to prove it. Over several months she'd lost only three pounds, and was very frustrated. Her cholesterol and blood pressure were lower, likely due to the patent medications, but she "just didn't feel right" and wanted to know if there were any vitamins, minerals, or herbs that would control her cholesterol and blood pressure just as well.

I asked her if any of her relatives had type 2 diabetes, and she said yes, her mother's sister, but her own blood sugar was normal, so that wasn't her problem. Then I asked her if the doctor who'd prescribed the patent medications had checked her for insulin resistance or explained "Syndrome X" to her. She looked puzzled, and said "no"—he hadn't mentioned diabetes at all.

So I explained to her that her high cholesterol, high blood pressure, and even her obesity were probably "secondary" problems, and that her primary problem was very, very likely a case of undiagnosed and mistreated insulin resistance. The patent medications she'd been given made as much sense as clamping a lid on a pot of hot water to prevent it from boiling over, instead of turning down the heat.

But there are better solutions for alleviating these symptoms—ones that address the underlying cause safely and naturally. When her test results came back positive for insulin resistance, Mrs. Williams started using them: I'm happy to report that she's already making great progress. And so can you. In fact, implementing these strategies now will not only lower your cholesterol, blood pressure, and weight, but they'll also reduce—even eliminate—your risk of type 2 diabetes.

Getting rid of the problem
that just won't go away

We've covered insulin resistance in bits and pieces before, but since cases are increasing rather than decreasing, and since mainstream physicians simply won't diagnose it (or perhaps don't know how to), it's time to go over it more completely.

Like many other health problems, insulin resistance has both a genetic and an environmental component. If you have these genetics (and estimates are that over 90 million Americans do), and you eat sugar on or in anything, your body responds—and not favorably.

Let's go over some of the mechanics involved:

When you eat or drink refined sugar—especially fructose, high fructose corn syrup, sucrose, and dextrose—your blood sugar goes much higher than it does when you eat the sugar as part of its "original package" (whole fruit, whole corn, or sugar cane). Your pancreas "cranks up" in response to this sugar overload and makes an overly large quantity of insulin to help clear the excess sugar from the blood stream. Nearly everyone's metabolic response to refined sugar follows this pattern.

People with a genetic disposition towards insulin resistance and type 2 diabetes also have an extra burden in terms of diet: Simply eating too many carbs overall—even if they are from whole, natural sources—can lead to insulin resistance, too, even though it definitely takes longer than it would from eating sugar and refined carbohydrates.

If you've inherited the genetics for insulin resistance, and this pattern happens over and over again, your cells that receive insulin become resistant to repeated exposures. Because of this resistance, as the years go by, your pancreas is forced to make more and more insulin to keep your blood sugar levels under control. Those higher levels of insulin "work" for a while, but then the receiver cells become even more resistant, so your pancreas must make even more insulin, and the "more insulin/more resistance/even more insulin/even more resistance" spiral continues ever upward, until the insulin simply can't overcome the resistance at all. At that point, the blood sugar can't be regulated, and type 2 diabetes is the ultimate result.

While they're on the way up, those ever-increasing levels of insulin can cause other problems as well: They can cause your liver's production of LDL (bad) cholesterol to increase and it's production of HDL (good) cholesterol to decrease. They can also prompt the kidneys to retain sodium, or the adrenal glands to secrete too much adrenalin, (or both), resulting in higher and higher blood pressure. Most noticeably, the combination of refined sugar and carbohydrate—or simply carbohydrate—consumption and the excess insulin secretion commonly results in increased synthesis of triglycerides (the fat inside body cells), resulting in obesity.

You could wind up with just one of these problems, a combination, or, like Mrs. Williams, all of them.

Mainstream treatment is masking the problem— not solving it

But instead of looking at these conditions as symptoms of one overall condition and addressing them at the source, nearly all mainstream doctors respond by prescribing patent anti-hypertensive and statin medications, as if high blood pressure and cholesterol are always due to patent medication deficiency.

Then, when type 2 diabetes ultimately shows up in these individuals, they prescribe yet another patent medication to "control" blood sugar, usually adding it to the "diet" of anti-hypertensive and lipid-lowering patent medications already prescribed.

Patent medication companies are increasing the pressure on mainstream doctors to prescribe in this way. In July, a panel of "experts" from the American Heart Association and the National Institutes of Health issued new guidelines for the use of cholesterol-lowering drugs that would increase the number of Americans "eligible" for them from approximately 36 million to approximately 43 million. But the nine-expert panel neglected to disclose that eight of them had received money from some of the biggest patent medicine companies, for other projects, including Pfizer, Merck, Squibb, and AstraZeneca. Disclosure of these ties came only after an outcry by consumer groups.

Similarly, "experts" are also urging mainstream physicians to prescribe ever-increasing quantities of patented anti-hypertensives, as "guidelines for healthy blood pressure" call for lower and lower blood pressure readings.

And the pressure isn't just on physicians: Who hasn't seen a TV commercial (usually featuring smiling senior citizens) telling us that the way to control cholesterol or high blood pressure is the patent medication they're touting?

Your step-by-step guide for changing the channel on insulin resistance

So it's time to change the channel once and for all and get to the root of the problem. Here are the steps for doing just that:

1.) Diagnosing insulin resistance

You've probably heard of the glucose tolerance test. It's the standard tool used to diagnose diabetes. Insulin resistance is diagnosed in exactly the same way, but with an extra step taken by the laboratory. Each time one of the blood specimens is tested for glucose, it's also tested for insulin, which is why it's called the glucose tolerance insulin resistance test (GT-IRT). The lab technicians look for several different patterns of higher insulin that are unique to people with insulin resistance.[1]

If your GT-IRT shows you do have insulin resistance, that means you're also at an increased risk for type 2 diabetes. Type 2 diabetes is <u>always</u> preceded by insulin resistance. But it takes decades before it results in the actual onset of the disease: I've seen positive insulin resistance tests in teenagers, and children as young as eight. So there's absolutely no reason at all for type 2 diabetes to "sneak up" on anyone; it can always be predicted by a positive insulin resistance test. And you can avoid it altogether by implementing the next few steps.

2.) Toss the sugar and refined carbs

Eliminating all refined sugars is priority No. 1. Although refined carbohydrates don't cause damage as fast, they still cause the same problems, and must be eliminated too. Even if you don't have the genetics for developing insulin resistance, refined sugar will cause your health problems— at the very least accelerated aging. Remember, humans are "designed" to digest and metabolize whole, natural foods, not refined foods. All of our ancestors for hundreds of thousands of years ate absolutely no refined food of any kind.

Admittedly, these are probably the hardest steps of the bunch: Over the years, refined sugar and flour have made their way into more foods than you can even imagine. But it is possible, and there are a few "tricks" you can use to make it a bit simpler.

First, reading labels—and knowing what to look for on them—is crucial. Look for ingredients like high fructose corn syrup, dextrose, and enriched flour. If the product contains any of these, don't buy it. In fact, you'll be better off avoiding packaged foods altogether, which explains why this step can be so difficult: Supermarket shelves are stocked primarily with processed, packaged foods, and I'd be willing to bet that 90 percent of them contain some sort of refined sugar or carb.

Shopping along the outer edges of the grocery store—where fruits, vegetables, and meats are usually located—will make avoiding the packaged stuff a little easier. And you may also want to find a natural food store in your area. While not everything these stores carry is truly healthy, they often have more options in terms of products made without refined ingredients. These methods of shopping will also help you transition into the next step:

3.) Eat a high-protein, low-carb diet

My No. 1 recommendation is the "original human diet," or the versions of it explained in the books, *The Paleo Diet* by Loren Cordain, Ph.D., and *The Paleolithic Diet Prescription* by S. Boyd Eaton, Ph.D., Marjorie Shostak, and Melvin Konner, Ph.D.

"Regular" high-protein, low-carbohydrate diet plans are OK too. The point is to regulate your blood sugar swings to avoid the release of excess insulin. Limiting your carb intake is the best way to do that—no matter which specific diet plan you choose.

4.) Take your vitamins

I wrote about supplements to reduce insulin resistance at length in the August 2001 *Nutrition & Healing* issue. Each of them should be taken daily.

However, you probably won't need to take each of these items separately, since many of them can be found together in good multiple formulations. Two formulas I have recommended to patients with success are *Glucobalance* and *Blood Sugar Improvement Formula*, both of which are available from the Tahoma Clinic Dispensary. There are other good multiple formulas available too; check your natural food store to see what they carry and compare the labels to the list of nutrients to the right to find the best one. So far, I haven't seen any single formula that contains all of the items listed in the amounts noted, so you'll probably need to take at least a few of them separately to make up for the ones your multi doesn't contain (or doesn't contain enough of). Please refer to the box on the next page for the complete list.

5.) Get moving

Last, but not least, don't forget to exercise. After all, you can't expect eating right and supplementing to do all the work: Giving your food and supplements a fit, healthy environment to do their jobs will help your progress along even more. And you don't have to devote hours on end each day to high-impact aerobics classes. Even a 30-minute walk three times a week may be enough to make a difference. Check with your doctor about the right amount of exercise for you.

Find the real problem and eliminate many others

Unfortunately, the word just doesn't seem to have gotten out about insulin resistance—even though it was first described over 20 years ago. I'm seeing more people than ever who've been given patent medications to treat its symptoms (high blood pressure, high cholesterol, high triglycerides) with no attention paid at all to the diagnosing and treating the real problem. And symptom treatment just doesn't cut it when it comes

Your guide to beating insulin resistance in one, easy-to-follow outline

Here's what you need to do:

- Have a glucose tolerance insulin resistance test (GT-IRT) done. (The results will tell you for sure whether or not you have this condition.)
- Eliminate refined sugar and refined carbohydrates from your diet.
- Adopt a high-protein, low-carb diet.
- Begin an exercise program—even a low-intensity one, like walking for 30 minutes—several times a week.

And here's what you need to take:

- Chromium—1,000-2,000 micrograms
- Niacin—15-25 milligrams
- Niacinamide—50-100 milligrams
- Biotin—8 to 16 milligrams
- Alpha-lipoic acid—300 milligrams
- Co-Enzyme Q10—60 milligrams
- Vitamin K—5-10 milligrams daily
- Vitamin D—2,000 IU daily
- Vitamin E (as mixed tocopherols)—400 IU
- Vitamin C—2,000-3,000 milligrams
- Magnesium—300-400 milligrams
- Vanadium—1-2 milligrams
- Zinc—30 milligrams
- Copper—2 milligrams
- Manganese—5-10 milligrams

Look for a good multiple formula that combines many of these individual supplements. Check your natural food store to see what they carry, or try one of the following:

- Glucobalance
- Blood Sugar Improvement Formula

to preventing the ultimate onset of type 2 diabetes—and stopping the burgeoning epidemic of this disease.

So take a minute to see if any of the following criteria apply to you: High cholesterol, high triglycerides, high LDL cholesterol, low HDL cholesterol, or high blood pressure; overweight; a personal history of hypoglycemia (low blood sugar); a family history of type 2 diabetes; or any combination of these problems.

Of course, there are other reasons besides insulin resistance for elevated blood pressure, cholesterol, triglycerides, weight, and so on. But since insulin resistance is at the top of the "cause list" for these problems, it should always be checked. The more of these problems you have, or are in your family, the more likely it is you have insulin resistance. So don't let your doctor shrug you off with prescriptions for patented anti-hypertensive or statin medications. Look for a doctor skilled and knowledgeable in nutritional and natural medicine, who can help you with the GT-IRT test and any necessary recommendations. If your test is positive, diet, exercise, and appropriate supplementation will help you control or eliminate all these problems—and may just help prevent many others, too.

Chapter 2:

Do-it-yourself pain relief for diabetic neuropathy: Even the "last resort" is natural and side-effect-free!

When you're dealing with the numerous complications that come along with diabetes, the best place to start is getting the diabetes itself under control as best you can. But that's not to say there aren't additional things you can do at the same time to help relieve those complications even more.

Take neuropathy, for example. It's one of the most common complications of both type 1 and type 2 diabetes and its main symptom is nerve pain that ranges from slight to intense. At the Tahoma Clinic, we've recently been part of an IRB (Institutional Review Board) supervised double-blind, placebo-controlled trial on the ability of magnetic energy (MME) to relieve the pain. Although we don't have those results yet, three out of the five patients who previously underwent MME treatment for neuropathy experienced significant pain relief.

But since MME treatments are more expensive than nutritional and other natural therapies, my colleagues at the Tahoma Clinic and I always recommend trying those first. The natural neuropathy treatments with the most published success include primrose oil, lipoic acid, capsicain, biotin, vitamin B12, and vitamin B6. And very recently, vitamin D has joined the list too.

Natural neuropathy relief backed by science

In a double-blind, placebo-controlled research trial using 4 to 6 grams of primrose oil daily, diabetics with peripheral neuropathy experienced significant pain relief after six to 12 months.[1]

Another study showed that alphalipoic acid taken both intravenously[2] and orally[3] for three weeks in 600-milligram daily doses was significantly more effective than placebo in relieving symptoms of diabetic neuropathy.

And research also showed that a topical cream containing .075 percent capsaicin (an active ingredient from pepper) cut diabetic neuropathy pain in half for 50 percent of the patients using it.[4] (One note of caution: Capsaicin can cause burning initially, but that usually subsides with persistent use.)

"Uncontrolled" reports (not double-blind, placebo-controlled studies) have noted diabetic neuropathy relief from injections of biotin and vitamin B12, and oral vitamin B6. Since these nutrients are all safe and easy to group together, we generally combine them into a single injection at the Tahoma Clinic. The combination injection we typically use contains 10 milligrams of biotin, 1,000 micrograms of vitamin B12, and 50 milligrams of vitamin B6. These injections—which can be self-administered after a simple "how-to" lesson—should be given every day for six weeks, then tapered to every other day for another six weeks. If they're effective after 12 weeks, then the dosage can be adjusted according to response.

If you're nervous about self-injection (which is considerably less expensive than a doctor or nurse giving you the shot), it's also reasonable to try swallowing these vitamins according to the same schedule first, and moving on to the injections if the "oral route" doesn't work (which isn't unusual with vitamin B12, especially for individuals past age 50).

And just this year, researchers reported that 100 percent of the type 2 diabetics with peripheral neuropathy they examined had low serum 25-hydroxyvitamin D levels. So they instructed everyone to take approximately 2,000 IU vitamin D daily (a relatively low quantity in view of recent research).

After three months, the participants reported 40 to 50 percent less pain.[5] The researchers concluded: "Vitamin D insufficiency is under-recognized and may be a significant contributor to neuropathic pain in type 2 diabetes. Vitamin D supplementation may be an effective 'analgesic' in relieving neuropathic pain."

Find the natural combination that works for you

You may not need every item listed above to relieve your pain. The point here is that if you have diabetic neuropathy, there's hope besides taking patent medicine for pain relief. Try one or all of the nutrients and natural substances listed above (just remember that, depending on which one you're trying, you may need to give it anywhere from three weeks to a year to determine how well each one may work for you).

And if none of them help, there's always the "energy medicine" approach of MMF, which does cost more, but can be a very effective option for relieving the pain of diabetic neuropathy.

It's always a good idea to work with an M.D., D.O., or N.D. skilled and knowledgeable in nutritional and natural medicine to get your diabetes under the best possible control you can. This may help the pain of diabetic neuropathy, too, and will very likely slow its progression considerably.

Chapter 3:

Beat diabetes with this miracle spice!

Diabetes is in the news quite a bit these days. It's becoming more and more common, and odds are you know at least one person with the disease and may very well be at risk yourself. Finding effective methods of treatment and prevention for diabetes in the face of this potential epidemic is more important than ever.

Luckily, there's an all-natural, great tasting, completely underused treatment that can help prevent type 2 diabetes as well as help treat existing type 1 and type 2 diabetes (both of which are often treated with either an oral medication and/or insulin). Don't expect to hear about it from your "friendly" neighborhood patent medicine salesman or, in all likelihood, even from your doctor. It's non-prescription, cheap, unpatentable cinnamon! The risks involved with this treatment are small, and it's well worth considering both for current diabetics and for those with a high risk of developing the disease.

Just a spoonful of this common spice can help stave off type 2 diabetes

A few years ago, a small flurry of news reports (many found on the Internet) revealed that a research team led by Dr. Richard Anderson had isolated a part of cinnamon (a flavonoid called "methylhydroxychalcone polymer," or MHCP) that closely mimics insulin activity. The researchers observed that a combination of MHCP and insulin worked synergistically (meaning they were more effective when used together than when either one was used on its own) in regulating glucose metabolism.

The research team worked with cell cultures to examine the effects of MHCP on a series of enzymes known to be affected by insulin. Results showed that MHCP affected these enzymes in a very similar (although not precisely the same) way as insulin. The researchers concluded that although there were noticeable differences between the responses MHCP and insulin can have on regulating sugar metabolism, the benefit of combining the two therapies is clear. They also noted that MHCP does mimic insulin and that, in most instances, MHCP can work alone—without the presence of insulin. (For more information on Dr. Anderson's MHCP research, refer to the *Journal of the American College of Nutrition*, volume 20, issue 4, pages 327-356.)

One of the possibly overlooked but successful areas for cinnamon/MHCP use is in preventing type 2 diabetes before it ever begins in those who are considered at increased risk.

Cinnamon may eliminate the need for diabetes drugs

Cinnamon/MHCP might not only help control blood sugar but also, when combined with appropriate diet, exercise, and other supplementation, make patent medications and their myriad adverse effects (including significantly increased cardiovascular mortality and occasional deaths from other causes) totally unnecessary.

Individuals with type 2 diabetes who aren't using patent medications should also consider this addition to their diet, exercise, and supplement plan. If you have a mild case of diabetes, it's quite possible that your blood sugar level will normalize simply by using cinnamon or MHCP. At the very least, it should improve. And in either circumstance, using cinnamon or MHCP should postpone or even help prevent progression of type 2 diabetes and its complications. Of course, it's wisest to always work with a physician who can monitor your progress and help you withdraw from any patent diabetes medication you may be taking. For

---

Seeing is believing

How do you know if you're at risk for type 2 diabetes? Well, here are some of the physical symptoms to look for on your body that might be trying to warn you that diabetes is on its way.

- Shin spots. Slow-spreading, brownish-red (occasionally yellowish) discolorations on the shins are often an early warning sign of impending adult onset (type 2) diabetes.

- Skin tags. As the name aptly describes, they're "tags" of skin most frequently found on the neck, under the arms, and in the groin area, and they're a common occurrence on adults.

- Dupuytren's contracture. This condition occurs when the connective tissue under the skin of the hand begins to thicken and shorten. As the tissue tightens, it may pull the fingers down towards the palm of the hand.

- Excess weight. Obesity is probably the most widely known physical symptom for type 2 diabetes, and it's usually the easiest to spot. If this is a problem for you, make sure to carefully examine your body for the other symptoms as well.

In addition to the symptoms you can actually see on your body, you should also be aware of some internal risk factors for type 2 diabetes—namely, high blood pressure, elevated cholesterol and triglyceride levels, and, of course, family history of the disease. While these factors may not put you at risk on their own, combined with the other physical signs they can be additional clues as to whether type 2 diabetes may be in your future.

a referral to such a physician in your area, contact the American College for Advancement in Medicine (800-532-3688; www.acam.org).

Type 1 diabetics can reduce insulin dependence

Since insulin and MHCP have been found to be synergistic, taking MHCP or whole cinnamon should make it possible to regulate blood sugar with less insulin. Some complications of type 1 diabetes may come from insulin use itself, so using less insulin while maintaining blood sugar control could be beneficial. In cases of type 1 (insulin-dependent) diabetes, it's definitely wisest to work with a physician whenever trying to taper down insulin usage.

Before you start sprinkling it on...

Dr. Anderson noted in his research that all species of cinnamon and numerous bottles of commercial cinnamon were tried and that they all worked to help regulate glucose metabolism in his research teams' experiments.

Coupled with the widespread availability of self-monitoring devices for blood sugar measurement, it isn't hard to tell if cinnamon or MHCP is helpful. However, keep in mind that whole cinnamon, like most plants and other living things, has both fat-soluble and water-soluble fractions. There is some evidence that high levels of the fat-soluble fractions of cinnamon could be cause for concern. Some researchers have found that substances in the fat- (and oil) soluble fractions of cinnamon may be both carcinogenic and genotoxic (damaging to genes, and leading to an increased risk of both cancer and birth defects). Fortunately, these risks are easily avoidable, and you can still get all the benefits of cinnamon just by taking a few simple steps.

Dr. Anderson has observed that essentially all toxic materials in cinnamon are fat soluble. He simply recommends that, to be safe, anyone using more than 1/4 to 1 teaspoonful of whole cinnamon daily first boil it in water, then pour off the resulting watery solution for use, and discard the solid remainder, which would contain the fat- and oil-soluble fractions. Since MHCP is water-soluble, it's still readily available in the watery solution poured off after boiling the cinnamon.

A helpful hint for actually going about separating the oils and fats on the surface of the water: Try pouring the water through a cheesecloth (cheesecloths are available in many supermarkets and other cooking supply stores).

If you prefer not to take these steps, but still want to try this natural approach to controlling diabetes, you can avoid the potential hazard of whole cinnamon by using the cinnamon derivative, MHCP.

Since I've needed this tool for many individuals with diabetes or those at risk for diabetes, and since the long-term risks (if any) of whole cinnamon aren't known, I've worked with the Life Enhancement Foundation to make MHCP available in supplement form as a product called Insulife. A daily amount of Insulife combines approximately the amount of MHCP found in 1 teaspoonful of whole cinnamon with chromium and other nutrients shown to help reduce insulin resistance. Insulife is available through natural food stores, compounding pharmacies, and the Tahoma Clinic Dispensary (425-264-0059, www.tahomadispensary.com).

Taper down your medications with caution: Work with a physician

If you're already taking insulin or a patent medication for diabetes and you want to try cinnamon or MHCP, it's important to work with a physician who can assist you in safely tapering down the amounts of medication you're using.

Since many conventional physicians may not be familiar with (or may resist) the idea of using even a well-researched natural product (in combination with diet, exercise, and other specific supplementation) while reducing or completely eliminating the need for a patent medication, you may want to consult one of the following groups for a referral to a skilled alternative physician in your area: The American

College for Advancement in Medicine, (800)532-3688, www.acam.org; the American Academy of Environmental Medicine, (316)684-5500, www.aaem.com; or The American Association of Naturopathic Physicians, (866)538-2267, www.naturopathic.org.

Chapter 4:

Get your type 2 diabetes under control...without a single drug

B est known for its natural antibiotic activity, berberine deals a serious blow to common infectious organisms—organisms like "staph," "strep," Chlamydia, diphtheria, salmonella, cholera, diplococcus pneumoniae, pseudomonas, gonorrhea, candida, trichomonas, and many others. Berberine is a component (for the technically inclined, a "plant alkaloid") of the commonly used herbs goldenseal and Oregon grape, and of several other less well-known botanicals. A 0.2 percent solution of berberine has been found effective against trachoma—in "third world" countries, a major infectious cause of visual impairment and blindness, as well as many other types of conjunctivitis.

It's less well known that berberine has been found more effective than aspirin in relieving fever in experimental animals, and is able to stimulate some parts of the immune system. It's also a stimulant for bile secretion.

And it's not at all well known that research published in well-known, respected, "peer-reviewed" medical journals in 2008 found that berberine is just as effective—and of course much safer—than metformin, the formerly patent medicine most commonly now prescribed to help re-regulate blood sugar in type 2 diabetes!

Another cover-up?
That won't stop the truth

Where has this information been? I suspect that *Nutrition & Healing* readers know the answer…so let's move on to review the research, and then what's known about how berberine does this job.

Two studies were reported in one of the 2008 research reports.[1] In the first study, 36 adults with newly diagnosed type 2 diabetes mellitus were randomly assigned to treatment with berberine or metformin (500 milligrams of either, three times a day) in a three-month (13-week) trial.

At the end of three months, average fasting blood sugars in the berberine group dropped from 191 to 124 milligrams per deciliter, average post-prandial blood sugar (blood sugar after eating) dropped from 356 to 199 milligrams per deciliter, average hemoglobin A1c (a measurement of longer-term blood sugar control) dropped from 9.5 percent to 7.5 percent, and fasting triglycerides dropped from an average 99 to 78 milligrams per deciliter.

The researchers wrote, "Compared with metformin, berberine exhibited an identical effect in the regulation of glucose metabolism, such as HbA1c, FBG [fasting blood glucose], PBG [blood sugar after eating], fasting insulin and postprandial insulin [insulin level after eating]. In the regulation of lipid metabolism, berberine activity is better than metformin. By week 13, triglycerides and total cholesterol in the berberine group had decreased and were significantly lower than in the metformin group (P<0.05)."

Insulin resistance dropped by 45 percent

The second study in this same publication involved 48 adults already under treatment for type 2 diabetes with diet and one or more patent medications and/or insulin. Despite these various treatments, their type 2 diabetes was still poorly controlled. Diet and all medications had been the

Are you a type 2 diabetic taking one of these medicines?

The Lancet, considered to be one of the world's "top" medical journals, published an editorial titled "Individualized incretin-based treatment for type 2 diabetes" in the August 7, 2010 edition. The author wrote, "All GLP-1 receptor agonists [molecules which stimulate the receptor for the incretin hormone GLP-1, which helps regulate blood sugar] that are "approved" [quotation marks added] or in development for the treatment of type 2 diabetes cause nausea, vomiting, and sometimes diarrhea in a substantial proportion of patients."

He continued by observing that GLP-1 can help regulate blood sugar without these effects—which should be rather obvious because our own internally secreted GLP-1 doesn't cause any of these problems! But rather than recommend that natural GLP-1—or berberine, which stimulates GLP-1—be used instead of "approved" or "under development" patent medicines, he instead suggests that researchers look into why the patent medications cause these problems, as this would "pave the way to an even more impressive exploitation of the incretin-based treatment strategy."

Exploitation is exactly the correct word to describe this point of view, which ignores completely the much safer and considerably less expensive molecules found in our bodies and in Nature, and continues to pursue the development, sale, and use of prohibitively expensive patent medicine substitutes with much greater incidence of so-called "side" effects—which are actually part of the real effects of these never-before-found-on-planet-Earth (extraterrestrial, space alien) molecules.

But it's your body and your health! If you have type 2 diabetes and are being "treated" with Byetta®—which all affect the incretin-driven blood sugar regulatory system—consider switching to berberine at 500 milligrams three times daily. There's ample scientific evidence to support such a change! Make sure to work with a physician skilled and knowledgeable in nutritional and natural medicine.

same in each individual for two months before berberine treatment was added, and remained unchanged for the three months of this second study.

After just 7 days, the added berberine (500 milligrams thrice daily) led to an average reduction in fasting blood sugar from 172 to 140 milligrams per deciliter, and average post-prandial blood sugar had declined from 266 to 210 milligrams per deciliter.

During the second week of added berberine, average fasting blood sugar dropped to 135 milligrams per deciliter, and postprandial glucose to 189 milligrams per deciliter. The researchers reported that these improvements were maintained for the rest of the three-month study.

In addition, hemoglobin A1c decreased from 8.1 percent to 7.3 percent, fasting insulin decreased by 28 percent, insulin resistance was reduced by 45 percent, and total and low-density (LDL) cholesterol were both significantly reduced.

The researchers wrote that in their study of newly diagnosed diabetics who took berberine or placebo alone, "[n]one of the patients suffered from severe gastrointestinal adverse events when berberine was used alone."

By contrast, the researchers wrote about the poorly controlled diabetics who added berberine to their on-going patent medication treatment: "Incidence of gastrointestinal adverse events was 34.5 percent during the 13 weeks of berberine…combination therapy."

These adverse events included diarrhea in 10 percent, constipation in 7 percent, flatulence in 19 percent, and abdominal pain in 3.4 percent. The side effects were observed only in the first four weeks in most patients. In 24 percent, berberine dosage was decreased from 500 to 300 milligrams thrice daily because of gastrointestinal adverse events, and all of these side effects disappeared within one week.

The researchers concluded, "In summary, berberine is a potent oral hypoglycemic [blood sugar lowering] agent with modest effect on lipid metabolism. It is safe and the cost of treatment by berberine is very low."

Better blood sugar control
...and a few pounds shed

In a second publication, other researchers described results achieved by 116 individuals with type 2 diabetes and cholesterol and triglyceride abnormalities who participated in a randomized, double-blind trial that compared 500 milligrams of berberine taken twice daily with placebo, also taken twice daily.[2] In the berberine group, average fasting blood sugar decreased from 126 to 101 milligrams/deciliter.

Two hours after a standardized glucose challenge, blood sugars decreased from an average 216 to an average 160 milligrams per deciliter. Average hemoglobin A1c decreased from 7.5 percent to 6.6 percent, average triglycerides decreased from 221 to 141 milligrams per deciliter, average total cholesterol decreased from 205 to 168 milligrams per deciliter, and average LDL-cholesterol ("bad" cholesterol) decreased from 125 to 97 milligrams per deciliter.

These researchers also reported "secondary outcomes." Body weight decreased from an average 151 pounds to an average 146 pounds with berberine, a significantly greater fall (five pounds) than in the placebo group, who went from an average 158 pounds to an average 155 pounds, a loss of three pounds. A greater reduction of body mass index (BMI) was also found at three months in the berberine group than in the placebo group. Systolic blood pressure decreased from an average of 124 to 117 and diastolic blood pressure decreased from an average of 81 to 77 in those treated with berberine, exceeding the fall from 126 to 123 systolic and from 83 to 80 diastolic in those who took the placebo.

Side effects were few and mostly transient in the berberine group. Tests were done for kidney and liver function, as well as blood counts and electrolytes. Mild to moderate constipation occurred in five participants receiving berberine and one participant in the placebo group. Constipation "cleared up" in three of the five taking berberine and the one in the placebo group. The other two in the berberine group reduced their quantity of berberine by half to 250 milligrams twice daily, which relieved the constipation. Three measured liver enzymes (for the technically inclined AST, ALT, and GGT) all decreased to within the normal range.

How berberine does the job

So how does berberine improve blood sugar control? Much of the answer involves the effect of berberine on insulin and insulin regulation. Some of the rest is explained by berberine's indirect effect on blood sugar regulation through its effect on little-known (to non-researchers) gastrointestinal hormones termed "incretins."

Berberine improves the action of insulin by activating an enzyme (for the technically inclined, AMP-activated protein kinase, or AMPK) which helps regulate the cellular uptake of glucose, the oxidation ("burning") of fatty acids and the synthesis of glucose transporter 4 (GLUT4), the insulin-regulated glucose carrier found in fat and skeletal and cardiac muscle that is responsible for moving glucose from the bloodstream into cells.[3-6] GLUT 4 is found only in muscle and fat cells, the major tissues in the body that respond to insulin.

Berberine increases the "expression" (number and activity) of insulin receptors.[7,8] The increase in number and activity of course enables the same amount of insulin to be more effective than before. Another way of describing this activity of berberine is "decreasing insulin resistance." Other researchers have reported that berberine inhibits an enzyme (for the technically inclined, protein tyrosine phosphatase 1B, or PTP1B) which in turn inhibits the insulin receptor.[9] When the insulin receptor isn't inhibited as much, it can of course function better, and the net result is that insulin can "work" better.

"Incretins" are hormones secreted by our stomachs and intestines that simultaneously increase the amount of insulin and inhibit the amount of glucagon (a pancreatic hormone which "opposes" insulin) released from the pancreatic islet cells after eating, even before blood sugar levels rise. (It's like an "anticipatory" action so more insulin—and less glucagon—will be immediately available when the glucose starts to rise in the blood.) Incretins also slow the rate of absorption of nutrients into the blood stream by slowing stomach emptying; this may indirectly reduce food intake. Another way in which berberine regulates blood sugar is by increasing the secretion of one of the major incretins, glucagon-like peptide 1 (GLP-1).[10]

However, the actions of GLP-1 and other incretins to increase insulin release, lower glucagon release, and help regulate blood sugar are normally rapidly negated by another enzyme called DDP-4 (for the technically inclined, dipeptidyl peptidase 4). Yet another aspect of the blood sugar regulating action of berberine is its ability to inhibit DDP-4.[11] When DDP-4 is inhibited, GLP-1 and other gut-secreted incretins aren't broken down as rapidly, so they can continue to stimulate insulin and inhibit glucagon release significantly longer.

Thousands of years of use, and still largely ignored

Berberine is a major active component of the herb Coptis chinensis (Huang-lian), which—according to one research group—has been used in China to treat what is now identified as type 2 diabetes for literally thousands of years.

According to another research group, its blood sugar lowering effect was noticed when it was given to type 2 diabetic individuals to treat diarrhea. After the isolation of the berberine molecule itself, one of the first publications describing its use to lower blood sugar in type 2 diabetics was published in China in 1988.[12] This and two subsequent research papers published in 2004[13] and 2005[14] found significant reductions in fasting and after-eating blood sugar control, and one also found significant reductions in cholesterol and triglycerides. Only one case of constipation (but no other adverse effects) was reported.

However, despite the safe and effective results reported, these studies suffered from the "defect" of not being placebo-controlled, and were (and are presently) only available in Chinese, so no one noticed them—with the possible exception of patent medicine companies working to make a patentable un-Natural molecule "analog" to berberine, and they won't tell!

But the research studies you've already read about were "controlled," and compared berberine directly with placebo or the number one established patent medication, metformin (Glucophage®, Glucophage XR®, Glumetza®, Fortamet®, Riomet®), or used berberine in addition to patent medication treatment—and all proved berberine to be clinically effective.

If you have type 2 diabetes and are using any patent medication, consider consulting a physician skilled and knowledgeable in natural and nutritional medicine and switching to berberine. Of course, there are many other natural techniques which can also be used to regulate and even normalize blood sugar in type 2 diabetes, including diet, exercise, vitamins, minerals, and other botanicals. It appears, however, that berberine can be a major tool, with fewer and less severe adverse effects than patent medications.

Tahoma Clinic physicians presently recommend Berberine Advantage (Tahoma Clinic Dispensary) or Berberine Plus™ (True Botanica™), 500 milligram capsules, each of which contain 485 milligrams of berberine itself. They are available at natural food stores, compounding pharmacies, and the Tahoma Clinic Dispensary. Although I work with Tahoma Clinic Dispensary, I am not affiliated with True Botanica™.

Thank you to Ronald Steriti, N.D., who researched and organized the material used in this report!

Part V

Digestion

Chapter 1:

Poor digestion shows its colors: The story of "The Gray Man"

At the Tahoma Clinic, he was known as the "Gray Man." He got the nickname after our staff agreed it had never seen anyone with his skin tones. His visible skin was devoid of any pink tones, had scarcely any brown, and instead was a peculiar whitish-gray. I've not seen anyone like him before or since.

The Gray Man hadn't come in to find out why he looked gray—although his wife had mentioned it to him "a time or two." Actually, he explained, he didn't have any symptoms or illnesses but was just plain tired. Really tired!

Further questioning turned up little but the fatigue. In the past, he'd had chronic indigestion and intermittent but persistent heartburn. He noted that both symptoms had gone on for over 20 years and that he'd taken "plenty of those Tums and Rolaids and other antacids" since his 40s. However, he reported he hadn't had any indigestion or heartburn problems at all since he'd started taking Tagamet every day since it came out. Now that I mentioned it, he guessed he had been taking Tagamet for seven years by now.

"You know that stomachs are naturally designed to secrete enough acid to turn even large meals into the equivalent of soup?" I asked.

"Yeah, I know that in general, but all the doctors told me that indigestion and heartburn are due to too much acid," he replied.

"Did anyone ever actually measure your stomach-acid production?"

"No…but the symptoms sure have gone away since I blocked all that acid out."

"And a river will dry up if we stop all the rain," I said. "Maybe that's an advantage for a little while if the river has been overflowing, but what happens if we stop the rain permanently?"

He thought for a moment. "Permanently?"

"At least seven years."

"Quite a drought. Nothing would grow."

"Right. And if we shut off or neutralize our stomachs' natural acidity for more than brief intervals, there are similar consequences. First, we don't break down foods as well, and many nutrients, especially essential amino acids, certain minerals, and at least two B vitamins, aren't made as available by natural acid digestion as they usually are and aren't properly absorbed into our bloodstreams. So our cells don't have the normal amounts of nutrients for nourishment."

"Second, when that acidified soup empties out of our stomachs into the upper small intestine—the duodenum—it triggers the secretion of hormones that in turn stimulate the pancreas and gallbladder to make or release their own digestive secretions, such as enzymes, bicarbonate, and bile. Without the acid "trigger," these hormones are under produced, and the next stages in digestion don't work as well as they should either. This makes another whole group of nutrients less available to our cells."

"So it's like a cascade of events. If the acidity isn't there, then other parts of digestion aren't triggered properly either."

"Exactly. And we don't even know if we know absolutely all the 'cascades' in the digestive stream."

"No wonder I'm tired. I've literally dried up a lot of my digestion for years. Why didn't anyone tell me about this?"

"Don't know. It's all right there in the basic textbooks for medical students. But that's not all: The same basic textbooks list a third consequence of low or no stomach-acid production. Let's think about it this way: What happens if I put bacteria or parasites into an acid in a test tube?"

"Not sure, but I'd guess a lot of them die."

"Right. They die and turn into a minor protein supplement. Textbooks of gastroenterology actually call stomach acid the acid barrier to intestinal tract infection. Also, everyone knows that farther down the intestinal tract is home to a wide variety of micro-organisms—sometimes called intestinal microflora—that help with digestion, secrete a few important vitamins, and generally behave themselves. But if the acid-alkaline balance, technically called the pH, isn't just right, then many of the friendly micro-organisms literally die out and are replaced by not-so-friendly germs. At best, these unfriendly micro-organisms aren't as helpful to us as the friendly ones. Worse, some of them excrete substances toxic to our own body cells, that are absorbed and spread all around our bodies."

The Gray Man shifted uncomfortably in his chair. "So not only have I been semi-starving myself but also maybe encouraging toxins from my gut to enter my system?"

"Afraid so."

"Could blocking my normal stomach function be the basis for this incredible fatigue?"

"Very likely. Let's work on restoring normal digestion as much as possible, make up for at least seven years of unintended malnutrition, and, if necessary, work to restore normal gut flora. Then we'll see."

"I guess the first thing is to stop this Tagamet. But then I'll have indigestion and heartburn all over again, won't I?"

"Most of the time there are natural ways to stop indigestion and heartburn without blocking stomach acid."

"How?"

"First, we need to find out if your stomach really does make too much acid. Chances are very high—over 90 percent—that it doesn't, and that the real culprit is likely *underproduction* of stomach acid, along with some of that small amount of acid turning up in the wrong place, causing burning. Let's wait until we do a test or two."

You can eat all the right foods but still slowly starve to death

Like the overwhelming percentage of individuals with indigestion and heartburn, the Gray Man found, after some testing, that his stomach had actually been under producing acid for all those years. *Hypochlorhydria* (low or no stomach acid) is one of the most common digestive malfunctions, and it's often accompanied by other, seemingly unrelated, health problems. Unfortunately, inadequate digestion becomes even more frequent with age. So, even if you're following the best possible diet plan in general or for a particular ailment, if the food you're eating is incompletely digested or assimilated, your body won't get the nutrients possible from it and it won't be effective.

Think about it. Our bodies are made up of 60 or so essential nutrients (*essential* being defined as nutrients without which we'd sooner or later drop dead); how healthy can you be if your body isn't absorbing even one of those nutrients? And what if a dozen or more nutrients are in short supply? If our foods and supplements don't encounter the proper acid and enzymes, they won't digest and absorb, which will cause malnutrition. In essence, you could be eating all you need but still starving yourself.

Antacids may be squelching the only stomach acid you have left

Many people who have too little stomach acid are being treated as if they have too much—probably because the symptoms are similar. Ten to 15 percent of the population suffers from hypochlorhydria, and most people are being misdiagnosed and mistreated. A full 50 percent of people over 60 are hypochlorhydric, and most of them are being treated for the opposite problem.

Why in the world would you want to take antacids or acid blockers when your stomach is already weak and not digesting adequately? It's easy—SYMPTOM RELIEF. It also just so happens that this phenomenon is making drug companies very rich! If doctors aren't prescribing high-strength antacids, people are just getting them over the counter and often popping several a day. Multimillion-dollar promotions to the public were launched to drive home the point that "heartburn" and indigestion are caused by too much acid, which can be blocked by antacid products with minimal risk. Oddly enough, the FDA has never required the companies advertising these products to document their claims that indigestion is actually caused by over acidity.

This disease is testable and treatable— but your doctor may not know it

You can be tested for hypochlorhydria and other possible stomach malfunctions. I recommend direct measurement of gastric acidity by radio telemetry using the Heidelberg capsule. At present, it's the best test available for functional determination of the stomach's ability to secrete acid normally.

I also use other laboratory clues to help my diagnosis. One is a mineral analysis of a hair specimen. If six or more nutrient minerals are low, excluding sodium and potassium, your stomach-acid level should be checked. The other test routinely done in our laboratory is on a stool specimen, to check for completeness of digestion. It's not unusual to find an excess of undigested meat fiber in such an analysis. And measurement of the stomach acid in those cases usually discloses an insufficiency.

Once the problem is found, I recommend treatment with hydrochloric acid (**which can be dangerous, however, and should be used only with careful supervision**). I've found that hydrochloric acid when used in conjunction with pepsin usually gives the best results. And unless you're sensitive to it, pepsin is usually recommended with hydrochloric acid. Powdered preparations of HCL in capsules are much more effective than the solid tablet forms. Some individuals may have pain, burning, or additional stomach problems when using HCL; when that's the case, I find that small, gradually increased quantities of lemon juice or vinegar can usually do the same job.

To minimize even minor side effects, I always start with just one capsule (5, 7.5, or 10 grains) taken just before meals. After two or three days, if there are no problems, I suggest increasing the dosage to two capsules before meals for another two or three days and then to three capsules. The dose is gradually increased in this fashion until the recommended amount is reached. The amount of hydrochloric acid that's usually effective for adults is at least 40 to 70 grains of betaine hydrochloride (or glutamic-acid hydrochloride) with pepsin per meal. That's about four to seven 10-grain (8 to 14 5-grain) capsules per meal.

The "Gray Man" followed this type of treatment program and as long as he kept it up controlled his indigestion and indigestion symptoms. His program also included replacement digestive enzymes, intestinal flora "normalizers" (also called probiotics), and supplements of amino acids, vitamins, and minerals.

The Gray Man's skin color slowly returned to the normal brown and pink skin tones. As his grayness turned to normal, his nickname faded away too, and was replaced by only his first name, John. His fatigue also waned and was replaced by increased energy. His wife noted improvements in mood and attitude. Six months later, he declared himself "back to normal."

The only thing entirely atypical about the Gray Man's—John's—case was his skin color. As noted above, I've never seen anything like it before or since. But the rest of the story—indigestion and heartburn caused by underproduction of normal stomach acid—is absolutely typical.

If your doctor cannot offer help for hypochlorhydria, or is not willing to test you, call the American College for Advancement in Medicine, tel. (800)532-3688, to find a doctor in your area who can help. If your doctor would like more information on how to test/treat you for this problem, have him/her call the Tahoma Clinic; tel. (253)854-4900.

Parts of the above chapter are excerpts from the book, "Why Stomach Acid Is Good for You: Natural Relief from Heartburn, Indigestion, Reflux & GERD" written by Lane Lenard, Ph.D., and Jonathan V. Wright, M.D.

Chapter 2:

Age and antacids—a double whammy against your body's optimal health

A nti-aging enthusiasts will all tell you that eating a whole-food, organic diet is a necessary part of staying younger longer—and I agree
with them. But such a diet won't do you much good if you're not digesting and assimilating the nutrients from the food you eat. That's why good
digestion and assimilation are equally important factors in maintaining
optimal health. Yes, you've read this from me before, but I'll repeat it
from time to time until every anti-aging physician and enthusiast gets it.

The main causes of poor digestion and assimilation are age-related
gastric hypochlorhydria (more commonly referred to as low stomach
acid) and age-related gastric achlorhydria (which is no stomach acid at
all). Like it or not, the older you get, the more likely you are to develop
these problems.

According to research conducted in the early 1900s, approximately
50 percent of people over the age of 60 had significantly low stomach
acid due to age. But if stomach acid tests conducted at the Tahoma Clinic

are any indication, that number has jumped considerably since the initial research was done. (We use the extremely accurate "gastric analysis by radio telemetry," also called the "Heidelberg capsule test.")

Unfortunately, doctors rarely recognize the seriousness of this problem and treat the underlying cause. Instead, many doctors today are only making the problem worse by putting people on patent medications specifically designed to suppress stomach acid production.

This could all be changing in the near future, though, as doctors are slowly becoming aware of the fact that low or no stomach acid can literally influence the health of the entire body. Not surprisingly, this "discovery" is coming about in a backward way: By observing the negative effects of patent medications that induce low levels of stomach acid—and even worse, ones that wipe it out altogether.

But whether your low stomach acid is caused by age, by certain acid-suppressing patent medications, or by both, the end result is the same: Poor digestion and assimilation of nutrients that are vital for your body's ultimate health and longevity potential. And this isn't just theory: Published research shows that both patent medication induced gastric acid suppression and age-related lack of gastric acidity have the same effect on your body's ability to absorb nutrients.[1]

The good news is that whatever the underlying cause of low stomach acid is, the condition is easy to treat.

An open invitation for unfriendly intestinal bacteria

Low stomach acid levels lead to alterations in your intestinal microflora. Friendly intestinal microorganisms are dependent on the natural intestinal pH balance that results when all digestive organs are working well. When the major source of intestinal acidity (the stomach) fails or when it's suppressed by patent medications, intestinal contents become too alkaline, allowing unfriendly microorganisms to enter the scene, including Candida albicans (yeast) and many others.

The *Journal of the American Medical Association* (JAMA) published the results of a study demonstrating that two different types of patent medications known to suppress stomach acid are both associated with a significantly increased risk of overgrowth of a potentially serious intestinal micro-organism called clostridium difficile.[2] This antibiotic-resistant bacterium produces a toxin that causes watery diarrhea, which can occasionally lead to hospitalization and sometimes even death.

Low stomach acid linked to hip fractures, pneumonia, macular degeneration, and more

The increased risk of infection that goes along with low gastric acidity isn't limited to the intestinal tract, though. Other studies have shown that when patent medications suppress stomach acid, many seemingly unrelated parts of the body are affected. And it makes sense when you think about it since individual nutrients are vital for maintaining all sorts of body functions.

For example, a study published in JAMA, which involved 150,000 individuals followed from 1987 to 2003, demonstrated that people who are on proton pump inhibitors (patent medications that totally shut off stomach acid production) have a significantly higher risk of a hip fracture. The researchers reported that the risk of hip fracture steadily increased with the length of time the patent medication was taken, as well as with higher doses.[3] They suggested that the hip fractures were caused because of poor calcium absorption caused by the stomach acid suppression.

Having low stomach acid also increases your risk of developing pneumonia. When researchers studied 364,683 individuals—5,551 of whom developed community-acquired pneumonia—they found that those on acid-suppressing meds were four times more likely to develop pneumonia.[4]

And in 2005 researchers noted once again[5] the finding that antacid use significantly increases the risk of age-related macular degeneration.[6]

Recently, researchers found that the suppression of gastric acidity also interferes with the absorption of vitamin C (although at this point they don't know what causes this to happen). In research involving a commonly prescribed acid-suppressive patent medication, they reached the following conclusion: "We have shown that a short course [only 28 days of the patent medication] will cause a reduction in the plasma vitamin C level of healthy volunteers. This decrease in plasma vitamin C is independent of dietary intake of the vitamin and indicates reduced bioavailability."[7]

Vitamin C isn't the only nutrient affected by low or absent gastric acidity. Older research demonstrated that iron, calcium, folic acid, vitamin B12, and zinc are all poorly absorbed when your stomach acid is low.[8]

Step up your anti-aging routine

If you're seriously into health maintenance and anti-aging, you should work with your doctor to monitor your stomach acid. If you do have age-related gastric hypochlorhydria or achlorhydria—and we all develop one or the other sooner or later—the problem is fairly easy to treat. Talk to your doctor about taking hydrochloric acid and pepsin capsules to improve your digestion and balance the pH of your gastrointestinal system.

Although it's not as common, poor digestion and/or absorption can also be caused by low levels of pancreatic enzymes and by hidden gluten/gliadin sensitivity. So your doctor should check those levels as well.

In the meantime, I also recommend reading the book that Lane Lenard, Ph.D., and I wrote about the causes and consequences of low stomach acid levels. *Why Stomach Acid Is Good for You* is available through compounding pharmacies, natural food stores, and the Tahoma Clinic Dispensary. (See the Alternative Health Resources section on page 485.)

Chapter 3:

The 99.9-percent effective technique for eliminating gallbladder attacks forever

If you still have your gallbladder, you probably don't spend much time thinking about it, even if you're very health conscious. If you don't have your gallbladder anymore, you probably think about it even less. The only time you might consider your gall-bladder is when it's hurting bad—a situation usually called a "gallbladder attack."

And why should you? After all, nearly a million people every year have their gallbladders removed, and they all appear to go on about their lives just as healthy as anyone else. Doctors don't seem to care about gall-bladders much; if yours is subject to "attacks" of pain, they don't try to help you keep it. If it hurts too much or too often, the nearly universal prescription is "just get it out." Even though it requires surgery and a hospital stay—not to mention thousands of dollars—just go ahead and do it. Besides, it's "covered" by your insurance.

After the surgery, you're not advised to do anything in particular to make up for the loss of your gallbladder. So it's no wonder most people are under the impression that it's just not that important.

But if you've read this far, I'm sure you've guessed that I'm about to tell you that there's much more to the gallbladder story than that. Your gallbladder performs some important functions in your body that make it well worth keeping. Possibly the most important is to regulate bile flow to optimize fat, oil, and fat-soluble nutrient absorption. Without your gallbladder, mechanically, this just can't happen properly.

If you've already had your gallbladder removed, there are some simple steps you can take to keep nutrient deficiencies from happening. But before I tell you what to do if your gallbladder's already gone, let's cover a more urgent question: How can you keep your gallbladder in the first place, and get those "attacks" to disappear for good? If it was used as a first line of defense, this technique would make 99.9 percent of all gallbladder surgeries—including yours in particular—totally unnecessary. That's right, 999 of 1,000 gallbladder surgeries are entirely preventable, and without patent medications, vitamins, minerals, or herbs. This procedure works so well that I haven't needed to refer anyone for gallbladder surgery for over 30 years.

Hospitals already use this technique— without even realizing it

It may sound like I'm making a totally unsupportable claim, but research about "how to prevent gallbladder attacks" was actually published back in the 1960s and '70s by Dr. James C. Breneman, who, at the time, was chairman of the Food Allergy Committee of the American College of Allergists, or ACA (now called the American College of Allergy and Immunology, or ACAI). Ironically, if you've ever been hospitalized with a severe attack of gallbladder pain, but your gallbladder wasn't removed, and the pain subsided, you've very likely had "Dr. Breneman treatment."

So what is Dr. Breneman's secret for preventing attacks of gallbladder pain? It's simple: Don't eat or consume anything you're allergic to.[1]

And that's exactly what the doctors do when you're hospitalized with a severe gallbladder attack—they take away all your food, you're given IV fluids, and you're not allowed to eat anything until the pain subsides. It's a "perfect" food allergy avoidance strategy, and works nearly every time. Unfortunately, the doctors who order this procedure every day still don't realize why the strategy works. But back to Dr. Breneman…

Back in 1968, he asked 69 individuals suffering from recurrent attacks of gallbladder pain to go onto an elimination diet to determine their food allergies.[2] Six of these individuals had already had their gallbladders out, but were still having attacks of gallbladder pain, a situation termed "post-cholecystectomy syndrome," or, as I like to call it, "my gallbladder's gone, but I'm still hurting anyway." Dr. Breneman reported that all 69 people (100 percent!) were completely free of gallbladder attacks when they avoided their individual food (and other) allergies. And all 69 had their symptoms return when they ate the foods they were allergic to once more.

The primary offending foods were eggs (92.8 percent), pork (63.8 percent), onions (52.2 percent), chicken and turkey (34.8 percent), milk (24.6 percent), coffee (21.7 percent), and oranges (18.8 percent). Corn, beans, nuts, apples, tomatoes, peas, cabbage, spices, peanuts, fish, and rye accounted for between 14.5 percent and 1 percent of gallbladder attacks. In addition to foods, 14 of the 69 study participants—just over 20 percent—had gallbladder attacks caused by medications.

Food, medication, and other allergies vary from person to person, and the same allergen can cause different symptoms in different people, so it's best to work with a physician skilled and knowledgeable in nutritional and natural medicine to determine what your allergies might be. In addition to the American College for Advancement in Medicine noted on page 485, you might want to contact the American Academy of Environmental Medicine (316-684-5500, www.aaem.com), for help in determining which foods or medications may be triggering your gallbladder attacks.

Gallbladder removal could send your health on a downward spiral

This approach is so simple, and yet no medical school to this day teaches how to prevent gallbladder attacks by avoiding your food allergies and (in some cases) other allergies. Instead, they continue to recommend unnecessary gallstone removal surgery. But the truth is, gallstones don't even cause 99.9 percent of gallbladder "attacks": Allergies do. Avoid allergies, stop "attacks" of pain, and keep your gallbladder! That's it—that's all there is to it. And believe me, it's worth it. Because without your gall-bladder, your absorption of vitamins A, D, E, K, and essential fatty acids is very likely to be impaired.

Let me give you a specific example of what can happen if your body isn't absorbing enough of these essential nutrients. Several years ago, a woman contacted me with a question about a very specific problem she was having. Every time she drove the Los Angeles freeway system, she experienced recurrent breakdown of the tissues covering the cornea of her eyes. Her ophthalmologist attributed the "spontaneous corneal breakdown" to air pollution and told her not to drive when pollution levels rose. She didn't argue with the diagnosis but wondered why everyone else she knew could drive those same freeways with intact corneas.

When she asked me that question, I admitted I didn't know either but suggested that she try extra vitamin A (not beta-carotene) to try to stop the problem. She pointed out that she was eating carrots and "yellow vegetables" and taking a multiple vitamin containing vitamin A. But since insufficient levels are one definite cause of corneal damage, I told her it was still worth trying, especially since it's relatively difficult for an adult to overdose on vitamin A, and since any possible overdose is easily reversible if the vitamin A is promptly stopped. (This does not include women who are pregnant or might become pregnant: Even small excesses of vitamin A can raise the risk of birth defects.)

So we went over vitamin A overdose symptoms that she should look out for, just in case. They include headache, progressively drier skin, loss of hair (especially eyebrows), cracked lips, and pain in "long bones" (upper arms, upper legs). I recommended she start with 25,000 IU of vitamin A daily and gradually increase the amount toward a maximum of 100,000 IU daily, keeping a close watch for both favorable results and any possible symptoms of excess.

When we next talked, she had very good news: When she'd gotten to 80,000 IU of vitamin A daily, her corneas stopped giving her so much trouble. They were healthy once again, with no further break-down, and she could drive the freeways as much as she wanted.

She'd also had no signs at all of vitamin A excess. However, when she told her ophthalmologist the good news, he panicked and sent her immediately to have a vitamin A blood test, telling her to stop taking vitamin A right away as she might be "poisoned."

However, she knew that she wasn't having overdose symptoms, and that her eyes were staying intact for the first time in several years, so she decided to wait a few days for the results of the test before stopping. The test report showed her vitamin A level to be well within normal limits, but, to her surprise, she was told she should stop the extra vitamin A anyway, since it was "just too much." Sensibly, she declined to stop, pointing to her now-normal eyes, and instead decided to investigate why she might need so much vitamin A to produce normal blood levels and maintain eye health.

She remembered she'd had her gallbladder removed a few years before her eye problems started. Researching that, she discovered that normal absorption of fats and oils is very dependent on bile—which is made by our livers, but "stored for use" in a normal gallbladder. She knew that vitamin A is a "fat-soluble" vitamin (as are vitamins D, E, K, and the essential fatty acids) and wondered if perhaps her missing gallbladder might account for her high vitamin A requirement.

I told her she was probably right and asked her a question that I ask all my patients who've already had gallbladder surgery. The question was (and is): "After your gallbladder was removed, did your surgeon or any other doctor explain what you should do to insure normal absorption of fats, oils, and especially fat-soluble vitamins?" Of course, her answer, like that of every other patient I've asked over the last 30 years, was "no."

But despite most doctors' sins of omission on this topic, it's important for you to understand that without your gallbladder, your body just doesn't generate enough bile to break down and absorb many essential nutrients.

Protecting your body's nutrient-absorption team

You might ask why this is, since bile is made in your liver and the liver is still completely intact after gallbladder removal. To understand the relationship between the two, you need to know a bit about how your gallbladder works.

When your liver secretes bile, a relatively large quantity is "captured" by your gallbladder and stored there for use. When you eat certain fatty or oily meals—a fish dinner, perhaps, with lots of heart-healthy omega-3 fatty acids—and all the incompletely digested oils and fats are passed from your stomach into your duodenum (the uppermost portion of your small intestine), the fats and oils trigger the release of the hormone "cholecystokinin" (CCK). CCK travels to your gallbladder, telling it "oil's coming, fat's coming!" In response to CCK, your gallbladder contracts, pushing out just the right quantity of stored bile. The bile arrives in your intestines at the exact time it's needed, in the exact quantity needed. Working with your pancreatic fat- and oil-digesting enzymes, the bile digests and emulsifies those oils, making them "just right" to be absorbed.

Marvelous how it all works together, isn't it?

But without your gallbladder, most of that marvelous coordination is lost. The small, steady trickle of bile from the liver is still there, but it's no longer "matched" to the amount of fat or oil you've eaten in either quantity or timing. The resulting "mismatch" inevit-ably affects your digestion and absorption and puts your fat-soluble nutrient status at risk.

Fortunately (or unfortunately), the symptoms of inadequate vitamins A, E, D, K, and essential fatty acids are rarely as dramatic as the case mentioned above; instead they often take years to develop. When they do, they're usually not identified (except by nutritionally aware physicians) and hardly ever traced back to gallbladder removal.

The missing ingredient for missing gallbladders

And that brings us back to the question: "What should I do if my gallbladder's already gone?"

First, you'll need a bottle of "bile salts" (basically, bile in tablet or capsule form). After any meal containing more than a tiny bit of fat or oil, take one to three tablets or capsules.

Some physicians think that trying to reproduce a more normal bile flow with bile salts is too much trouble and advise taking large extra quantities of all the fat-soluble nutrients daily instead. But even those who choose this option need some bile to achieve optimal fat-soluble nutrient assimilation, so I continue to recommend copying nature by taking bile salts if your own gallbladder is gone. You'll never be able to exactly match the amount of bile you take to the oil or fat you eat the way your gallbladder did automatically, but taking bile salts will go a long way in helping the process along, and it's much better for your health than not taking them at all.

Fortunately, there are very few potential adverse effects of taking replacement bile salts. Too much, and bowel movements become abnormally dark and sometimes loose. Conversely, too little, and bowel movements are very light in color—nowhere close to a "normal" medium to dark brown.

Bile salt replacements are available in natural food stores, compounding pharmacies, and at the Tahoma Clinic Dispensary (see Alternative Health Resources on page 485). I recommend the formulas Cholacol, manufactured by Standard Process Laboratories, and Bile Salt Factors, by Jarrow Laboratories. (I'm not associated with either of these companies.)

For further guidance about bile salt replacement, check with a physician skilled and knowledgeable in nutritional and natural medicine.

The bottom line is, you should do everything you can to keep your gallbladder. If you're having gallbladder attacks, find out what you're allergic to, and deal with it. And if your gallbladder is already gone, follow nature's lead and replace the bile and nutrients your body needs.

Chapter 4:

Soothing the symptoms of IBS and colitis

The major problem with irritable bowel syndrome (IBS)—aside from the obvious ones it presents to people suffering from it—is that it's sort of a "last ditch" diagnosis, meaning you're only told you have it if and when everything else has been ruled out.

Clinical trials suggest that peppermint oil may be beneficial in the treatment of some symptoms of IBS. In the most recent one, 110 IBS patients took either a placebo or a capsule containing 187 milligrams peppermint oil three times per day, 15 to 30 minutes before each meal for one month. Patients taking the peppermint experienced improvements in abdominal pain, abdominal distension, stool frequency, and flatulence that were significantly better than those in the placebo group. If you decide to try peppermint oil, look for capsules that are enteric-coated. This sort of coating won't allow the capsule to break down until after it has passed through the stomach and into the small intestine. Without a protective coating, peppermint oil capsules can cause heartburn.

Ulcerative colitis is often referred to in conjunction with IBS. It's a chronic inflammatory disease of the colon. My colleague and regular contributor to *Nutrition & Healing*, herbalist Kerry Bone has had a great deal of experience—and success—treating colitis with herbal remedies. His approach is based on the evidence linking ulcerative colitis to the nature and quantity of your gut flora (the friendly bacteria that live in your digestive tract). In fact, in cases of ulcerative colitis, the immune system is actually attacking the gut microflora, as opposed to the gut itself. This means that it's not strictly an autoimmune disease as such, because autoimmune diseases attack the body's own tissues. Basically, the gut inflammation in ulcerative colitis is collateral damage.

So having healthy bowel flora will decrease your chances of stimulating an attack from the immune system. And you can promote healthy bowel flora by reducing your intake of processed foods, by keeping fat and protein to a minimum, and by taking in lots of natural fiber and raw, organic fruits and vegetables.

It's also important to reduce your intake of sulfur-containing foods, which feed sulfur-reducing bacteria. These produce hydrogen sulfide, which is toxic to the already damaged gut lining. A pilot clinical study found that subjects who stuck to a low-sulfur diet for 12 months experienced a remarkable clinical improvement in their colitis symptoms. Patients in the study reduced their intake of red meat and completely avoided eggs, cheese, milk, ice cream, mayonnaise, soy milk, mineral water, and sulfated drinks (wines, cordials, syrups, and the like). They also avoided nuts, cruciferous vegetables, garlic, onions, and food that contained sulfur additives (such as dried fruit).

In terms of herbal supplements, Kerry recommends garlic and goldenseal because they reduce levels of harmful bacteria in the gut. Use either a freshly crushed clove of garlic or a garlic powder product (which mimics in the digestive tract what happens when you crush a fresh clove). These can be taken about two days per week.

But the top three herbs on Kerry's colitis-fighting list are St. John's wort, echinacea, and Boswellia. St. John's wort is extremely effective against viruses that have an envelope around them, such as cytomegalovirus (CMV), which is a virus related to herpes. More than 40 years of studies have linked ulcerative colitis with CMV. And echinacea root helps fight any viruses or bacteria that are feeding the immune imbalance that creates gut inflammation.

A group of Indian and German scientists conducted a study to test the effects of the herb Boswellia in treating ulcerative colitis. For the study, 34 patients were given 350 milligrams of Boswellia resin three times a day while eight other patients were given the drug sulfasalazine (1 gram, three times a day). Symptoms like abdominal pains, loose stools, mucus, and blood improved in both groups, and about 80 percent of the patients receiving Boswellia went into remission.

Toxicity studies show that Boswellic acids don't cause adverse effects even after repeated administration. The dosage of Boswellia should be 200 to 400 milligrams of extract three times a day. The extract should be standardized to have a Boswellic acid content of about 60 percent.

Part VI
Immune System

Chapter 1:

Dangerous grains linked to serious disease!

There is no food that's good for everyone. We've all heard the old adage "One man's meat is another man's poison." Well, it's true! And the ever-touted "healthy" whole grains that we're often told by nutrition "experts" to load up on are no exception.

While whole grains *are* good nutrition—*for some of us*—the fact is, for years we've known that grains cause digestive disorders that can lead to gas, bloating, and even malnutrition in some people. More recently, we've learned that allergic reactions to grains could actually cause several different types of autoimmune disease. And now, in a new book being published this year, two experts share eye-opening evidence that undiagnosed sensitivities to certain grain proteins can be the route to some very serious—even deadly—diseases including cancer, chronic pain, psychiatric disorders, infertility, liver disease, and osteoporosis. And the frightening list goes on and on.

Sensitivity may start in your intestinal tract

Experts have known for years that certain whole grains (wheat, rye, barley, spelt, triticale, kamut, and possibly oats) are the cause of celiac disease in some people. Celiac disease affects the intestinal tract, and its symptoms can vary from mild gas, bloating, and loose stools to life-threatening conditions like malabsorption of essential vitamins and nutrients, weight loss, and malnutrition. But celiac disease is somewhat rare. Fewer than one in 100 Americans are diagnosed with it. So why should the rest of us worry?

Because for the past two to three decades, at an accelerating pace, researchers have demonstrated that the offending proteins (including gluten, gliadin, and glutenins) found in the above-mentioned grains can cause symptoms and sometimes full-blown diseases that reach far beyond celiac disease. These diseases can affect nearly any area of the body, not just the intestinal tract. They are often called "non-celiac gluten sensitivity symptoms and diseases," or "gluten sensitivity symptoms and diseases," or simply "gluten sensitivity."

Cure so-called "incurable" autoimmune disease by cutting out grains

I first became aware of the wide reach of gluten sensitivity when I read the book *Relatively Speaking*, originally published in Australia and then re-published in the USA under the title *Your Family Tree Connection*. (This book is now out of print, but it can still be found on-line through used book sources.) The book, written by Dr. Christopher Reading and Ross Meillon, describes Dr. Reading's detective work as he unravels the causes of many supposed "undiagnosable" symptoms by closely examining a family health history.

Years later, during a trip to Australia in the 1980s, I got to visit Dr. Reading's office in Sydney. On one wall was a chart that listed over 100 individuals who had initially consulted Dr. Reading about a common so-called "incurable" disease called lupus (systemic lupus erythematosis or SLE). All the patients on the list had suffered the symptoms (fever, joint pains, and skin rash are among the most common symptoms) and had tested positive for lupus in blood tests. However, everyone on this particular list had been symptom free, with negative blood tests for five years or more! It's true. Over 100 people were *cured* of so-called "incurable" lupus in the 1980s. Even today, just about any "lupus specialist" in the U.S. will say that's impossible…and then resume writing prescriptions for prednisone, the most commonly prescribed patent medication used to treat the disease.

How did Dr. Reading do it? Through complete elimination of all grains except rice and corn. (Note: His treatment also excluded milk and other dairy products from his recommended diet and included heavy nutritional supplementation, both orally and intravenously.)

Autoimmune disease is linked to genetics

When I got back to the United States, I headed for the university medical library where I found a short but very intriguing article in the *Lancet*[1]. The author points out that many people suffering from autoimmune diseases share a genetic marker called HLA-B8; much more commonly than would be expected by chance.

The author's point is that every one of these diseases *except* for celiac disease is an autoimmune disease thought to be caused by an internal reaction by the body against itself. But celiac disease was known to be caused by an external phenomenon, gluten sensitivity to certain grains. The author asks: "Could this external agent, gluten sensitivity, also be involved in causing the rest of these diseases linked to HLA-B8?"

I figured that Dr. Reading had already proven this by helping over 100 people to cure their lupus (SLE) by (among other things) totally eliminating all gluten-containing grains from their diets. So, since the 1980s, every time I'm consulted regarding any of the conditions mentioned in the list below, I recommend absolute avoidance of all gluten-containing grains.

The results I've seen have been fantastic. This is especially true when they are compared with the results of conventional treatment, which usually consists of prednisone prescriptions and other dangerous patent medicines. Although not everyone has been cured, many patients have seen major improvements or complete remission from their auto-immune diseases, with the exception of patients with established type-1 diabetes, where already-destroyed islet cells cannot be brought back to life, even by a gluten-grain free diet. In these cases, insulin treatment needs to be continued.

When treating autoimmune illnesses, I also recommend several other steps along with advising patients to completely avoid gluten-containing grains. First, stop consuming milk and other dairy products. The next step is to undergo comprehensive allergy testing and desensitization, along with gastric analysis. Digestion is abnormal in much more than 50 percent of all problems linked to HLA-B8. Once those steps have been taken, patients usually need to work with their physician to plan an individual treatment regimen, which usually involves taking large quantities of omega-3 fatty acids and many other oral and intravenous vitamin and mineral supplements. Often, hormone level testing and subsequent treatment with DHEA and testosterone can also offer significant benefit.

Dangerous grains are linked to many of today's top illnesses

With their new book, *Dangerous Grains*, James Braly, M.D., and co-author Ron Hoggan, M.A., have reminded me of the still-growing volume of gluten sensitivity research. Dr. Braly estimates that 90 million Americans may suffer from non-celiac gluten sensitivity. In fact, he and Mr. Hoggan report that undiagnosed sensitivities to gluten, gliadin, and other grain proteins are "the root cause of many cancers, autoimmune diseases, neurological diseases, chronic pain syndromes, psychiatric and other brain disorders, and premature death." Furthermore, they claim, "there is also a clear causal connection with some cases of osteoporosis, epilepsy, learning disorders, attention deficit disorders, infertility, miscarriage, premature births, chronic liver disease, and short stature."[2]

Dr. Braly is a long-time clinical investigator into allergy, sensitivity, and health. He warns that *anyone who has gluten sensitivity also has other food sensitivities, frequently many of them.*

I agree with Braly's view that gluten/gliadin/glutenin sensitivity and dairy product sensitivity are among the more common sensitivities that can lead to the development of many allergies. When gluten sensitivity (or dairy product sensitivity) is found, comprehensive allergy testing should always be done. Keep in mind, however, that <u>although successful desensitization techniques can eliminate other allergies and sensitivities (and allow you to reintroduce certain foods back into your diet), you shouldn't even try to desensitize gluten/ gliadin/glutenin sensitivity</u>. It, along with dairy product sensitivity, is one of the root causes of allergies, and if you're sensitive, the offending grains and dairy products should be permanently eliminated from your diet.

The first step is to determine your own gluten sensitivity

The most sensitive and specific blood test for gluten/gliadin sensitivity that's presently available is called the tissue *transgluaminase* (tTG) test. It's the one I've used since it became available. Others include the *endomysial antibodies* (EMA) test, which checks mostly "short-lived" antibodies and the *antigliadin antibodies* (AGA) test, which checks "longer-lived" IgG antibodies as well as IgA antibodies. [Note: You will not have antibodies to anything you haven't previously been exposed to. So if you've been avoiding all gluten grains, the test will be negative even if you are truly gluten sensitive.]

Fortunately, these newer blood tests for gluten sensitivity have made diagnosis much easier and have greatly facilitated research. But, keep in mind that the standard test for celiac disease is an intestinal tissue biopsy, followed by a probe for characteristic changes in the biopsied tissue. And since most gluten-sensitivity-linked symptoms and diseases (such as those listed in *Dangerous Grains*) are *not* accompanied by changes in the intestine, this older test may not be appropriate. Please make sure your doctor uses the test that's applicable to your specific situation.

Also keep in mind that before the blood tests were available, Dr. Reading figured out many of the disease and symptom connections with gluten sensitivity by examining family trees for various symptoms and diseases. Armed with a copy of *Dangerous Grains* for a comprehensive list, you can examine your own family tree and make a very educated guess as to whether or not you have a gluten sensitivity problem. Dangerous Grains is available in bookstores and through the Tahoma Clinic Dispensary.

If you have any suspicion that gluten grains may be contributing to your symptoms or illness, check with a health care practitioner skilled and knowledgeable in nutritional medicine, and have testing done, especially the tTG determination. (Remember that the test is only accurate if you've been eating "gluten grains.") To locate such a physician in your area, contact the American College for Advancement in Medicine (1-800-532-3688, 1-714-583-7666, www.acam.org), the American Association of Environmental Medicine (1-316-684-5500; www.aaem.com), or the American Association of Naturopathic Physicians (1-703-610-9037, www.naturopathic.org).

225 reasons to steer clear of dangerous grains

Dr. Braly and Mr. Hoggan have compiled a list of 225 symptoms and disease conditions either linked to or caused by gluten sensitivity. The list includes symptoms and diseases in the following areas:

Gastroenterology: Recurrent canker sores, chronic diarrhea, constipation, gas, bloating, abdominal pain, celiac disease, and ulcerative colitis

Hepatology (Liver disease): Autoimmune hepatitis, gallbladder malfunction, primary biliary cirrhosis, and elevated liver-function problems thought to be "of unknown cause"

Hematology (Blood diseases): Iron and vitamin-deficiency anemias, vitamin K coagulation disorders, low white-blood cells (due to autoimmunity), and idiopathic thrombocytopenic purpura (ITP, a low platelet count again thought to be of "unknown origin")

Internal medicine: Unexplained weight loss, chronic fatigue syndrome, IgA nephropathy (an autoimmune kidney disease), kidney stones, and recurrent urinary tract infection

Pneumonology (Lung diseases): Bronchiectasia (a disorder of small "bronchial tubes")

Dermatology: Vitiligo (an auto-immune depigmentation disorder), alopecia ("patchy" or complete hair loss), hives, and dermatomyositis

Obstetrics/Gynecolgy: Infertility, amenorrhea (a lack of menstrual periods), recurrent spontaneous miscarriage, low birth weight, and vulvodynia (a painful vulva)

Rheumatology: Rheumatoid arthritis in adults and children, Sjogren's syndrome, autoimmune connective tissue disease, systemic lupus erythematosis ("lupus"), scleroderma, and polymyositis

(continued on next page...)

Neurology: Seizures accompanied by brain calcifications, cerebellar ataxia, brain atrophy, neuromuscular disorders, and peripheral neuropathy

Psychiatry: Depression, schizophrenia, and autism

Dentistry: Defects in dental enamel

Immunology: IgA deficiency (IgA is an immune globulin.)

Oncology (Cancer): Cancers of the mouth, pharynx, and esophagus; intestinal lymphomas; other intestinal cancers; sarcoidosis; kidney adenocarcinoma; and rhabdomyo-sarcoma (a muscle cancer)

Orthopedics: "Spontaneous" fractures, osteoporosis

Parasitology: Giardiasis

Infectious diseases: Delayed recovery from infectious disease

Endocrinology: Type 1 diabetes, autoimmune thyroiditis (Hashimoto's), Addison's disease (weak to very weak adrenal functioning), and Graves' disease (another autoimmune thyroid problem)

Genetics: Down's syndrome, Turner's syndrome, and other chromosome problems

Pediatrics: Unexplained weight loss in children over 2 years of age, dirt eating, recurrent infection, failure to thrive, and short stature

This is only a partial list. The entire list is printed in *Dangerous Grains*. Remember, gluten sensitivity is one possible cause of each of these symptoms or diseases; it's not necessarily the entire or only cause.

Chapter 2:

Forget the flu shot!
Three natural flu-fighters
you can rely on

I'm sure you've seen the news footage of the seemingly endless lines of people waiting and hoping to get one of this year's scarce flu vaccines. The shortage has created alarm and fear among those who rely on their yearly shot.

The advice from the Centers for Disease Control is that the current vaccine stocks are only to be used for those at highest risk—the elderly, the very young, and those with compromised immune function. But there's so little of the vaccine to go around, even people in these priority groups may "miss out."

The good news is that there are herbs available that can help to prevent and treat the flu. The even better news is that there are clinical trials supporting their efficacy. Let's go over three of the most effective: Echinacea, Andrographis, and Eleutherococcus.

Natural immune boosters you can use all year long

Echinacea is already the best-known herbal product for colds and flu. But recently it has suffered from well-publicized problems involving poor product quality and ineffective clinical trials. These problems can really be traced back to the fact that the Echinacea supplement market has become crowded, generic, and dominated by cheap, poor quality products.

So the key to the successful use of Echinacea to prevent winter illnesses is to know which form to use and how to use it. I believe that, as a preventative, the best form of this herb is the <u>root</u>, which is rich in phytochemicals known as alkylamides.

There is good clinical evidence for Echinacea root's cold and flu preventative effects. In fact, several years ago, I consulted on a randomized, double-blind, placebo-controlled trial, which demonstrated that a liquid extract of Echinacea root significantly reduced the incidence of winter infections in medical students. Med students tend to be highly stressed and more susceptible to illness during the winter.

The Echinacea liquid consisted of a flavored blend of *E. angustifolia* and *E. purpurea* roots (in equal quantities) standardized to contain at least 1 mg/mL of alkylamides.

Over the course of the trial, researchers tested three dosage protocols on the volunteers: High (4 mL twice/day, corresponding to a daily dose of 4 g of the Echinacea root combination), followed by medium (3 mL twice/day) followed by low (2 mL twice/day). The control group had about a 10 percent infection rate, but in the highest dose Echinacea groups, only 2 to 3 percent of the volunteers got sick.

The baseline preventative dose, which must be taken every day, should contain around 2.5 g of Echinacea root. When you feel a cold coming on, temporarily increase your dose to 7.5 to 10 g per day to ward off the infection, then resume your baseline dose. Contrary to what some reports have said, there is no harm from taking this form of Echinacea every day: It will <u>not</u> wear out your immune system.

The traditional Chinese way to fight the flu

In addition to Echinacea, the traditional Chinese herb Andrographis is emerging as another important immune-enhancing herb. A recent review of many published studies found that Andrographis was more effective than placebo in the treatment of respiratory tract infections. Andrographis helps prevent winter infections too.

In a randomized, double-blind, placebo-controlled clinical trial, 107 healthy children received either Andrographis extract tablets (200 mg per day of extract, standardized to 11.2 mg andrographolide) or placebo for three months during the winter "cold and flu" season. This dose corresponds to about 1 g of the actual herb.

By the end of the third month, there was a significant decrease in the incidence of colds in the Andrographis group compared to the placebo group: The relative risk of catching a cold was 2.1 times lower for the Andrographis group. This study was done in children, so the dose is smaller than it would be for adults.

Adults need to take the equivalent of around 3 g per day as a preventative or about 6 g per day when you're at risk of infections or when you're actually sick.

The Siberian secret to boosting your immune system

The final key flu preventing herb is Eleutherococcus, previously known as Siberian ginseng. In one double-blind study of 1,000 workers in a Siberian factory who received Eleutherococcus daily for 30 days, researchers observed a 40 percent reduction in lost work days and a 50 percent reduction in general illness over a one year period. Another placebo-controlled, double-blind German study demonstrated a strong enhancement of immune function, showing an increase in both natural killer cells and T-helper cells in healthy volunteers. These studies all confirm that Eleutherococcus can be considered a powerful, effective immune booster.

The optimum flu-prevention dose of Eleutherococcus is 3 to 4 g. One key point though, is to <u>stop</u> taking Eleutherococcus if you do get sick, because high doses during an acute infection are thought to make the illness worse. Instead, you should up your Andrographis or Echinacea (or both if you're taking them together).

You do have to take these herbs year-round to get their full infection-fighting benefits, but that means they'll already be active—and you'll be protected—well before flu season sets in. It also means you'll be protected from colds at other times of the year—like the ones that always seem to come on just as the weather finally gets nice in early summer.

While you may not be able to get your annual flu shot this year, you can get all of these herbs fairly easily from healthcare professionals and pharmacies and natural food stores stocking professional herbal lines. So thanks to Nature's own flu-fighters, there's no need to panic—or to stand in line.

Chapter 3:

The common health problem that's more serious than you think

Part I: Uncovering the hidden cause of your nagging symptoms

For most of us, allergy isn't a *serious* problem. A little antihistamine for the nose and sinuses, some cortisone for the skin—case closed (at least until the next time). If the reaction keeps coming back, some people see an allergist, have "skin tests," and get allergy shots, or rely on prescription antihistamines and/or inhalers. And if it's really, really bad, well, there's always Prednisone—a steroid often given to people whose allergy symptoms are too stubborn for the other methods. What else is there to know?

Well, as you might suspect, there's a lot more. In fact, there's so much to say about allergies I had to break it up in two parts. In this part, I'll cover testing and prevention. Next, I'll talk about treatments. But by the time you've finished this two-part series, you may well be reassessing your own nagging health problems (or those of a family member) from a new "allergy point of view."

Putting 30 years of allergy research to work

Let's start with James Breneman, M.D., who first published the widely ignored but brilliant book Basics of Food Allergy back in 1978. When he published his book, Dr. Breneman was the Chairman of the Food Allergy Committee of the American College of Allergists (later re-named the American Academy of Allergy and Immunology), the most prominent organization for MDs specializing in allergy.

But even the other physicians specializing in the field were taken aback when Dr. Breneman wrote that <u>60 percent</u> of all undiagnosed symptoms are due to food allergy or intolerance. After more than 30 years of medical practice, I think Dr. Breneman's estimate is a little too high—but not by much.

The following is a partial list of symptoms that Dr. Breneman identi-fied as often (but not always) caused by allergy:

- **asthma**
- **bedwetting (enuresis)**
- **recurrent bladder infections**
- **recurrent bronchitis**
- bursitis
- **canker sores**
- celiac disease
- chronic low back pain
- depression
- diarrhea
- **recurrent childhood ear infection**
- **eczema**
- edema
- fainting
- fatigue
- **gallbladder "attacks"**
- **gas**
- **gastritis**
- headache
- **hives**
- **hyperactivity (ADHD)**
- hypoglycemia
- **irritable bowel syndrome**
- **itching**

- joint pain and swelling

- personality changes

- **recurrent infection (any type)**

- **sinusitis**

- **ulcerative colitis**

- learning disabilities

- protein in urine

- seizures

- **skin rash**

Two important points to remember: Allergy is a <u>common</u> cause of these problems, but it's not the only cause. The conditions in **bold type** above are ones in which allergy is involved at least 70-80 percent of the time in the individuals I've worked with. Second, and even more important—this is only a <u>partial</u> list of the problems that may be caused by allergy. As Dr. Breneman wrote, with the exception of symptoms from accident or injury, any symptom at all might possibly be "triggered" by allergy.

Dr. Breneman focused primarily on food allergy, but "conventional" allergists focus the majority of their efforts on diagnosis and treatment of allergy symptoms caused by dust, pollens, molds, grass, trees, flowers, and other growing things. But there's more to the environmental allergy equation than just those factors.

In 1962, Dr. Theron G. Randolph published <u>another</u> brilliant but widely ignored book: *Human Ecology and Susceptibility to the Chemical Environment.* In it, he discussed his 20+ years of observation of allergies caused by chemicals. These include chemicals contained in outdoor air pollution (industrial emissions, microscopic airborne particles from automobile tires, etc.), indoor air pollution (gasses emitted from plastics and particle board, etc.), agricultural and horticultural chemicals (herbicides, pesticides, insecticides), food chemicals (synthetic colorings, flavorings, preservatives, etc.), water contaminants (fluoride, chlorine, etc.), and synthetic drugs.

Allergies become a sensitive subject

The reason most conventional allergists overlook so many potential allergy triggers is that they can't be identified by "objective" testing. In other words, if it doesn't show up on a blood test or skin test, they don't consider it a real allergy. Any other evidence of an adverse reaction (such as "I get dizzy, a headache, and almost pass out every time I smell that perfume") was—and still is—usually dismissed as "not an allergy" (at best) or "all in your head" (more usual). So Dr. Breneman, a board-certified allergist himself, compromised and wrote that allergic reactions that couldn't be "objectively proven" might be called "sensitivity reactions" instead.

But he also pointed out that the person suffering the "sensitivity" feels just as bad as if it were an "allergy." Basically, an allergy by any other name feels just as bad.

Are allergies to blame for your nagging symptoms?

Here are a few clues to help you figure out whether your own symptoms or those of a family member may be partly or even completely due to allergy.

Personal history of allergies. This is as good a spot as any to contradict all the pediatricians who tell moms that "children grow out of allergies." It isn't true! The symptoms of allergy may change: The recurrent ear infections, bedwetting, and eczema you had when you were a kid may give way to the migraines or gallbladder attacks you're experiencing now—but they're all caused by allergy.

If you've ever had any symptoms identified as allergy, even when you were a child, and you're having difficulty diagnosing or treating any symptoms now, there's a good chance your current symptoms are (at least partly) caused, aggravated, or triggered by allergy.

Allergy is a condition, not just a symptom or group of symptoms. The bottom line: Once allergic, always allergic!

Family history. Even if you've never had symptoms officially identified as allergy, if another family member has, then it's also quite possible that any undiagnosed but persistent symptoms you're having now are due to allergy. Members of "allergic families" usually inherit the condition and do have allergic symptoms to some degree, even if they're not severe enough to be classified as a full-blown allergy.

Physical signs. Sometimes allergies are physically obvious. This is especially true in children, especially smaller ones, but it is possible (though much less likely) for adults to have these indicators too.

In my experience, any child that has dark circles under the eyes is allergic. Horizontal creases in the lower eyelids (Dennie's lines) result from allergy too, as does a horizontal crease across the lower end of the nose. My friend and colleague Doris Rapp, M.D., and other allergists have also pointed out that children's ears suddenly turning bright red is another physical sign of allergy. Colic in infants and unusual gassiness in children are also almost always physical reactions to allergy.

Scratch, patch, and drop

Skin testing is one of the oldest forms of testing for allergy. There are several varieties, including scratch tests, patch tests, serial dilution titration, and provocative neutralization.

Scratch tests are the oldest of the four types. In this technique, a drop of an extract of a potential allergen is placed on the skin, and a "scratch" is made in the skin under the drop. The allergist determines if the person is allergic to the substance (and how severe the allergy is) based on whether or not a red bump forms and how large it is.

Scratch tests are generally accurate for inhalant allergies (dust, pollen, mold, etc.) but aren't very accurate for food allergies. Many allergists won't even do skin tests for food allergy.

Patch testing is basically another version of skin testing. The allergist puts a drop of an allergen directly on the skin and covers it with a Band-Aid. Then the skin is observed for redness and/or swelling. Unfortunately, patch testing isn't very effective for inhalants and is virtually useless for foods.

Dilution/titration and provocative neutralization are much more accurate and can diagnose both inhalant and food allergies. These techniques, particularly provocative neutralization, can be used for both testing and treatment. In fact, they can actually "shut off" many allergy symptoms entirely.

In both tests, patients are given a series of very carefully measured amounts of allergens, which are injected under the skin. The allergist follows a pre-set schedule and observes the patient's reactions to each dose.

Both these techniques do take a considerable amount of time. Depending on the individual's reactions, a test for one allergen can take from a few minutes to over an hour, or occasionally even longer. So testing for a number of potential allergens could take up most of the day. But the hundreds of thousands of individuals who have been successfully tested and treated using these techniques since the 60s would probably tell you it's worth the time and effort.

Unfortunately, most board-certified allergists won't do dilution/titration or provocative neutralization. To have this type of testing done, contact a physician-member of the American Academy of Environmental Medicine. (See the Alternative Health Resources section on page 485.)

Allergies in the blood

Blood tests come in several different forms—most of them with confusing acronyms for names, like "RAST" and its variant "MAST," "ELISA," and its variation "ELISA/ ACT." Most of them measure antibodies specific to individual inhalants, foods, and (in some cases) other substances.

The problem is, many allergens don't cause antibody formation or white blood cell damage, so blood tests will miss those potential triggers. But even if they can't find everything, these tests can find a lot and can be very helpful in determining a wide variety of allergies—definitely enough to make a significant difference in an individual's symptoms and over-all health.

It's usually necessary to work with a physician skilled and knowledgeable in natural medicine and allergy/sensitivity to have any of these blood tests done. ("Conventional" allergists sometimes do these tests too, but most don't.) To find such a physician (M.D., D.O., or N.D.), contact one of the organizations listed in the Alternative Health Resources section on page 485.

Uncovering your "virtual allergens"

Electrodermal testing is one of the more controversial approaches to allergy testing. It's also called Electroacupuncture According to Voll (EAV) and Meridian Stress Analysis (MSA). This technique was invented by Dr. Reinhold Voll of Germany, who observed that "acupuncture points" conduct tiny electrical currents differently than the rest of the skin.

Dr. Voll noticed that the current flow at acupuncture points varies if an allergen or toxin is placed near (though not necessarily in direct contact with) the person being tested. Eventually, Dr. Voll and his successors found that even a computerized representation of an allergen (a "virtual" allergen) would cause the same variation in current flow as the actual allergen itself. This allows physicians to test patients for hundreds of items in just an hour or two.

In my experience, this is by far the best and least expensive way to test for sensitivity to synthetic chemicals.

Unfortunately, electrodermal testing is the subject of intense controversy. Many states (most notably California) have persecuted and prosecuted physicians using the technique. Left to politicians, it'll take decades before electrodermal testing is widely available. It may not be widely available, but it is available. It might take some hunting and possibly even some traveling, but if you have nagging symptoms that aren't associated with any specific condition, finding a source for electrodermal allergy testing could very well be worth it.

Subjective but effective

Kinesiology tests the "baseline" strength of a specific muscle or muscles. The person being tested is then put in direct contact with a potential allergen, and the muscle strength and resistance is tested again.

One of the most common ways this is done is to have the person being tested hold out their arm. The clinician instructs the patient to resist any force placed on the outstretched arm with all of their strength, and then he pushes down on the patient's arm. The clinician takes note of how much the person's arm moved and uses this as the baseline.

Then the practitioner gives the person being tested a vial containing a potential allergen and tells him to hold it while they repeat the previous step. If the person's arm goes down more easily when pushed this time, it's likely that the contents of the vial he's holding are an allergy or sensitivity trigger for him.

Kinesiology is criticized as being much more "subjective" than other allergy testing techniques, since it's entirely dependent on the skill and education of the individual doing the testing. It's done by various health care practitioners, most often chiropractors (D.C.s) and naturopathic doctors (N.D.s), but sometimes M.D.s or D.O.s, too. I've seen both excellent and not-so-good results from kinesiology.

Lengthy testing, lasting results

Elimination diets are one of the oldest techniques for allergy testing. They obviously only detect allergies to foods and other ingestible substances (like medications).

During the testing process, the patient has to eliminate all but a few foods (ones unlikely to be allergens) from his diet for at least a few days. If his or her symptoms improve or disappear, chances are they were due to one or more of the foods (or chemicals in those foods, such as colorings, pesticides, herbicides, etc.) previously being eaten. The foods are then added back one at a time, and very careful observations are made to see which ones cause symptoms to resurface: Those that do are the person's allergens.

When properly done, this method is very accurate. The major drawback is the amount of time it takes to do an elimination diet: They can last anywhere from a few weeks to a few months depending on how quickly the allergens are identified.

Mysterious methods offer accurate diagnosis

I once sent an unmarked Polaroid photograph of an allergic individual (no name, address, or other identifying data) from Washington state to a practitioner of radionics over 2,000 miles away. Back came an accurate diagnosis of the person's condition (rheumatoid arthritis) as well as a list of food items the person should avoid. The "radionics" list contained most (although not all) of the same items found by the "RAST" blood test.

Radionics is based on the concept that all living organisms are surrounded by an electromagnetic energy field. Practitioners diagnose allergies and other health problems by "reading" those energy fields and detecting abnormal vibrations.

It sounds a little "out there," but radionics can be a useful diagnostic technique. Useful or not, though, most radionic practitioners keep a very low profile, or practice outside the USA. No wonder: In 1951, Dr. Ruth Drown had her radionics practice raided, her equipment smashed, and was charged by the FDA and California medical "authorities" of fraud. After numerous appeals, Dr. Drown was actually imprisoned for her so-called "offense."

Some people have also effectively determined their allergies by using a pendulum. They've observed on their own that the pendulum swings very differently when exposed to something they're allergic or sensitive to. (In fact, I know a "board certified allergist" who sometimes uses this technique.) Although I don't use this testing method myself, it appears to work well in some cases.

I'm sure there are many other "unconventional"—but very useful—allergy-diagnosing techniques that the AMA and each state medical board would just love to try to persecute/ prosecute, but, for the sake of all the people those techniques are helping, I'll end the list here.

Prevention and treatment go hand in hand

It's hard to separate allergy prevention and allergy treatment sometimes, since they're often the same, especially when it comes to alternative approaches. In this part I'll focus more on prevention in terms of how to control the factors that contribute to your allergies. In Part 2, I'll go over some of the specific nutrients and other steps you can take to treat your allergic symptoms and even eliminate them altogether.

The first method of prevention is reducing the total allergic burden. This is one concept shared by both "conventional" and "natural medicine" practitioners and basically just involves limiting exposure to your known allergens.

For example, years ago, I had a patient come to my office with severe pollen and grass allergies. Since he was a landscaper, this was obviously a big problem. So we went through the list of possible triggers that could be making his symptoms worse, and when we got to dairy products, he admitted that they usually gave him a bit of gas, but he ignored it because he liked eating cheese, ice cream, and other dairy foods. I convinced him to try eliminating them to see if it made a difference in his symptoms.

On his next visit, he told me that his allergy symptoms were much, much less—even nonexistent some days—as long as he strictly avoided drinking milk and eating dairy products. Within an hour or two of drinking or eating any dairy, his grass and pollen symptoms ("totally stuffed sinuses") returned in full force.

The "threshold effect," or "overflow effect," is another variation of the "total allergic burden" concept. Like a partially full cup or glass, our immune systems can handle a certain amount of allergy without reacting. But once the cup or glass is full, a few more drops can make it overflow. Similarly, once the immune system is "full," another allergen or two can cause the immune system to react—and not just to those last two items but to any number of allergens that never caused problems before the cup overflowed.

The key to preventing allergies using the threshold effect is to identify and deal with your allergens. You don't necessarily have to find and eliminate all of them—just enough to drop below the threshold again.

Take control of your surroundings

Environmental control is another effective prevention technique used to reduce the overall allergic burden and to control symptoms. Environmental control is recommended more often for people with obvious inhalant allergy symptoms, but it's actually helpful in reducing the total allergic burden for anyone who's allergic. In other words, it may not directly help combat food allergies, but it can minimize exposure to other allergens, which can help you deal with any potential food allergies more effectively.

Indoor environmental control involves outfitting your house with allergy-resistant materials and devices. Special filters are placed in furnaces and in all the ducts of heating and air-conditioning systems. Carpets are replaced with hardwood, tile, or other hard floor surfaces with only a few (if any) area rugs. Central vacuum cleaner systems, again with special filters, are installed. And "regular" vacuum cleaners are replaced by "hypoallergenic" versions that have HEPA or other special filters.

Environmental medicine physicians often make additional recommendations like replacing synthetic materials (textiles, plastics, etc.) with natural materials.

Negative ion and ozone generators go a step further to reduce airborne allergens. In its most natural state the "electrical balance" of air is slightly negative. Unfortunately, airborne allergens (both natural and industrial) are almost entirely positively charged, and positive electrical charges are very irritating to respiratory membranes.

Negative ions, on the other hand, help counteract the swelling and inflammation brought on by the allergy-triggering positive ions. Negative ion generators are sold in electronic specialty stores. They're quite safe and can be left on 24 hours a day. However, the generators do need to be cleaned regularly.

Ozone is highly negatively charged and does all the same things that "regular" negative ions do. But it has its pros and cons. On the "plus" side, ozone kills any micro-organism it contacts. Mold, bacteria, virus... it doesn't matter. With ozone, they're all dead. So your chances of infection are reduced. But very much on the minus side, ozone is very bad for respiratory membranes. If exposed for very long, delicate lung membranes can be temporarily or even permanently damaged. (Negative ions on their own will not do this.)

My recommendation: If you have allergy symptoms, particularly respiratory allergies, buy a negative ion generator and keep it on permanently. If you buy an ozone generator too, only turn it on as you're leaving the house, and turn it off immediately on returning home. It's best to stay out of the room containing the ozone generator, or even step outside, for about five minutes until the airborne ozone is almost entirely gone.

All these strategies can cut down your risk of encountering your allergens and triggering an attack. In part II, we'll talk about how to stop those attacks when and if they do happen.

Part II: Simple solutions for treating—even eliminating—your allergies

You may not be able to prevent all allergies, but you can cut them way down and even eliminate them in some cases. We just went over some prevention strategies, so now let's move on to treatment.

It's worth a shot

Allergy shots are one of the most common tools used by mainstream allergists. Patients are given very tiny quantities of the very items to which they're allergic. Quantities are slowly increased over time until the person builds a resistance to the allergen and it no longer causes an adverse reaction. No one knows for sure how these injections "switch off" the allergic response, but they usually do.

In most cases, conventional allergists only use allergy shots to treat inhalant allergies, but physician-members of AAEM have developed very effective injectable techniques to treat food allergies: Provocative neutralization and serial dilution titration. While they're very effective, the major drawback to these techniques is the amount of time spent in the doctor's office. It's not unusual for it to take a week or more of all-day sessions, which may need to be repeated every few weeks, to make a significant difference in allergy symptoms.

Allergy "drops" use even smaller homeopathic dilutions of the substances to which an individual is allergic. One of the biggest differences is that the drops are taken under the tongue rather than by injection. Most of the time, precise dosages of these drops are determined with electrodermal testing.

The drops are taken under the tongue two to four times daily and usually need to be continued for six to 12 months. Every six to eight weeks, the patient returns for follow-up testing and dosage adjustments.

As is the case with "conventional" tiny-dose allergy shots, there's no explanation as to how even-tinier-dose homeopathic drops work, but once again, they usually do. And they appear to be effective for both food and inhalant allergies

I've used both electrodermal testing and homeopathic allergy drops as treatment since the 1980s (in fact, these techniques were part of the FDA's "excuse" for their armed raid of our clinic in 1992) with considerable success.

Nutrients can help—but they're not cure-alls

Vitamins, amino acids, and botanicals can all help reduce—and in some cases eliminate—inhalant allergy symptoms. However, keep in mind that they're only "symptom relievers" and aren't nearly as effective for food allergies as they are for environmental allergies.

Vitamin C is always the first vitamin to try. It's been shown to reduce bronchial, nasal, and sinus allergy symptoms. I recommend the "bowel tolerance" quantity of vitamin C. Basically, this means using as much vitamin C as possible, every three to four hours, without causing gas or loose bowels. For some people, this is 1,000 milligrams (1 gram) three to four times daily; for others, it can be 4 grams or more three to four times daily.

Years ago, nutritionist Adelle Davis recommended the use of 1,000 milligrams of pantothenic acid (vitamin B5) along with vitamin C. Some people with inhalant allergies find taking this combination three to four times daily helps relieve their symptoms more so than vitamin C on its own; others don't. Fortunately, it's harmless at these quantities.

Sometimes it's better to take a step backward

Allergic reactions, particularly more serious ones, have been treated with adrenaline injections since the 1930s. But one group of researchers took this approach a step backward and tested the effects of natural adrenaline precursor molecules on allergy symptoms.

The body makes adrenaline from the amino acid tyrosine, with the help of pyridoxine (vitamin B6) and niacinamide (a form of vitamin B3). So the researchers asked 492 individuals with hay fever, allergic headaches, and "poison oak" allergy to take these supplements.

In mild to moderate cases, quantities were 200 to 600 milligrams of tyrosine along with 2.5 to 7.5 milligrams of pyridoxine and 10 to 30 milligrams of niacinamide four times daily. In more severe cases, quantities were 1,200 milligrams of tyrosine along with 15 milligrams of pyridoxine and 60 milligrams of niacinamide four to six times daily.

The study participants reported that their itching seemed to be under control within four to 16 hours and that their hay fever symptoms, allergic headache, and poison oak were better in two to five days. Although there weren't any reports of side effects of any type, the research did note that symptoms were sometimes aggravated in the first few days—especially in chronic disorders. They also emphasized that the treatment only worked if all three nutrients were taken at the same time

Although apparently harmless, these are very large quantities of tyrosine for a 24-hour period, so not many of the people I've worked with have tried this treatment. But those who have all say it's helped, from a little to a lot. The only side effect I've heard of is insomnia from larger quantities, particularly if the person takes the combination late in the evening.

Two non-Ephedra herbs just as effective for combating allergies

Like nutrients, herbs are most effective for inhalant allergies. Unfortunately, the most effective one is also the most controversial. Ephedra sinica (also known as ma huang) is the "prototypical" decongestant herb. It also acts as a bronchodilator, opening up airways and allowing people to breathe easier during allergy or asthma attacks. Contrary to the media hype surrounding it, when it's used in traditionally recommended quantities (125 to 250 milligrams of a 10% "standardized" extract three times daily), Ephedra is safe and usually quite effective for the majority of people who tried it before the FDA ban. The ban has since been overturned, and products containing 10 mg of Ephedra or less (per serving) are legal, but it will probably take quite a while for it to become common again.

In the meantime, 300 milligrams of Urtica dioica (stinging nettle) and 1,000 milligrams of quercitin (sometimes with bromelain) three to four times daily can also alleviate hay fever and other nasal/sinus allergies. Both are quite safe, but I've found that the results aren't very consistent: Some individuals find substantial relief when taking one or both of these herbs, others try and find it very little help.

The drug-less drink that can halt acute allergy attacks

Most over-the-counter and prescription drug treatments for inhalant allergies include antihistamines (most of which are synthetic, patentable versions of flavonoids) and decongestants (most of which are synthetic, patentable versions of Ephedra).

Other major categories of prescription drugs for inhalant allergy include higher-potency bronchodilators and synthetic versions of cortisone. Try to avoid cortisone whenever possible and never use it long-term: Possible adverse effects include an increased risk of cataracts, even in young people, along with suppressed immunity, and increased susceptibility to infection.

Drug treatment of food allergies is almost non-existent unless it's a very serious acute situation. In those cases, adrenaline, prednisone, and other synthetic cortisone preparations are usually used—often justifiably. When a child's kidneys are shutting down due to allergy, prednisone can be life-saving. If breathing is seriously impaired because of a reaction to peanuts, an injection of adrenaline can stop the reaction in its tracks.

However, if an allergic reaction is serious but not yet an emergency requiring a trip to the hospital, sodium bicarbonate stirred into water and drunk as rapidly as possible can bring the reaction under control in a relatively short time—often in less than an hour. The "bicarbonate in water" remedy (1 to 2 teaspoons stirred into 6 to 12 ounces of water) can be repeated as often as necessary until the symptoms are gone.

This method works because acute allergic reactions bring on a rapid acidification of the bloodstream. Bicarbonate neutralizes the rapidly growing acidity and usually reverses the allergic reaction.

Two specific formulas called TriSalts and Alkala are even more effective than sodium bicarbonate in emergency situations, but they aren't as readily available. If you have frequent serious allergic reactions, it's a good idea to talk to your doctor about these products.

Some physicians prefer sodium ascorbate (an alkaline form of vitamin C) to sodium bicarbonate, since it combines alkalinity with vitamin C, which fights allergy in its own way. I personally recommend taking the sodium bicarbonate (or TriSalts or Alakala) first, followed within an hour by 1 to 2 teaspoons (4 to 8 grams) of the sodium ascorbate form of vitamin C dissolved in 6 to 12 ounces of water.

Keep in mind, though, that this method should <u>not</u> be used as an "everyday" remedy for chronic allergy. It could ultimately lead to excess alkalinity in the blood, which can cause its own set of problems.

Have your allergies and eat them too

There are some treatments that are helpful specifically for food allergies. The first is to pay close attention to digestion. The relationship between digestion and food allergy is really a "chicken and the egg" situation: Food allergy can impair digestive function, and faulty digestion can cause food allergy. It's usually impossible to say which is the cause. So the most practical and effective approach is to always consider, test, and treat both conditions at the same time.

At a minimum, you should have a Heidelberg capsule test done to measure your stomach acid production.

Also consider having a comprehensive stool and digestive analysis, which evaluates the adequacy of pancreatic digestive enzyme output and other aspects of digestive function. If you do have digestive abnormalities (usually underproduction of one or more "digestive secretions"), taking supplemental digestive aids with each meal will not only improve your digestive function and the assimilation of nutrients, but it will also slow down or prevent the development of additional food allergies.

Elimination diets are the time-honored method of uncovering food allergies. They're also an effective treatment, particularly if impaired digestion isn't a factor. Not eating the foods you're allergic to for long enough usually allows you to re-introduce them back into your diet gradually without re-activating your symptoms.

Elimination diets can be very time-consuming and restrictive. But on the "plus" side, they're quite inexpensive and effective.

Sometimes, just following a "rotation diet" is enough to help manage food allergies without employing other techniques. But more often, they're combined with food allergy desensitization for faster results. In a rotation diet, the patient can't eat any of his or her particular food allergen more than once every four to five days. This minimizes the impact of each individual allergen and doesn't let them build up in the system, magnifying symptoms. Since only the "major" allergens are completely eliminated, and then only for the first 30 to 60 days, rotation diets are easier to manage than elimination diets (although still not easy) and are most effective if the patient can fully eliminate the major allergens for a month or two before re-introducing them.

Nambudripad Allergy Elimination Technique (NAET) is a "body work" or "body energy" procedure that's actually very difficult to describe in just a few words. In very simplified terms, it involves mildly stimulating a patient's central nervous system while he is being exposed to an allergen. This stimulation "reprograms" the brain and energy flow in the body so that it doesn't recognize the allergen as a threat anymore. It usually requires weekly visits to an NAET practitioner for several months. Each visit takes about 10 to 20 minutes.

NAET is most often used for food allergy elimination, but it can also be effective for inhalant allergies.

Although NAET is very controversial with conventional allergists and medical doctors, it's helped tens of thousands of individuals eliminate multiple allergy symptoms.

Reversing the trend

While no one can say for certain why cases of allergies appear to be on the rise, the evidence does seem to point to industrial pollution and other man-made substances, which have altered the normal functioning of human immune systems.

An article published in the British medical journal Lancet years ago pointed out that while asthma was written about in ancient Greek and Egyptian medical writings, the very first cases of "rose fever" (now called "hay fever") and upper respiratory allergy weren't recorded until the early 1800s.

The first cases occurred in the immediate vicinity of Britain's first major industrialized city, Liverpool. At first, there were so few cases that most doctors refused to believe them and actually ridiculed the doctors who published the case reports (sound familiar?).

But the *Lancet* authors hypothesized that this first concentrated center of industrial pollution (at that time, smoke, dust, and soot from coal were the major culprits) caused a few very sensitive individuals' immune systems to malfunction, developing adverse reactions to many other items, both natural and man-made.

The authors went on to track the spread of rose fever across Britain and found that it directly correlated to the spread of industrialization. And the process repeated itself in other countries as they also underwent industrialization.

Since that time, literally millions of unnatural, man-made molecules and compounds have been released into the air, soil, and water. The widespread use of herbicides, pesticides, and insecticides started in industrialized nations in the early 20th century and has since spread around the planet. There's no doubt that many of them cause immune system malfunction and a tendency toward allergies (among many other problems).

But industrial pollution and agricultural chemicals are only part of the picture. Health care practitioners and parents have observed that immunizations can also trigger allergies in children. The number of immunizations and vaccinations made with live viruses has increased dramatically in the last two decades, and human immune systems, particularly immature human immune systems, just aren't designed to handle the load.

Then there's the absolutely irresponsible practice of filling dental cavities with mercury-silver amalgams. Numerous studies have shown that mercury compounds cause immune system malfunction.

It's also true that allergy (like any other health problem) runs in families.

The list goes on and on…and it's a trend that's probably not going to be reversed any time soon. But with the strategies for detecting, preventing, and treating your allergies we've gone over in the past two issues, you can reverse your own allergy trend.

The best single resource for a very strong focus on allergy testing and treatment is the American Academy for Environmental Medicine (AAEM). This group of physicians investigates and treats all aspects of allergy, "conventional" allergy, chemical allergy and sensitivity, and food allergy. This is the first group I recommend contacting for "all things allergic." AAEM may be reached at (316)684-5500, www.aaem.com.

However, many members of other natural medicine organizations (the American College for Advancement in Medicine, the International College of Integrative Medicine, and the American Association of Naturopathic Physicians) are also very good at allergy testing and treatment. See the Alternative Health Resources section on page 485 for these organizations' contact information. It's best to speak to each individual doctor's office about how much and what types of allergy/sensitivity testing and treatment are done there.

Chapter 4:

5 ways to make sure you've had your last bout with the common cold— And 3 cures you never knew could work so well

If you, your children, or grandchildren never get colds or the 'flu, then you can safely skip this chapter. Still reading? I thought so. But there's a lot you can do keep yourself and your family from catching those occasional—or not so occasional—colds. In fact, there's a good chance that if you follow the steps I'm going to outline you may have had your last bout with these all-too-common nuisances.

And if you do come down with one at some point, there are several research-proven things to do to make colds go away a lot more quickly. Some of them, like vitamin C and zinc lozenges, are things you've likely heard of and probably even tried at some point or another. Whether or not they were effective, though, depends on some important details.

But before we get into the details that will help make those old standbys work as effectively as they should, let's talk about how you can keep from needing them in the first place.

Give your white blood cells a (germ) fighting chance

The first step in beating cold and flu season once and for all is the same first step I recommend for preventing many illnesses—get rid of the sugar!

Decades ago, Professor Emanuel Cheraskin and his colleagues demonstrated that refined sugar significantly impairs the ability of white blood cells to fight germs. To reach this conclusion Professor Cheraskin drew blood samples from research volunteers, and then observed under a microscope how many germs the average white blood cell could destroy per minute. One hour after each volunteer swallowed approximately 1 teaspoonful of refined sugar, his or her white blood cells could only destroy half as many germs as before. And the white blood cells didn't recover their full "germ-eating" capability until four to five hours later.

So as Professor Cheraskin observed at subsequent lectures, if an individual ate a sweet roll or doughnut for breakfast (or even just sweetened his or her coffee or tea with sugar), then had a soft drink or candy bar at lunch, ate a piece of pie or other sugared dessert at dinner, and perhaps had some ice cream before bedtime, the only time he or she should ever expose him- or herself to germs should be between 2 AM and breakfast time. Otherwise the likelihood of catching an infection would be significantly greater since the person's white blood cells would be impaired from sugar all day long.

Granted, the "germs" Professor Cheraskin's team observed were bacteria, not "common cold" viruses. But it's been my experience in over 36 years of practice that eliminating refined sugar (as well as refined carbohydrates) is absolutely necessary to minimize or eliminate colds.

Uncovering and eliminating (or desensitizing) allergies is a close second to eliminating sugar when it comes to cold prevention. For my first 25 years of practice, I worked with children (and their parents) quite frequently. I saw hundreds of children for recurrent colds, sore throats, ear infections, bronchitis, and 'flu. If the recurrent infection didn't subside after the parents got rid of all the refined sugar in the child's diet, we then checked the kids for allergies, particularly food allergies. Every single one of these children had significant food allergies, and if the offending foods were eliminated (or in the long run, desensitized), the recurrent colds and infections always vanished (or nearly so, except perhaps for the very infrequent case of sniffles).

The same strategy applies with adults, although in general adults have a greater proportion of inhalant allergies than children, which can only be dealt with by total removal from the environment, or desensitization.

Build your body's store of "natural human antibiotics"

Taking care of sugar and allergies will give your immune system a solid foundation for fighting all kinds of infections, including colds and the flu. But there are also a few supplements that can support your efforts even further.

Some of the most exciting recent vitamin D research has demonstrated its ability to prevent viral and other infections by stimulating the production of "natural human antibiotics" in your body. (For the best discussion of recent vitamin D research available anywhere, see www.vitamindcouncil.com.)

For adults, I recommend 3,000 to 4,000 IU of vitamin D daily, for children, from 1,000 to 3,000 IU, depending on size. (It's certainly best to check with a physician skilled and knowledgeable in natural and nutritional medicine for recommendations for children.)

Many people still believe that long-term use of Echinacea can have adverse effects. The truth is that there is solid evidence showing this herb's ability to increase the production of natural killer (NK) cells in the body. NK cells are a critical part of fighting off any type of infection. To help prevent colds Kerry recommends 1 to 3 grams of dried Echinacea root per day. Echinacea is available in all natural food stores, compounding pharmacies, the Tahoma Clinic Dispensary, and even many national supermarket and pharmacy chains.

A product called "Cold-fx," a standardized extract of American ginseng (panax quinquefolius) was touted as the "official cold and flu remedy of the National Hockey League and the National Hockey League Players Association." Double-blind, placebo-controlled research showed that regular use of a single 200-milligram Cold-fx capsule daily significantly reduced the incidence of colds, and that when colds did occur, their duration was significantly shorter.

The evidence is convincing enough that the Canadian equivalent of the FDA recently "approved" Cold-fx and allows it to bear the therapeutic claim that it "helps to reduce the frequency, severity, and duration of cold and flu symptoms by boosting the immune system."

Cold-fx is available at some compounding pharmacies, natural food stores, the Tahoma Clinic Dispensary (see "Alternative Health Resources," page 485), and in some national pharmacy chains.

The germ-killing duo you need at the first sign of a sniffle

One of the things that makes Cold-fx unique is that it works for both treatment and prevention. Most people think that the next item on the list does so as well. But research on vitamin C done decades ago showed that this nutrient doesn't actually help prevent the common cold. It does, however, reduce the severity and duration of colds that do occur.

At the very first sign of a cold, I recommend taking a minimum of 1 gram of vitamin C four times daily, and if the vitamin C is tolerated well (meaning it doesn't cause loose bowels or diarrhea), considerably more is safe and even more effective.

Next to vitamin C, one of the most effective germ- and infection-fighting treatments available is something that I covered in detail in the September 2006 issue of *Nutrition & Healing*. You might recognize it by its more common name, colloidal silver, but I prefer to use a slightly more technical name, nano-particulate silver. The "nano-particulate" part is very important because the smaller the particle size of the silver, the greater the germicidal effect.

I recommend Argentyn 23™ and Sovereign Silver™, both of which are available at natural food stores, compounding pharmacies, and the

Tahoma Clinic Dispensary. At the first sign of a cold, use 1 tablespoonful to start, and then continue to take 1 teaspoonful on an empty stomach every 3 to 4 hours while you're awake until the infection is gone.

Unlike vitamin C, nano-particulate silver should not be used every day (unless recommended for a very particular reason by a physician skilled and knowledgeable in nutritional and natural medicine), but reserved only for treatment of active infections.

Forget what you've heard: Zinc can knock out colds in half the time

Some individuals I've worked with have sworn that zinc lozenges are "almost miraculous" for treating colds. Others swear they're useless. Research studies have been equally conflicting. The answer to this apparent contradiction is that *certain types* of zinc lozenges are indeed very effective, while other types are not very effective at all.

Ananda Prasad, Ph.D. (professor at Wayne State University School of Medicine) is widely recognized as one of the leading researchers and authors on zinc. This month, he gave a presentation at the meeting of the International Society for Trace Element Research in Humans (IS-TERH) about a randomized, double-blind, placebo-controlled study he and his colleagues conducted to examine the effects of zinc acetate lozenges against the common cold.[1]

Fifty research volunteers took either zinc acetate lozenges (which contained 13.3 milligrams each of elemental zinc) or placebo every three hours while awake, starting within 24 hours of the onset of cold symptoms. In the zinc acetate lozenge group, the subjects' colds lasted an average of 3.5 days versus 7.4 days in the placebo group. Coughs lasted a mean 2.1 days and nasal discharge 3.0 days in the zinc acetate lozenge group versus 5.3 days and 4.7 days in the placebo group. In essence, the zinc cut the amount of time the subjects spent sick in half—that's quite a significant reduction (just ask anyone suffering a cold).

This was actually Dr. Prasad's second positive research report about zinc acetate lozenges shortening the mean duration of the common cold and its symptoms. Seven years ago, he published similar results in the *Annals of Internal Medicine.*[2]

As in his recent study, Dr. Prasad enrolled 50 volunteers who each took zinc acetate lozenges (these ones containing 12.8 milligrams each of elemental zinc) or placebo, every 2 to 3 hours while awake, within 24 hours of the onset of cold symptoms. Compared with the placebo group, the zinc group experienced results similar to those seen in the recent study: Shorter overall duration of cold symptoms (4.5 vs. 8.1 days), cough (3.1 vs. 6.3 days), and nasal discharge (4.1 vs. 5.8 days) and decreased total severity scores for all symptoms.

A tasteful solution to zinc's spotty reputation

But despite the fact that Dr. Prasad's two research reports (as well as several others) have been very positive, there have been almost as many negative reports about zinc lozenges' ability to treat colds—including first-hand accounts from many people who have tried them and say they had no effect. So what's the real answer?

The real answer is that the zinc itself isn't what's contributing to the conflicting results: Zinc has been proven to interfere with virus replication by direct contact, as well as in other ways. So there's no doubt that the zinc itself works. To sort out which zinc lozenges are actually effective, you have to look at the "rest of the story," meaning all the other things going into the various zinc lozenge products that have been put on the market since the first positive research on zinc and colds was published back in 1984.[3]

When you buy a mineral supplement, you never just buy just the mineral itself. The mineral is always attached to something called a "binding ligand" which makes it stable, and (in some cases) easier to absorb. For example, calcium tablets or capsules don't contain just calcium; they contain calcium carbonate, calcium lactate, calcium citrate, or some other "form" of calcium. Similarly, magnesium is sold as magnesium oxide, magnesium citrate, magnesium glycinate, magnesium taurate, and many other forms. Zinc is sold as zinc picolinate, zinc citrate, zinc aspartate, and—in lozenges—zinc acetate.

Making zinc lozenges to treat common colds is particularly tricky for manufacturers. First, the goal of the zinc lozenge isn't absorption of the zinc as it is with capsules or tablets. The goal of the zinc lozenge is to rapidly release the zinc so it can come into contact with both the cold virus itself and the mucous membranes of the mouth, throat, and surrounding areas.

But while it's doing that, the zinc lozenge must also achieve its second goal—to taste good, or at least acceptable, even to small children. Unfortunately, anyone who's ever tasted an "elemental" liquid zinc solution in chemistry class (usually zinc chloride) knows that zinc tastes terrible!

As George Eby, one of the original zinc lozenge researchers, explained: "[Manufacturers] found that zinc gluconate forms very bitter complexes with all sweet carbohydrates (except fructose) upon aging for a few days to a few months, depending on the exact formulation… Manufacturers and researchers alike in desperation to solve the taste problem added metal chelators, reduced [zinc] dosage or used other non-ionizable zinc compounds, resulting in a loss of Zn2+ ions and efficacy, with at least two formulations actually making colds worse in clinical trials; reports of which temporarily discredited this major medical discovery."[4]

But sometime before 1990, Mr. Eby found that zinc combined with acetate could be made into compressed tablets or hard candy lozenges that were both stable and pleasant tasting. When the lozenges dissolve, the zinc and acetate rapidly break apart, releasing the ionic (positively charged) zinc to come into contact with both the viruses and mucous membranes where it can "do its job." Research continued until zinc acetate lozenges were proven to be effective when mass produced. And this technology still holds today: As noted above, Dr. Prasad's very positive work used zinc acetate lozenges.

At present, to make certain of effectiveness against the common cold virus, I recommend only the zinc acetate lozenge formula designed by George Eby, called Zinx™. You should start taking it within 24 hours of the onset of cold symptoms, and continue with another dose every two to three hours while you're awake until the cold symptoms are completely gone.

Zinx™ lozenges are available through a few natural food stores and compounding pharmacies, and the Tahoma Clinic Dispensary (see "Alternative Health Resources," page 485). (I have no business connection with George Eby or the company which manufactures and sells Zinx™.)

How to juggle that ounce of prevention and pound of cure

Obviously, prevention is always best. Your chances of eliminating or at the very least minimizing your bouts with the common cold are excellent if you follow the preventive measures noted above. But just in case, and particularly if you have children at home, it's a good idea to have some nano-particulate silver (Argentyn 23™/Sovereign Silver™) and zinc acetate lozenges (Zinx™) in your pantry, along with a powdered form of vitamin C, which can be stirred into liquids to make it easier to take larger doses.

Of course, while getting better as quickly as possible is the ultimate goal when you come down with a cold, there are a couple of precautions to bear in mind before bombarding your system with all of these treatments at once.

Certainly eliminating sugar and allergies, and taking vitamin D, Echinacea, and Cold-fx are all compatible with each other and can be taken together safely. Vitamin C can be used with all of these, too, but at higher (treatment) quantities it's best taken with food to reduce chances of gastric irritation. By contrast, nano-particulate silver should be taken on an empty stomach, with no food for at least one hour before or after. And, as I mentioned above, nano-particulate silver isn't a preventive measure to be used on a daily basis. It should only be used when you're actually sick.

And last but not least, make sure you don't swallow those Zinx lozenges. To get the germ-killing effects, you should let the lozenge dissolve completely under your tongue. After that, you might gargle the resulting liquid or otherwise "swoosh it around" your mouth to try to contact as many infected surfaces as possible. If there's any liquid left after doing all this, it won't hurt to swallow it—after all, it's a low quantity of zinc—but it does the most good against the "common cold" by contacting the lining of your mouth and throat.

Chapter 5:

Fight lupus without dangerous prescription drugs

DHEA supplementation has shown to be effective in decreasing the need for prednisone (a cortisone-like drug often prescribed to patients with this disease) in people with lupus. It also appeared to have a beneficial effect on overall well-being, fatigue, and energy levels.

Some recent research has also uncovered a connection between the 2/16 ratio and lupus that could open up a whole new avenue of treatment for people suffering from this painful condition.

Researchers measured the "2/16" estrogen metabolites in 32 people with lupus and 54 healthy individuals. They reported that although all groups had very similar levels of 16-alpha-hydroxyestrogen (a "bad" estrogen), the healthy individuals had 10 times more 2-hydroxyestrogen (a "good" estrogen) compared to the individuals with lupus. That's as far as the study went, but if you have rheumatoid arthritis or lupus, it suggests another possible way to improve your symptoms.

First, you should have your own "2/16" ratio measured. It's a simple process you can do at home by ordering a test kit, collecting urine samples for 24 hours, and sending them back in to the lab. If your results aren't good (meaning you have more 16-hydroxyestrogen than 2-hydroxyex-trogen), following the steps for correcting the imbalance may help ease your symptoms.

But since lupus is well known to be accompanied by numerous allergies to both foods and supplements (as well as other things), it's also a good idea to have a thorough allergy screening for both foods and potential supplements done before you get started with treatment.

Once you've gotten the "green light" to move forward, start adding more Brassica vegetables—broccoli, cabbage, cauliflower, bok choy, Brussels sprouts, etc.—to your diet. These vegetables contain a substance called indole-3-carbinol (I-3-C), which can help improve your 2/16 ratio.

You may also want to consider taking supplements of another 2/16-regulating nutrient called di-indolylmethane (DIM), 60 milligrams three times daily.

I-3-C also comes in supplement form, but, more often than not, individuals with autoimmune disease also have hypochlorhydria, a condition in which the stomach doesn't produce enough hydrochloric acid to effectively digest and assimilate foods and supplements. I-3-C needs stomach acid to help it work, so DIM supplements are a better choice. But, once again, determining whether or not hypochlorhydria is a problem for you—and treating it if it is—is a good idea in general: It will improve your overall health and your current symptoms by helping your body get the most benefit from the foods and supplements you take.

As you can tell, these suggestions can get a bit complicated, so it's wisest to work with a physician skilled and knowledgeable in natural and nutritional medicine to help you navigate through the tests, allergy screening, and anything else that may occur.

Contact the American College for Advancement in Medicine (800)532-3688; www.acam.org) for a list of physicians in your area.

Part VII
Women's Health

Chapter 1:

Forget your annual mammogram! New tool offers better, earlier breast cancer detection (and it's pain-free, too!)

Over the years, my colleagues at the Tahoma Clinic and I have heard from many women who have reservations about mammography for breast cancer, and some who just refuse to get mammograms altogether—especially every year for a decade or more. Their concerns are understandable: While it's true that mammograms have increased the detection of breast cancer, more and more flaws associated with this screening tool have come to light too.

Some studies have found the sensitivity of mammography to be as low as 25 percent. In other words, it only detects about one quarter of breast cancers. Mammograms' "specificity" (accurately identifying an area as cancerous) is even worse: It can be as low as 17 percent—which means that as many as 83 percent of areas deemed "suspicious" from mammogram images actually turn out not to be cancerous after further checking. Obviously, this puts many women and their families through a great deal of unnecessary worry and emotional turmoil.

In addition, a little-publicized Canadian study of over 70,000 women found that mammograms done between ages 40 and 50 actually did not increase the breast cancer detection rate! The researchers attributed this finding to the fact that women's breast tissue is denser between ages 40 and 50 (after age 50 breast tissue "thins out" due to menopause). Even though this study is well-known among medical "authorities" in these United States—and has never been refuted—these same "authorities" rarely mention it, and continue to recommend annual mammograms to all women over the age of 40.

But besides the general lack of accuracy, there's an even darker side to mammography. It involves radiation, which (if repeated) actually contributes to breast cancer risk. In fact, each mammogram increases risk of breast cancer by 1 percent. So if you follow the "expert" recommendation to get a mammogram every year after you turn 40, by the time you're 50, you'll already have increased your chance of getting breast cancer by 10 percent.

And a follow-up to the Canadian study mentioned above disclosed that the women in the 40 to 50 year age group who'd had annual mammograms actually had a slightly higher death rate from cancer than women who only underwent manual breast exams.

Certainly doesn't seem like a very good trade off!

All this probably leaves you wondering if there isn't something else you can do to detect breast cancer—especially early cases. We've been wondering the same thing for a long time! Fortunately, there is equipment that can do the job.

Detect cancer without increasing your risk

In the 1950s it was discovered that cancerous tissue maintains a steady temperature independent of cooling or heating the surrounding tissue—and the concept of thermography for breast cancer screening was born. Thermography has been researched since then, gaining FDA "approval" in 1982 (the same year "regular" mammography was approved, incidentally). Many versions of thermography (with variable reliability) have existed, leading up to this latest version, called infrared thermography, which has proved to be very reliable: It only misses 5 to 10 percent of cancers and the number of false positives is equally low.

Infrared thermography detects differences in heat given off by the body (in this case, the breasts) by precise measurement of infrared frequency wavelengths. These wavelengths are very close to visual frequencies, and measuring them doesn't involve radiation like what is used in mammography, x-ray, CAT scans, and other tests. So thermography won't increase cancer risk, since nothing is "beamed" into or at the body.

In addition to not using radiation, thermography has other advantages too. First of all, there is no compression of the breasts, which is good news for at least three reasons: 1.) It's painless; 2.) Women with implants can relax; and 3.) It eliminates the concern that preexisting cancer will be spread by the compression of the tissue.

Another benefit of thermography is that it's very likely—although not yet proven—that it's more accurate for women ages 40 to 50, since breast tissue density makes no difference to heat emissions.

Thermography can also tell you and your doctor other important things about your breast health in addition to assessing the possibility of cancer. It's also possible for it to identify fibrocystic breast disease and hormone imbalances.

Of course, at the Tahoma Clinic, our goal is always to prevent breast cancer.

Prevention is even more important than detection—even early detection—and thermography can help with that, too. In contrast to mammography, which detects only anatomical changes in the breasts, thermography detects functional changes in breast tissue. It finds areas of abnormally increased or decreased blood flow. This is a huge advantage, since cancer takes approximately 5 to10 years to reach a size detectable with mammography or physical exam. With thermography, we're able to monitor functional changes associated with very early breast cancer and possibly even changes which precede breast cancer. Although it's too soon to say for certain, it's very possible that appropriate treatment may reverse those risk-associated changes.

So with the goal of prevention in mind, my colleagues at the Tahoma Clinic and I now recommend that all of our female clients have a yearly breast thermogram starting at age 40, or age 30 if you have a family history of breast cancer.

What to expect from the breast thermography "experience"

To make sure thermography is as accurate as possible, temperature reading is the "name of the game," so the procedure is performed in a room kept at 68° F. You sit in this cool temperature wearing the infamous "examination gown" (definitely not Dior!) for 15-20 minutes while your breast health history is reviewed. After you've acclimated to the temperature, a set of three pictures is taken—one frontal and two oblique (an angle between front and side)—followed by a one-minute "autonomic nervous system stress test" and another set of three images.

The autonomic system stress test involves placing your hands in cold water for exactly one minute. This challenge tells your body to send all the available heat via the blood from the surface of the body, inward. Any breast tissue that isn't functioning properly will not be able to do this and will then be highlighted on the second set of images.

Your appointment is finished with a manual breast exam, the findings of which are included in the notes that are sent with the thermographic images to be interpreted. (All thermographic images are sent electronically via the Internet to a qualified expert in thermographic image interpretation.)

Buyer beware

Although thermography is FDA "approved" it is still in the early stages of organization, so the facilities offering it may or may not have kept up with the many advances in thermographic technology. A high quality thermographic imaging facility should at least include the following four things:

- **Temperature-controlled room:** This is a must, since you're measuring temperatures! If the room is too hot, the results won't be accurate.

- **High-definition radiometric camera:** This kind of camera measures actual temperatures, not temperatures calculated from colors on the image or averaged temperatures from a video card. With this type of camera, temperature measurement is much more accurate and can be repeated and compared with even more accuracy.

- **Autonomic challenge test:** As I mentioned above, the autonomic challenge is usually done by having the client place her hands in cold water for 60 seconds. Although it's not the most pleasant experience, it's vital to a complete infrared thermogram and greatly increases the accuracy. Without it, the number of abnormal results are often much higher than they actually should be and cause unnecessary follow-up testing and considerable worry. (As a side note, non-radiometric cameras will not be able to detect the changes caused by the autonomic challenge test.)

- **Quantitative and qualitative interpretation:** This is the most up-to-date interpretation scoring system at this time. It includes both "qualitative" data—including hot spots, cold spots or irregular vascular patterns, along with "quantitative" data, which includes temperature readings from each of the 76,000 "pixels" recorded by the radiometric camera.

At present, there are many more practitioners offering mammograms than infrared thermograms, but the number of certified thermographers is growing. As you might have guessed, one of them practices at Tahoma Clinic (see Alternative Health Resources, page 485). Others can be located through by calling (760)494-5993. (Unfortunately, as yet there's no website listing all certified clinical thermographers.) At the Tahoma Clinic, infrared thermography is priced at $225; elsewhere, the price ranges from $200 - $500.

To read more about the thermography research discussed above, please refer to the following study:

Kuhl CK. "The 'coming of age' of non-mammography screening for breast cancer." *JAMA* 2008; 299(18): 2,203-2,205

I am very grateful to Olivia Franks, N.D., C.T.T (Certified Thermographic Technician) for much of the information contained in this chapter.

Chapter 2:

How women can be saved from congestive heart failure

By the time she came in to see me at the Tahoma Clinic, Helen's heart was so weak that she had to sleep propped up because of the fluid that was in her lungs. She had been taking three prescriptions to help her but still didn't feel right. She was taking the usual group of medications for heart failure: Digoxin, furosemide, and potassium.

I recommended a series of magnesium injections, taken intravenously, along with vitamin B6. It sounds expensive and troublesome, but it really is the best method: For congestive heart failure, magnesium frequently works better when given by relatively rapid IV injection. In heart failure, the heart muscle cells are sometimes too weak to extract all the magnesium they should from the blood stream.

A fairly rapid IV injection forces magnesium in to the heart muscle cells, helping them to work better and be stronger. The shots are a bit of a bother, but magnesium—even intravenously—is cheap. And once magnesium is forced into the cells, they continue to take up more magnesium on their own. So, you don't have to have this done on a regular basis.

The other recommendations I made for Helen were ones that she (and you) could take at home:

- Coenzyme Q10, 60 milligrams three times daily.

- L-carnitine, 250 milligrams three times daily. This takes care of congestive heart failure all by itself sometimes. It enables the heart muscle cells to use more sources of energy and to burn them all more efficiently.

- Taurine, another naturally occurring amino acid like L-carnitine. It's the most abundant amino acid found in the heart and is known to keep the electrical activity of the heart flowing smoothly. Take 1,500 milligrams twice daily between meals. The other supplements can be taken at any time.

- Hawthorn (the solid extract); take 250 milligrams of the standardized 10 percent proanthocyanidin extract three times daily. Hawthorn improves energy production in heart muscle cells and improves heart muscle contraction. It dilates coronary arteries, providing more blood flow. It also acts as a mild diuretic, can lower cholesterol, and can slow and possibly even reverse atherosclerosis a bit.

After three months, Helen reported "feeling much stronger, not taking water pills at all, and sleeping flat with only one pillow like when I was younger." At this point, I told her she could stop the magnesium injections and take magnesium capsules instead, along with the other minerals she'd been taking. When she came back for her second follow-up visit, she reported that she had all her strength back and was working hard around the house and yard.

Of course, Helen's exact treatment plan may not work for you. It's best to check with your doctor to determine a supplement program tailored specifically to your needs.

Chapter 3:

The only HRT solution used safely for 200,000 years

One day in July 2002, the phones at the Tahoma Clinic suddenly started ringing off the hook. The callers were almost all women wanting answers about the risks of hormone replacement therapy (HRT). At first, I wasn't sure where all the concern was coming from, since I usually don't get that many calls on the same topic in a whole month, let alone in one afternoon. But then I saw the front page of the newspaper: HRT had made national headlines. Directors of a national study known as the Women's Health Initiative abruptly stopped their research and instructed the women to discontinue taking HRT, because it increases the risks of breast cancer, blood clots, stroke, and heart attack.

Things have quieted down a bit at the Tahoma Clinic since that first frenzy of calls, but I've gotten so many letters from readers all over the world asking questions and expressing concerns about HRT, I wanted to take the time to go over this issue in detail so that you know exactly what's safe, what isn't, and why.

Why is HRT risky?

You've undoubtedly seen those TV commercials—with Lauren

Hutton and some other familiar celebrity faces—singing HRT's praises. The problem with the kinds of HRT you've seen advertised by celebrities on TV commercials and the kind used by researchers in the cancelled Women's Health Initiative study is that they don't replace human hormones with human hormones.

So HRT, especially long-term HRT, is risky for the same reasons any patent medication treatment is risky: It uses molecules never before found in human bodies! (At least not until patent medicine companies got a hold of them, synthesized and/or patented them, and then paid for FDA approval.)

Whenever you put molecules in your body that nature didn't intend to be there, you risk damaging the very precisely balanced biochemical system going on inside you—sometimes temporarily, sometimes permanently. And the longer you ingest any unnatural molecules the more likely it is that you'll have bad effects.

The most widely prescribed hormones used in conventional HRT, the same kinds used in the Women's Health Initiative study, are lumped together into a product called Prempro, a combination of Premarin and Provera (a form of progestin). But you're probably still wondering what exactly these substances are—this is the part of the story reporters and even experienced science writers just don't seem to want you to know (or just don't know themselves). So I'm going to give you the inside scoop.

Let's start with Premarin. Brace yourself for this one: Premarin is a combination of estrogens concentrated from horse urine. That's right, I said urine. Not exactly the most welcoming news to most women—I've seen more than a few grimaces of disgust from patients when they learn they've been ingesting the stuff. But disturbing as this thought might be, horses are natural, right? So shouldn't their hormones be safe? Well, horses are certainly natural, but there are some obvious differences between them and women. There are equally obvious differences between horse estrogens and human estrogens. The principal horse estrogen is called equilin, of which there is not a speck, not a nanogram, in any woman.

Equilin is much stronger than any type of human estrogen. Just to give you an example of this: Equilin's effects on the lining of the uterus are up to 1,000 times stronger than the effects of human estrogen (which gives us a clue as to why Premarin may increase the risk of uterine cancer).

Now, on to Provera (which makes up the "pro" part of Prempro). Provera is a synthetic type of progesterone molecule (officially known as medroxyprogesterone) invented and patented in the 1940s because the profit margin on selling natural, identical-to-human progesterone wasn't high enough. (I'm not just being cynical here. This is the motivation behind the entire patent medication industry!) Studies have shown Provera to be hazardous to heart health, and women who have taken it have had more heart attacks than those women not taking it.

So far, this seems awfully bleak, but bear with me—we're about to get to the good news. Though it hasn't made any national headlines, and probably won't anytime very soon, there is a safe, effective alternative to conventional HRT.

Real hormone replacement therapy has nature's stamp of approval—not the FDA's!

Of course, the "alternative" isn't really "alternative" at all. It's actually the real thing: Hormones present in women's bodies for at least 200,000 years (and probably a lot longer). Premarin and Provera are actually 20th century substitutes for the real thing, introduced and sold for all the wrong reasons. If you're going to use hormone replacement at all, wouldn't you rather use hormones "approved" by nature rather than those approved by the FDA for their profit potential?

Actually, this idea didn't originate in the 20th century. Hundreds of years ago, Imperial Chinese physicians appear to have been the first to use bio-identical hormone replacement therapy as an important part of overall anti-aging therapy for the emperor and his court. They evaporated urine from women in their late teens and early 20s, and combined the crystalline residue left behind with herbs and sweet gums to give to the empress and women of the Imperial Court. They did the same thing for the emperor and men of the Court using urine from young men. Those who took these preparations (all in older age groups) noted an anti-aging, rejuvenating effect on their skin, a major boost in their energy levels, and an improvement in their sex drives.

Before you get nauseated at this thought, remember that literally tens of millions of American women have been swallowing purified horse urine without a qualm for nearly 40 years!

Since all of the hormones found in human bodies are excreted in the urine, a "recycling" program from those whose bodies produce the most hormones—young people—to those who produce the least is actually the safest, most natural, and best-balanced way to go. But somehow I doubt this recycling approach will gain much public support, so the next best and safest method of hormone replacement is to use "bio-identical" hormones—estrogens, progesterone, and testosterone precisely identical to those found in human bodies.

Replacing the natural hormones your body needs

Bio-identical hormone replacement can be confusing, so it might help to know a bit about the basic biology behind it. Progesterone and testosterone are each individual molecules. "Estrogen" is actually a collective term used to refer to at least 20 to 30 distinct molecules all naturally present in human bodies. (To make it even more confusing, there are distinct animal estrogens, such as equilin, and a whole variety of plant estrogens, generally termed "phytoestrogens"—but for our purposes here, you don't need to worry about those.) Although researchers have started to sort out the roles of all the various estrogens, the job is nowhere near complete.

The three human estrogens studied the longest are estrone, estradiol, and estriol. Estrone and estradiol are generally considered slightly pro-carcinogenic; estriol is generally considered anti-carcinogenic, or at worst, neutral.

In the early 1980s, I had a patient who came to me after her doctor prescribed conventional HRT. She insisted she wasn't a horse (I'm not kidding!) and wasn't going to take horse hormones. I realized, obviously, that she was right, and that the point of HRT should be to replace the actual hormones your body would produce if it could. So I checked with several major clinical laboratories to find out the exact proportions of the three major estrogens circulating naturally in a woman's bloodstream. It took a considerable amount of inquiry and calculation before I finally found out the breakdown: It turned out to be approximately 10 percent estrone, 10 percent estradiol, and 80 percent estriol.

Once I had the proportions, I contacted a friend of mine named Ed Thorpe, a compounding pharmacist at Kripps Pharmacy in Vancouver. He assembled the three estrogens in their natural proportions into a compound, called Triple Estrogen. In the 20 years since Ed and I worked together to create that first batch of Triple Estrogen, its use, and the use of similar estrogen compounds, (both along with natural progesterone and testosterone) has spread from my patients at the Tahoma Clinic to tens of thousands of women all around the USA.

It's natural, but is it safe?

In the last 20 years, I have written several thousand Triple Estrogen prescriptions, along with prescriptions for natural progesterone and testosterone. But I'm always very careful to explain to my patients that no treatment, not even natural treatment, is perfectly safe, but bio-identical estrogens, progesterone, and testosterone are much safer than horse urine estrogen or medroxyprogesterone.

Here's how the "excess risks"—those of heart attacks, blood clots, strokes, and cancer—found to accompany horse urine estrogen and medroxyprogesterone pan out using natural HRT:

Natural hormones handle your heart with care

A few years ago, I returned to work after being away from the clinic for two weeks. I was greeted with the news that a patient named Fran had called to tell me she didn't have "that bad angina" anymore. Since she'd never complained of problems with angina previously, I asked for a bit more explanation. It seems that Fran, who was 63 at the time, had started having "just a little" chest pain several months before. The pain gradually got worse, but she hadn't done anything about it until two days before I left, when her husband "dragged" her to an emergency room because she couldn't walk more than a hundred yards without chest pain. She'd been given nitroglycerin to relieve the symptoms and referred to a local cardiologist, who had tests performed and then told her to check into a hospital for coronary bypass surgery.

Instead, Fran persuaded her husband to drive her to the Tahoma Clinic. One of the clinic nurses started her on daily intravenous magnesium injections along with Triple Estrogen and progesterone. Ten days later, she could walk as far as she wanted with no chest pain at all. A month after my first visit with her, Fran's HDL cholesterol was considerably improved.

While this doesn't prove that Triple Estrogen and progesterone prevented Fran's heart attack (intravenous magnesium likely helped a lot), it does show they didn't cause one, even in a "high risk" individual.

It makes sense when you think about it: Men start having a significant number of heart attacks in their 40s, when their testosterone levels take a nosedive. Women start having a significant number in their 50s, when menopause has deprived them of a good portion of their estrogen and progesterone levels. So if losing your natural hormones increases your heart attack risk, it's pretty safe to say that replacing those lost hormones with bio-identical versions will very likely reduce your heart attack risk.

An easy way to eliminate your risk of estrogen-induced blood clots and stroke

Even bio-identical estrogens, particularly large quantities of them, raise a woman's risk of blood clots. And, unfortunately, if blood clots form abnormally in the brain, a stroke follows.

But estrogen-related blood clots are entirely—and easily—preventable with omega-3 fatty acids and vitamin E. I recommend one table-spoonful of cod liver oil and 400 IU vitamin E daily.

DHEA: A vital but neglected part of natural hormone-replacement therapy

DHEA (dehydroepiandrosterone) is a hormone manufactured by the ovaries and the adrenal glands. It's been shown to have a bone-building effect. The decline in ovarian DHEA production at the time of menopause may be one of the factors contributing to postmenopausal osteoporosis. In fact, DHEA may be more important than estrogen for osteoporosis prevention.

DHEA is one of about 70 hormonal materials made in the cortex of our adrenal glands. It's actually the most abundant adrenal steroid hormone, and it was the first discovered.

We all peak in our DHEA production at about 25 to 30 years of age. It's supposed to drift gradually down after that, but some of us go "klunk" a little sooner, and the reversing of our well-balanced immune system, good tissue strength, a portion of our cancer protection, and so on begin to occur. And that leads to an acceleration and intensification of aging symptoms. If our bodies maintain, by supplementation if necessary, reasonably normal levels of DHEA, it may have an anti-aging effect. I'm not talking about using DHEA as a "wonder drug" to turn back the hands of time, but as a replacement therapy if you don't have a normal amount.

Furthermore, treatment with DHEA sometimes relieves hot flashes and other symptoms that have been attributed to estrogen deficiency. DHEA therapy is even more effective when used with natural progesterone. Most laboratories can measure serum DHEA levels. If your level is low (results vary from lab to lab, but the lab reports contain guidelines), you might want to locate an innovative physician who is willing to prescribe a small amount of this important hormone (5 to 15 mg/day is the usual dose).

Other potential benefits of DHEA are improved immune function, more energy, lower serum cholesterol, a better memory, and a longer life.

I admit that all those claims make DHEA sound a little bit like a "cure-all," but the research on this hormone really is solid.

How to check your levels of DHEA

Monitoring your DHEA levels should be done with the help of a physician who's knowledgeable in DHEA testing and use—especially the testing of DHEA metabolites, to guard against effects of excess.

There are two ways of testing for DHEA levels: The "serum DHEA" test and the 24-hour urine test that checks not only DHEA levels but also DHEA metabolites. The serum DHEA test is relatively inexpensive and especially suitable for initial screening.

Remember that since DHEA is a "precursor" hormone as well as being effective in its own right, it can't be safely taken over a long period of time without checking those metabolites. The lab I work with, Meridian Valley Clinical Laboratories in Kent, Washington, has taken the time and trouble to survey for accuracy all the commercially available test kits. It has also pioneered the study of DHEA, its metabolites, and all the steroid hormones by mass spectroscopy, a very advanced and much more accurate technique. Using this method, the lab has been able to bring costs down by over 50 percent, making the test accessible to many more people. For more information, call Meridian Valley Laboratory at (425)271-8689.

Even safe, effective, natural hormone treatments should be monitored closely

As I said, I've been prescribing this type of HRT for 20 years, and out of the thousands of women treated, only two have been diagnosed with cancer. And in one of those cases, it's very likely the cancer was present before the bio-identical hormones were started. Even in the other case, there's no evidence to support that the hormones had anything to do with her condition.

But as the saying goes, "better safe than sorry." In the last few years, it's become possible to estimate your risk of estrogen-related cancer with a simple urine test (FDA approved, no less—and something useful for once). So I insist that every woman who uses bio-identical hormones have this test done. It's called the "2/16a hydroxyestrogen test." It was first performed (at my request) by Meridian Valley Laboratories.

If test results are abnormal, it's possible to lower your estrogen-related cancer risk simply by eating vegetables in the "mustard family" (cabbage, broccoli, cauliflower, Brussels sprouts, bok choy, mustard greens, and many others). If eating these vegetables doesn't lower your risk enough, then supplements of indole-3-carbinol (I-3-C) or di-indolylmethane (DIM) have always done the trick.

Other foods and supplements that can lower your risk of estrogen-related cancers include flaxseed, selenium, folic acid, and soy (but no more than two or three times weekly, please!).

Sometimes even a little can go a long way

One thing to keep in mind: You may not need long-term bio-identical hormone replacement. Maybe just a little to "get you through" hot flashes, depression, sleeplessness, and irritability during menopause, but that's all. If you're healthy and your female relatives have lived to ripe old ages, free of heart attacks, osteoporosis, senility or Alzheimer's disease, then excellent diet, exercise, positive attitude, and non-hormonal supplementation may be the way to go.

But if you have any of these risk factors in your family, you may still want to consult your doctor about bio-identical hormone replacement therapy. After 20 years, it's obvious to me that among women who use bio-identical hormone replacement, skin aging and aging in general is less, strength and endurance is better, and mood and attitude are improved. And as an added benefit, many women have reported that their sex drive improves—and stays improved.

The proof is in the practice— 20 years of natural HRT success

I'm the first to admit that my 20 years of observation isn't the same as a placebo-controlled, double-blind study. But now the Women's Health Initiative study has confirmed my theories on the risks of conventional HRT, so maybe the so-called "experts" will finally start to eliminate the use of horse urine estrogen and medroxyprogesterone, and scientists will finally turn their attention—and their research funding—to bio-identical hormone replacement.

So when all is said and done, should you take conventional HRT? Given the risks associated with it, my answer is what it's always been—a resounding NO! Especially when there's a much safer alternative: Bio-identical hormone replacement therapy, using hormones identical to those found in women's bodies for at least the last 200,000 years. And it's not as difficult to get as you might think. Triple Estrogen is available from over 1,000 compounding pharmacies across the U.S. You'll need the help (and prescription) of a good physician who's knowledgeable in natural hormone replacement. Contact the American College of Advancement in Medicine at (800)532-3688, or www.acam.org for a list of doctors in your area who are skilled and knowledgeable in natural and nutritional therapies.

(For more details on bio-identical hormone replacement therapy, please refer to the book *Natural Hormone Replacement for Women Over 45* by John Morgenthaler and me, available through the Tahoma Clinic Dispensary.)

Chapter 4:

The natural secret to great sex after menopause

Over the years, I've noticed that much more attention has been paid to male sexual health and satisfaction than it has to female. Contrary to what the mainstream medical community might want to believe, I know (from the feedback we get from patients visiting the Tahoma Clinic) that women are interested in having fulfilling sex lives too—yes, even after menopause. But sometimes it just physically isn't that easy. Atrophic vaginitis can make sex downright unpleasant for many women. This condition is very common and includes symptoms like vaginal dryness, itching or burning, painful sexual intercourse, light bleeding after intercourse, and sometimes incontinence.

You may have all of these symptoms or just a few. But, since the usual treatment for this problem is hormone replacement therapy (HRT), you may have decided to "just live with it," rather than face the risks that have recently surfaced regarding synthetic hormone replacement.

Keep in mind you can take hormone replacement safely with all-natural, identical-to-human HRT (as I discussed in Chapter 3), but there may be an even simpler solution—all-natural ginseng.

Decades ago, a British researcher found that Panax ginseng can be used effectively to treat atrophic vaginitis. Women with a history of vaginal dryness and painful intercourse were asked to volunteer for biopsies of the vaginal mucosa. When examined microscopically, the biopsy specimens showed typical atrophy, with a thinner skin and little to no mucous production. Physical examination prior to biopsy showed the same changes.

The women were asked to take Panax ginseng for two to three months. Repeat biopsies showed significantly thickened mucosa with more normal surface mucous. Physical examination showed the same types of changes, and women reported disappearance of vaginal dryness and painful intercourse.

I've been recommending this same treatment to my patients for years, and they've reported great success. I usually advise 100 milligrams of a standardized Panax ginseng extract three times daily. After comfort has returned and symptoms have diminished, you can usually lower your dosage of ginseng to an appropriate maintenance level that works for you.

No one should have to give up hope, comfort, or great sex after menopause. If any of the symptoms listed above apply to you, Panax ginseng is certainly worth a try. It's available in almost any natural food store, as well as many pharmacies and supermarkets.

Chapter 5:

Breast cancer—stop the most feared disease among women from happening to you

It's no wonder that breast cancer is the biggest fear of so many women. All you hear about these days are the dismal odds: Currently, researchers expect one in eight women—that's 17 million—to be diagnosed with the disease. And the treatment options are nothing short of barbaric: Surgery that leaves you disfigured, radiation that leaves you swollen and tender, and chemotherapy that leaves you weak, bald, and nauseous.

Sure, there are a few brave women (like Suzanne Somers) who refuse the conventional recommendations and opt for alternative natural therapies. But even if they succeed in their fight against the disease, they have to endure the constant and critical questioning of their decision—not exactly the most supportive environment for a cancer patient (who needs it most).

But with all of the attention focused on breast cancer lately, I'm disappointed at how much of it is geared toward, basically, waiting until a woman actually has the disease and dealing with it then. Unfortunately, this has been the standard practice for years—though I'm sure you'd rather not become a part of that "standard." So why not focus on preventing breast cancer before it ever happens?

Most mainstream doctors would probably say that we just don't know enough about the causes of breast cancer to focus on prevention. That's partially true: Not all of the causes of the disease have been identified, so you can't completely eliminate the risk. But we do know about enough causes and risk factors to make it possible for you to cut your risk way back. First you have to determine just how at risk you are.

Measuring your levels of various estrogens is a simple technique to help predict if you're at higher risk for certain types of cancer (especially breast and uterine). Then, once you have that information, supplementing with the right kind of estrogen (along with other supplements and a diet rich in certain foods) can reduce your risk of ever getting those cancers—or possibly even help treat existing cases.

But since not all estrogen is created equal, let's take a few minutes to go over some of the intricacies.

Five estrogen metabolites you need to know about

The term estrogen doesn't actually describe a single molecule; instead, it's a "group word" covering two dozen or more molecules all built on a common framework. Since these molecules are transformed (metabolized) one into another into another, they're also all called estrogen metabolites.

The "early days" of estrogen research focused mostly on three estrogen metabolites called estrone, estradiol, and estriol.

Over the last three decades, with improved analytic techniques and evolving research interest, attention has turned to some of the other estrogen metabolites, including "good" and "bad" estrogens. The technical terms for these are 2-hydroxyestrogen (good) and 16a-hydroxyestrogen (bad), and together they make up what's known as the 2/16 ratio. High 2/16 ratios generally mean a lower risk of estrogen-related cancers (like breast, uterine, and ovarian). Low 2/16 ratios mean higher risk of these same cancers. (I've also observed an unusual number of low 2/16 ratios in men with newly diagnosed prostate cancer, and men with a strong family history of cancer.)

The good news is, testing your own 2/16 ratio couldn't be easier. You don't even have to leave home to do it. Some changes in the actual testing equipment have made the process a lot easier. In fact, the testing kits can be mailed to you at home, where you'll collect a urine specimen in the container provided. If you're pre-menopausal, try to collect the urine specimen during days 19 to 23 of your 28-day cycle, and be sure to note the cycle day and time, in case you need to take a repeat test or two. When you've collected your sample, just mail it back to the lab.

Once you send your sample back to the lab, it generally takes about two to three weeks to get your results.

Eat your way to a breast cancer-free future

You definitely want more "good" (2) estrogen than "bad" (16) estrogen—substantially more if possible. So when you get your results, check the proportion of these two substances: Any ratio below 1.0 is unfavorable. Although there's no consensus on an ideal ratio number, I recommend 2.0 or greater if possible.

If your 2/16 ratio is less than 1.0, there's a good chance you'll be able to boost it just by eating a few specific foods. Start with Brassica (or mustard family) vegetables. These include cabbage, broccoli, cauliflower, bok choy, Brussels sprouts and many others. You can also eat freshly ground flaxseed, 1 tablespoonful daily. You don't need to go overboard with Brassica vegetables. I know it seems odd for me to be warning you not to eat too many vegetables, but it is possible for Brassicas to cause suppressed thyroid function and even goiter if you eat a lot of them on a daily basis. Three to four servings a week is a good general range.

In a lot of cases, just eating these foods will bring a low 2/16 ratio to 1.0 or above in just four to six weeks without any other specific supplementation. But if you find you're still not getting sufficient improvement, you can also take di-indolylmethane (DIM) supplements to boost it even further. DIM is actually a substance found in Brassica vegetables, but it's also available in most health food stores in supplement form. If you need some extra help, take 60 milligrams three times daily, and check your 2/16 ratio again in another four to six weeks.

Should you or shouldn't you?
An answer to the soy question

When soy became a big-ticket item for American business giants, we were hit with an enormous wave of pro-soy promotion. Some of it is actually true. For example, in Asian countries where soy products are eaten regularly, the incidence of breast cancer is definitely lower.

But there's also been a "research backlash," including a recent study showing that former breast cancer patients who ate soy had a higher rate of cancer recurrence than a control group that ate no soy.

Despite the negative soy research, I'm not completely anti-soy. There is also a good deal of research about soy's health benefits. And incorporating soy products (tofu, tempeh, soy milk, etc.) into your diet is a good option for boosting 2/16 ratios. A little goes a long way though, and two or three servings a week is plenty.

When less isn't more:
Boosting a stubborn 2/16 ratio

The first woman to do the 2/16 test at Meridian Valley Lab was a Tahoma Clinic employee named Beth, the youngest of nine sisters. Her eight older sisters had all suffered breast cancer, so she was first in line for the test as soon as it became available. Her first 2/16 ratio was 0.5, so she made all the diet changes noted in the left-hand column. But her follow-up test was only 0.6—obviously not good enough. She added di-indolylmethane (DIM), 60 milligrams, three times daily. Much to her disappointment, her next test was still well below 1.0. But she didn't give up: With her sisters' health history in mind, Beth increased her dosage of DIM to 120 milligrams, three times daily. Finally, her next test was above 2.0.

After a few months, she decided to cut the DIM back to 60 milligrams three times daily, partly to cut costs. Unfortunately, her next 2/16 ratio dropped below 1.0 again, so she resumed taking 120 milligrams three times daily, and her ratio rose back up above 2.0.

While supplementing with DIM doesn't guarantee you'll never get breast cancer, it certainly lowers your risk—especially if you have a stubborn 2/16 ratio (like Beth). Even though this approach can be more expensive, the peace of mind it brings is well worth it.

Another do-it-yourself breast cancer risk test

There's another estrogen ratio that's just as important as the 2/16 for estimating your risk of estrogen- related cancer. It's called the estrogen quotient, or EQ.

As I mentioned above, early estrogen research focused mostly on three estrogen metabolites: Estrone (also labeled E1), estradiol (E2), and estriol (E3). Although it's only present in small quantities in the body, estradiol is the most "potent" estrogen, responsible for most of the feminizing changes of puberty. Unfortunately, estradiol and its nearby metabolite estrone were both found to be carcinogenic. Researchers found that the body treats these two hormones with extreme care, rapidly converting them to estriol. As far as anyone could tell, estriol didn't have any carcinogenic tendencies.

With all of this in mind, Henry Lemon, M.D. (a women's cancer specialist), came up with an equation that, like the 2/16 ratio, can estimate a woman's risk of breast cancer. He called this idea the estrogen quotient, or EQ, and formally it's the amount of estriol divided by the sum of the amounts of estrone and estradiol. In mathematical terms, it looks something like this: EQ = E3 / (E1 + E2).

If a woman's EQ is low, her risk of breast cancer is higher. Basically, the higher the EQ, the better.

Sounds too easy to be true, but time after time the EQ proved itself. Take a look at some of Dr. Lemon's EQ research:

In 34 women with no signs of breast cancer, Dr. Lemon found the EQ to be a median of 1.3 before menopause and 1.2 afterward. The picture was quite different in 26 women with breast cancer. Their median EQ was 0.5 before menopause and 0.8 afterward.

In another study, Dr. Lemon found that women with higher EQs survived significantly longer after cancer surgery than women with lower EQs.

So, knowing that women need more estriol to boost their EQs, Dr. Lemon also tried using estriol treatments for breast cancer. He asked a small group of women with untreatable breast cancer (because it had metastasized to bones) to take a large dose of estriol. By the end of the study, an astounding 40 percent of these women had their cancers go into remission.

Less estriol, more cancer

Of course Dr. Lemon's EQ and estriol findings met with their share of criticism, and some researchers did publish claims disputing Dr. Lemon's results. But there was also plenty of additional evidence supporting him. For example:

• In one study of 150 close relatives (sisters and daughters) of breast cancer patients, researchers found that the majority had lower levels of estriol and higher levels of estrone and estradiol than women without a family history of the disease.

• American women (who have higher levels of breast cancer) have lower levels of estriol than Asian women (who have lower levels of breast cancer). Asian women living in Hawaii had levels of estriol midway between American women and Asian women living in Asia…and their levels of breast cancer were also midway between American and Asian women.

• Estriol enhances the ability of white blood cells to consume viruses, bacteria, and cancer cells.

- Women who have had children have significantly lower risk of breast cancer than women who have never had a child. During pregnancy, estriol levels climb enormously—by 1,000 times or more. Even after childbirth, estriol levels usually remain higher than they were before pregnancy.

This last bit of "pro-estriol" evidence concerning pregnancies leads me to some recent estriol research, which is once again reviving the "more estriol, less cancer" hypothesis.

A one-time boost can protect you for up to 40 years

In this one, 15,000 women were studied during a pregnancy occurring between 1959 and 1967. Invasive breast cancer cases or deaths from breast cancer were tabulated through 1997. What makes this study so remarkable is the fact that it looked ahead so far into the future of such a large group of women. Prospective studies like this are considered much more reliable than retrospective studies (ones that look back on information after it has occurred). And the results of this particular prospective study make it even more impressive:

The researchers found a clear protective effect based on the amount of estriol the women produced during their pregnancies: More estriol, less cancer later in life. Women in the uppermost 25 percent of estriol production during pregnancy had 58 percent less breast cancer over the next 30 to 40 years than women with the lowest 25 percent of estriol.

The authors concluded (cautiously, of course—they'd be laughed out of their lab coats by mainstream medical "experts" if they didn't downplay findings that nature might know best after all): "If confirmed, these results could lead to breast cancer prevention or treatment regimens that seek to block estradiol estrogen action using estriol, similar to treatments based on the synthetic anti-estrogen, tamoxifen."

After a decade or two of neglect, the EQ and the "estriol hypothesis" of estrogen-related cancer prediction and prevention (and maybe even treatment, like Dr. Lemon's unpublished research) are back. And some researchers are even starting to admit that maybe, just maybe, estriol in its natural form might work as well as (or even better than) synthetic drugs like tamoxifen.

What's your EQ?

Dr. Lemon tested estriol along with estrone and estradiol by having women collect their urine for 24 hours, then measuring the hormone levels in the specimens. It's still done the same way, and, like the 2/16 ration test, you can have a kit mailed to you at home, which makes things much more convenient, since you'll need to collect all your urine for a 24-hour period (only a small portion of the total collected amount is actually mailed in for testing, though).

If you haven't gone through menopause yet, and you have a menstrual cycle that follows the typical 28-day pattern, pick a 24-hour period between days 19 and 23 of your cycle (day 1 being the first day of menstrual bleeding) to collect your sample. If you've already gone through menopause, you can collect your sample anytime.

Again, once you send your sample back to the lab, it generally takes about two to three weeks to get your results.

The virtually fail-safe EQ-booster: You may only need one drop a day

When your results arrive in the mail, you'll see all of your different hormone levels listed. The ones we're most concerned with for determining breast cancer risk via the EQ are estriol, estrone, and estradiol. Remember, it's not the absolute amount of estriol that appears to be the most important number but the relative amount of estriol compared with the sum of estradiol and estrone. Again, the equation looks like this: EQ= E3 / (E2 + E1).

The lab report might already have your EQ calculated and listed. Some labs today consider EQs of 0.4 to 0.6 as normal. But when Dr. Lemon did his research back in the 1960s and 1970s, he found that women need an EQ of at least 1.0 (this level or above was considered favorable; the further below 1.0, the more unfavorable). So was Dr. Lemon wrong?

Well, let's put it this way: If women only need an EQ of 0.4, why has breast cancer risk gone up? Not only do I think you still need an EQ of at least 1.0, as Dr. Lemon found 40 years ago, but in today's environment, with the amount of estrogen-mimicking carcinogens increasing dramatically, it's more important than ever to keep your level of estriol as high as possible. So I don't see any reason why we shouldn't still follow Dr. Lemon and shoot for an EQ of 1.0 or above.

If your EQ is below 1.0, there's a simple, almost fail-safe solution: SSKI. SSKI is a solution that combines iodine and potassium. It's the iodine that works to boost the EQ: Iodide (and iodine) reliably promote the metabolism of estrone and estradiol into estriol. Although (so far) there haven't been any official studies on this, I've observed these effects in hundreds of my patients' lab tests.

Take six to eight drops of SSKI mixed in several ounces of water daily for two to three months. Then repeat your test, doing the 24-hour urine collection at the same time of the month as your first one. More likely than not, your follow-up EQ will be above 1.0—sometimes considerably above. If it is, try tapering down the SSKI to the smallest amount that helps you maintain your EQ at 1.0 or above. Some women find that they only need one drop a day, though others need more.

Although SSKI is safe for the overwhelming majority of people, there are individuals who are very sensitive to it. On rare occasion, long-term use of larger quantities of SSKI may cause thyroid suppression. Thyroid blood tests always pick up on this if it occurs.

Start today to make sure you're cancer-free tomorrow

There's no reason to just wait and hope that you're not that one woman in eight who gets breast cancer. The 2/16 ratio and the EQ provide two easy ways to estimate your own risk of breast, uterine, and other estrogen-related cancers.

For more information on these tests, contact a physician-member of The American College for Advancement in Medicine (ACAM) at (800)532-3688 or www.acam.org, the International College for Integrative Medicine at (866)464-5226 or www.icimed.com, or Meridian Valley Laboratory at (425)271-8689 or www.meridianvalleylab.com. Meridian Valley is actually located in Washington state where, by law, individuals can order their own lab tests.

If your risk factor calculations are unfavorable, or even if they're just OK, there are things you can do yourself—starting today—to lessen your breast cancer risk. Cancer is a frightening thing, but don't let that fear paralyze you: Do something about it—and pass the information along to your daughters and granddaughters, too!

Chapter 6:

Little-known cures for those all-too-common PMS problems

Despite the fact that premenstrual syndrome is one of the most common problems experienced by women of childbearing age, we still have little idea of what causes it or how we can "fix" it. In fact, there are some "experts" (usually male) who argue that it doesn't really exist—obviously very brave people.

In the past, sufferers usually focused on symptom control and over-the-counter treatments to get through the roughest times: Diuretics to help with bloating, aspirin for muscle aches, exercise for mood, etc.

But recently a new strain of super-PMS has been "uncovered." It's called PMDD (premenstrual dysphoric disorder), and the symptoms are so strong that the traditional band-aids don't help. PMDD is basically the same as regular PMS, but the symptoms— breast tenderness, headaches, joint and muscle aches, bloating and weight gain, difficulty concentrating, and mood swings—are so intense that they markedly interfere with normal functioning in day-to-day life.

Surprise! Hand in hand with this "new" disease is a "new" treatment that popped up in TV advertisements. It's called Sarafem,™ and its active ingredient is fluoxetine hydrochloride. This product is prescription only, and the capsules are more attractive (pink and lavender)—but guess what...its original market name is the well-known SSRI (selective serotonin reuptake inhibitor)—Prozac!

But you don't have to rely on the prescription antidepressants that can have negative side effects or the only mildly effective over-the-counter PMS concoctions. There are a few natural therapies that can help. Here's what we know.

Menstrual cramps: Not a Motrin, Advil, or Midol deficiency

Over the last 30 years, I've been treating and relieving muscle spasms (and the accompanying pain) with intravenous magnesium (accompanied by vitamin B6, which appears to help improve magnesium's action) in many conditions—one being menstrual cramps. I've learned that a magnesium and vitamin B6 IV can lessen or even eliminate severe menstrual cramping as it's happening. (Taking these supplements orally won't relieve cramps immediately, but may help lessen them over several months' time.)

A series of these IVs frequently lessens the severity of the cramping until you may be able to manage your symptoms with oral supplements alone. Specific supplementation (of various nutrients, including omega-3 fatty acids and various botanicals) is usually necessary to completely eliminate menstrual cramps.

Say goodbye to mood swings, tension, and irritability with an old favorite—ultra-safe L-tryptophan

According to the TV commercials, Sarafem is meant to help women who suffer from the form of severe PMS, called premenstrual dysphoric disorder (PMDD). But with side effects ranging from weakness and nausea to hallucinations and has even been reported to cause violence, Sarafem is one of the last medicines I'd ever want to give a young woman. Luckily, there's a much safer treatment option available for women who suffer from this severe type of PMS: L-tryptophan.

L-tryptophan really is safe, although this essential amino acid was banned in the early 1990s. The FDA forbid over-the-counter sales of L-tryptophan but at the same time required it to be included in amino acid formulas for intravenous use and in infant formulas! The ban obviously wasn't logical 10 years ago, and it's still not.

As a quick recap, I should point out that the "problem" with L-tryptophan (which was indeed serious—38 people died) that prompted the FDA to make it unavailable was actually due to contamination. The contaminant was produced due to a mistake in genetic engineering. I won't deny that contaminated L-tryptophan was a problem; by contrast, uncontaminated L-tryptophan itself is not only safe in commonly used quantities, but it's also essential to life. So please don't worry about L-tryptophan's safety.

In one important study, 71 women with PMDD took either L-tryptophan or a placebo from the time of ovulation to the third day of menstruation for three consecutive months. Compared with a placebo, L-tryptophan resulted in significant improvement in mood swings, tension, and irritability. The researchers suggested that increasing the brain's production of serotonin (one of the effects of L-tryptophan) is responsible for this beneficial effect.

This research used 2 grams of L-tryptophan three times daily after meals. In my experience, that much L-tryptophan is hardly ever required to relieve PMDD if it's taken properly and is accompanied by additional nutrients that help relieve other aspects of PMS, including water retention, bloating, and headaches.

Keep in mind that since L-tryptophan competes with other amino acids for absorption, it's absorbed best if taken before or after meals (by at least an hour or more). But unlike most other amino acids, L-tryptophan penetrates into the brain (where it's the precursor for serotonin production); it therefore works best when it's accompanied by a small amount of carbohydrates, such as 2 or 3 ounces of orange juice.

For a combination that eliminates a large majority of PMS symptoms for most woman, take 1,500 milligrams of L-tryptophan (twice daily between meals with a small amount of juice), along with 50 to 100 milligrams of vitamin B6, 100 to 150 milligrams of magnesium, and for some, 2 grams of gamma-linoleic acid (GLA) daily.

Even though it's a nutrient essential to life, not a patent medication, L-tryptophan is still not available in natural food stores as it was for over 20 years prior to the genetically engineered contamination episode. However, L-tryptophan is available by prescription through compounding pharmacies. For a prescription, check with a physician skilled and knowledgeable in nutritional medicine. If you need a referral to such a physician in your area, contact the American College for Advancement in Medicine, (800)532-3688 or www.acam.org; the American Academy of Environmental Medicine, (316)684-5500, www.aaem.com; or the American Association of Naturopathic Physicians, (866)538-2267, www.naturopathic.org.

The vitamin cure for heavy menstrual bleeding most doctors don't even know about

If you're a woman who has abnormally heavy menstrual bleeding, you're probably all too familiar with the inconvenience caused by your period each month. The clotting and cramping that often accompany this heavy bleeding may be painful; there's a risk for anemia from the high blood loss; and, you may just feel weak, tired, or sick for days at a time every month.

Unfortunately, there aren't many effective or appealing treatments for this problem. And, in some cases, the mainstream recommendations just don't work. One option is to go on the birth control pill, which means pumping your body full of synthetic hormones. Another is to undergo dilation and curettage, often referred to as a "D&C." This procedure involves scraping the uterine lining: Not at all pleasant, and it doesn't even work in the majority of cases. A third option—if you can call it that—is to undergo a hysterectomy.

Obviously, most women would prefer to try a natural line of treatment before resorting to any of those mentioned above. But unfortunately, most doctors just don't know that there is one.

I've been using vitamin A with tremendous success to treat heavy menstrual bleeding since 1977. I recommend 50,000 units of vitamin A (not beta-carotene) daily, and have found that the majority of women return to a normal bleeding pattern in just one or two months.

Although the original research found that 50,000 units of vitamin A daily was effective when given for 15 days, I recommend at least 30 days at this amount. Then, you can reduce the amount to 15,000 to 25,000 units daily to prevent recurrence.

Of course, you should first be checked by a gynecologist or family doctor for fibroids and/or other structural or functional abnormality before trying any line of treatment.

Chapter 7:

Remarkable solutions to some of the most painful female problems

Many women develop fibrocystic breast disease, which is character-ized by painful cysts in the breasts. In the 1970s, I learned from Dr. John Myers (one of the pioneering researchers in the use of trace ele-ments) that iodine can minimize and possibly eliminate even the most severe cases of fibrocystic breast disease. In minor to moderate cases, 6 to 8 drops of SSKI taken daily in a few ounces of water will frequently reduce fibrocystic breast disease to insignificance within three to six months.

Painful breast lumps relieved in
10 minutes with two minerals

I've seen remarkable results even in patients with very severe fibrocys-tic breast disease—sometimes there's improvement in as little as an hour or two. In these very severe cases, I use a form of iodine called Lugol's solution, which is applied to the vaginal area and cervix. Then, the iodine application should be followed almost immediately by an injection of magnesium sulfate. In one particularly amazing case, a patient of mine named Jenny had her swelling and tenderness go down noticeably just 10 minutes after she received this treatment.

Of course, you'll need a doctor's help with both of these steps (for a referral, contact the American College for Advancement in Medicine at 800-532-3688 or www.acam.org).

If you have fibrocystic breast disease, the other thing you need to do is cut caffeine out of your diet entirely. It isn't enough just to cut back on coffee; you really need to completely avoid coffee, sodas, tea, chocolate, and even painkillers that contain caffeine. I also generally recommend taking vitamin E, extra vitamin B6, primrose or black-currant oil, and selenium. It's also a good idea to include a high-potency vitamin-mineral combination in this program too.

Testing for fibrocystic breast disease and treatment using SSKI requires the help of a physician skilled and knowledgeable in nutritional and natural medicine, who can also help with monitoring thyroid function. (Although problems occur rarely, SSKI can cause thyroid suppression when used over a long period of time.)

Shrink uterine fibroids and ovarian cysts without surgery or years of waiting

Over the past 30 years, I've also used SSKI to treat at least 30 women—one of them my own daughter—for ovarian cysts. These cysts usually disappear within two to three months using the same quantity of SSKI mentioned above for breast cysts (6 to 8 drops stirred into a glass of water).

Conventional medicine only offers two treatment options for patients suffering from uterine fibroids: "Wait until menopause and they'll go away," or have them removed surgically. Neither option offers much appeal or comfort. But there has been significant success with a treatment that consists of a traditional Chinese herbal formula known in Japanese as Keishi-bukuryo-gan (KBG) and in Mandarin as Kuei-chih-fui-ling-wan. The formula improved 47 out of 110 cases, and normalized 21 in a study conducted on premenopausal women ranging from 27 to 52 years of age. The women were treated with the equivalent of 22.5 grams per day for 12 weeks or more. These women had symptomatic uterine myomas all less than 10 cm in diameter. The authors concluded that in young women who wished to remain fertile, and in women just before menopause, KBG treatment may be a good first choice.

Any compounding herbalist can put this formula together for you, especially herbalists familiar with traditional Chinese medicine. It's also available through the Tahoma Clinic Dispensary (425-264-0059; www.tahomadispensary.com) as "Gui formula."

Part VIII

Men's Health

Chapter 1:

Drop the finasteride! The benefits—and risks—of natural prostate treatments

Prostate enlargement (benign prostatic hypertrophy or BPH) sometimes seems an inevitable hazard of male aging.

A small minority of men notice symptoms of hesitancy (taking longer than usual to urinate), one or more trips to the bathroom at night, and diminished force of the urine stream as early as in their 40s. Many more develop these symptoms in their 50s, and the numbers only increase with age. It's unusual to encounter a man in his 70s or 80s who's had no symptoms of prostate enlargement at all.

Zinc, essential fatty acids (including alpha linolenic acid), and saw palmetto are all helpful in reducing or eliminating symptoms of BPH. There's just no need at all to take a patent medication such as finasteride or its patent medication competitors!

But even natural substances can be overdone—and possibly increase your risk of prostate cancer—so it's important to understand the benefits and risks.

From ALA to zinc:
Natural treatments that work

In 1941, the Lee Foundation for Nutritional Research published a small study of 19 men who had all the symptoms of BPH. Each participant in the study had a prostate examination confirming an enlarged but not cancerous prostate gland. Each man then took six capsules of an essential fatty acid complex (10 milligrams linoleic acid, 10 milligrams alpha-linolenic acid or ALA, and 10 milligrams arachadonic acid per capsule) daily.

After three days at six capsules daily, the quantity was reduced to four capsules daily for several weeks, then maintenance quantities of two capsules daily. All 19 men had reduction in prostate size as determined by physical examination, and the majority had all other symptoms of BPH reduced or eliminated as well.[1]

In 1974, Dr. Bush, head of the division of urology at Cook County Hospital in Chicago, presented another study of BPH treatment in a "poster session" at the annual meeting of the American Medical Association. Curiously enough, he also worked with 19 men with BPH, this time confirmed not only with a physical examination, but also with X-rays and other means that were "high-tech" in 1974.

These 19 men took 50 milligrams of zinc (from zinc sulfate) three times daily for two months, then 50 to 100 milligrams daily for another two to three months. Fourteen of 19 had shrinkage of the prostate gland as shown by the same examination techniques.[2]

In his presentation, Dr. Bush also observed that 105 of 150 men with "chronic prostatitis" not caused by bacterial infection were cured with this same zinc treatment. In 1976, another group also reported that zinc treatment reduced the size of enlarged prostate glands.[3]

Since 1974, whenever I work with a man with BPH, I advise him to take one tablespoonful of flaxseed oil daily (along with 400 IU vitamin E), and 50 milligrams zinc (from sulfate) twice daily (later modified to

30 milligrams zinc from picolinate two to three times daily). After three to four months, symptoms are almost always improved and the prostate is usually smaller.

I then recommend reducing the zinc (from zinc picolinate) to 60 milligrams every other day or 30 milligrams of zinc (from picolinate) daily, along with one to two teaspoons of flaxseed oil daily (and vitamin E). Men who eat enough unroasted sunflower seeds or pumpkin seeds (for essential fatty acids and zinc) and oysters (mostly for the zinc) can sometimes cut the supplements back further or even eliminate them for weeks to months at a time.

Saw palmetto is not my first choice

As natural medicine became ever more popular in the last quarter of the 20th century, more and more herbal products were introduced—among them a "breakthrough" herbal treatment for BPH: Saw palmetto. Saw palmetto quickly became available in nearly all natural food stores, and almost immediately became a bestseller, as it is quite effective for reducing—sometimes dramatically—the symptoms of BPH.

But even though saw palmetto was usually effective for the symptoms of BPH, I continued to recommend using zinc and essential fatty acids first for at least three to four months, followed by saw palmetto only if zinc and essential fatty acids together weren't effective in that time.

My reasoning, admittedly theoretical (no money for controlled studies was or is available), is that zinc and essential fatty acids are essential to life and health, and saw palmetto isn't. Most Americans live entire lifetimes without even one microgram of saw palmetto, but no one can live long without zinc or essential fatty acids! So even though saw palmetto isn't thought to be harmful (more about this below), it's best to use zinc and essential fatty acids for BPH first.

If a man's prostate function improves with more zinc, then his retina and "hearing apparatus" (both of which normally contain more zinc than the prostate) will very likely benefit from some of that supplemental zinc, too—even if those areas aren't yet symptomatic. Similarly, if a man's prostate function is improved with additional essential fatty acids, then likely his cardiovascular health will be improved as well—as *Nutrition & Healing* readers know, in just the last few years many research studies have shown that essential fatty acids significantly reduce risk of atherosclerotic vascular disease.

Again, if after three to four months zinc and essential fatty acids aren't effective, saw palmetto can always be tried next.

Everything in moderation

But in the last few years, evidence has been accumulating that —like many other individual nutrients—both zinc and essential fatty acids can be "overdone" and that excessive quantities may increase a man's risk of prostate cancer. The same risk hasn't been reported for excess quantities of saw palmetto yet. However, my observations of the effects of saw palmetto in laboratory tests of steroid metabolism appear to also make increased cancer risk a possible effect of excessive saw palmetto use.

That's because zinc, essential fatty acids, and saw palmetto all share a common "mechanism of action" with finasteride, a patented "space alien" molecule frequently prescribed for symptoms of BPH. This mechanism of action is inhibition of a testosterone-metabolizing enzyme called "5-alpha-reductase." As might be expected, the patent medication is a much more potent inhibitor of this enzyme than the natural substances.

The 5-alpha reductase enzyme metabolizes testosterone into di-hydrotestosterone (DHT), which is a much more potent testosterone, but also has been termed a "bad testosterone" since it causes more cellular disorganization. Cellular disorganization increases the risk of cancer.

For many men, finasteride reduces the symptoms of BPH. The well-known (to many physicians, at least) Prostate Cancer Prevention Trial[4] demonstrated that finasteride also lowers prostate cancer risk—but at the price of spurring more aggressive cancer when it does occur. In this trial, 18,882 men with normal prostate exams and PSA below 3.0 (normal) took either finasteride or placebo for seven years.

At the end of that time, 18.4 percent of the men in the finasteride group and 24.4 percent in the placebo group had developed prostate cancer; the reduction of cancer occurrence (24.8 percent) was statistically significant. But 37 percent of the cancers occurring in the finasteride group were more aggressive types (translation: more likely to kill you) versus 22.3 percent more aggressive cancers in the placebo group.

This shows us that inhibiting 5-alpha reductase may not be entirely a good idea. Since alpha linolenic acid, zinc, and saw palmetto all inhibit 5-alpha reductase, could they also have this downside? This appears to be the case if the quantities used are too high.

Evidence for increased cancer risk

Evidence has been accumulating for over a decade that higher levels of a major essential fatty acid found in flaxseed oil, alpha linolenic acid— much smaller quantities of ALA are found in canola and soy oils—may be associated with higher prostate cancer risk.

A large case-control study from Uruguay found that men in the highest quartile of ALA intake had almost four times the risk of prostate cancer compared with those in the bottom quartile of intake.[5] In a recent dietary case-control study,[6] 217 Spanish men with prostate cancer were matched with 217 hospitalized men (with non-cancer diagnoses) and 217 healthy "controls."

The prostate cancer patients were three times more likely to be in the upper quartile of ALA intake. (Other findings from this study: Animal fat intake was positively correlated with increased prostate cancer risk, while vitamin C intake was correlated with decreased prostate cancer risk).

Although the preponderance of the evidence (so far) indicates caution about higher quantities of ALA-containing oils being associated with higher prostate cancer risk, a smaller amount of evidence is contradictory. One review article noted that five research studies were positive (including the two noted above), but one was negative. It also pointed out that one study using actual prostate cancer cells showed that ALA promoted their growth,[7] while another showed growth suppression.[8]

Zinc also reduces 5-alpha reductase activity, and excess zinc may also be associated with increased cancer risk. A research group at the National Institutes of Health9 reported data from a study of 46,974 U.S. men participating in the Health Professionals Follow-Up Study. They wrote: "Supplemental zinc intake at doses of up to 100 mg/day was not associated with prostate cancer risk." By contrast, men who took more than 100 mg/day of supplemental zinc had an increased risk of prostate cancer.

So far, there aren't any research reports that implicate excessively high doses of saw palmetto as possibly increasing risk of prostate cancer. But in doing very careful laboratory follow-up of men taking both bio-identical hormones and saw palmetto, I and other Tahoma Clinic physicians have observed too many instances of definite over-inhibition of the 5-alpha reductase enzyme by saw palmetto supplementation. In these cases, the men involved have reduced their saw palmetto intake and the laboratory signs of 5-alpha reductase over-inhibition have gone away.

So what do I do?

If you're a man starting to have symptoms of BPH or already taking zinc, and/or alpha linolenic acid-containing flaxseed oil, and/or saw palmetto to control BPH, the information above does not mean you should stop taking these substances.

Correct quantities are good for you, but correct quantities can vary from person to person. For example: I've seen just one man whose metabolism was so sensitive to saw palmetto (as shown on his lab test by severe 5-alpha reductase inhibition) that he had to quit it entirely before the test result normalized. But zinc supplementation didn't have the same effect on his lab test, and helped his BPH symptoms, so he used that instead.

Very few men are that sensitive to the effects of saw palmetto, but laboratory testing has led me to recommend reduction, although not elimination, of saw palmetto supplementation for a significant minority of the men I work with.

But over-inhibition of 5-alpha reductase doesn't have symptoms, and waiting to see whether you've possibly increased your risk of a more aggressive type of prostate cancer isn't a good idea, either. Check with a physician who knows how to monitor testosterone metabolism with appropriate laboratory testing! Whether 5-alpha reductase is over-inhibited isn't the only question that needs to be answered; you also need to know whether the enzyme "aromatase" is turning too much of your testosterone (or DHEA) into excessive (for a man) estrogen, which may be equally if not more hazardous to your prostate.

Find a physician who uses the "24-hour urinary steroid analysis" to monitor steroid hormone metabolism. At present, neither saliva testing nor blood testing has the "breadth" (total number of steroid metabolites) to follow these and other aspects of testosterone metabolism. The test follows estrogen metabolism much more completely, too, and allows your physician to keep both testosterone and estrogens as safe for you as is presently possible.

Chapter 2:

The male side of the Great Hormone Debate: Is testosterone dangerous?

Eventually, nearly every man reaches a point where his testosterone no longer drives his sex life as well as he might like. And testosterone also shares a large part of the responsibility for a variety of other symptoms and diseases thought to be part of normal aging, including heart disease, prostate disease, muscle and bone weakness, depression, high cholesterol, abdominal weight gain, and loss of mental acuity. But you don't have to just sit back and let these things happen. You can significantly reduce your risks of these and many other "normal" symptoms of aging by replacing the testosterone your body is missing.

Unfortunately, most mainstream doctors actually warn against testosterone replacement therapy, since this hormone has been blamed for all sorts of health problems, including prostate cancer.

But there's one question that always pops into my head when I hear warnings against testosterone: "If testosterone is bad for the prostate, why don't young men have more prostate disease?"

Older men get enlarged prostate glands (BPH); younger men don't. Older men get prostate cancer; younger men don't. Yet younger men have the highest testosterone levels. So why do the conventional medical community, patent medicine companies, and government "authorities" continue to warn us of the hazards of testosterone?

Don't let the artificial scare you away from the real deal

The warnings are due, in part, to a 1940s and 1950s disaster with a synthetic, patented form of testosterone called "methyltestosterone." This molecule was invented for the singular purpose of being patented and making a profit. And even though it had never been found on earth before it was invented, it was sold to literally hundreds of thousands of unsuspecting men as "testosterone." After an initial wave of favorable publicity, researchers observed that methyltestosterone caused (among other things) cancer and heart disease. Sales dropped to virtually nil for years, and research on real testosterone was neglected for more than 20 years afterward, since "everyone knew" that "testosterone" was dangerous.

Sounds familiar, doesn't it? Just change the names to "estrogen" and "horse estrogen (equilin)," "progesterone" and "medroxyprogesterones"... and the scientific community is repeating the same error all over again, only this time for women. But back to testosterone...

The fact is, testosterone—real, natural testosterone—is very safe, and can help you tackle all sorts of health problems associated with aging.

Natural testosterone replacement steps back into the spotlight after 60 years

In 1935, Leopold Ruzicka discovered that although the testes produce testosterone, they really contain very little of it. And, instead of extracting minuscule amounts from testicular tissue, he discovered that it is possible to produce testosterone from a much more abundant substance—cholesterol. In fact, that's basically how the body does it. The testosterone Ruzicka produced from cholesterol in his experiment had an identical molecular structure to the body's natural testosterone. Even though it was synthesized in a laboratory, the natural testosterone molecules couldn't be distinguished from human hormones, and the body treated them as such.

So natural testosterone replacement has been around and available for over 60 years, but pharmaceutical companies thought they could "improve" on nature (or at least find a way to profit from it) and wound up making such a mess of it that most men are still too afraid to use either type.

The good news is that research on real testosterone has finally revived. A recent report drives home the point: Testosterone is good for the prostate!

90 percent of men find relief in just six months

Researchers studied 207 men, ages 40 to 83. The first group of 92 men had low testosterone levels. They were treated with 80 milligrams of testosterone daily. The second group of 115 men had very low testosterone levels. This group was treated with 120 milligrams of testosterone daily.

Measurements were done at one, three, and six months. These included prostate volume (size), PSA (prostate specific antigen), lower urinary tract symptoms, and several hormones, including testosterone itself, di-hydrotestosterone ("DHT," a supposedly "bad" metabolite of testosterone), estradiol, and FSH and LH (LH stimulates testosterone in men; FSH stimulates estrogens in women).

Before treatment, LH was elevated in all the men. LH should go back down in men given testosterone, and it did in all men in the first group, and all but 20 men in the second group. (The decline in LH indicates successful testosterone treatment.)

All the men whose LH declined with testosterone treatment had marked decreases in the size of their prostate glands. They also had marked decreases in PSA levels and lower urinary tract symptoms, and striking suppression of not only LH but also DHT, estradiol, and FSH.

Although this is (so far) just one study, it's certainly convincing: Every one of 187 men whose tests indicated effective testosterone treatment had improvement in all parameters measured, including a decrease in prostate size! Given "younger" levels of testosterone, it appears the prostate gland gets "younger" too.

The more testosterone, the sharper your brain

Researchers also continue to demonstrate that testosterone is beneficial for male mental function. Here are a few excerpts from some of the recent studies supporting this conclusion:

- "short-term testosterone administration enhances cognitive function in healthy older men"

- "decreased serum testosterone levels...adversely affect verbal memory in normal young men. These results suggest that short-term changes in sex steroid levels have effects on cognitive function in healthy young men"

- "beneficial changes in cognition can occur in...men using testosterone replacement and di-hydrotestosterone [DHT] treatment..."

- "Positive associations between testosterone levels and cognition are consistent with an effect of androgen treatment..."

There's much more research showing that adequate bio-identical testosterone is important for male cognitive function. Hopefully the "experts" will get around to reading it someday. But in the meantime, let's move on and go over testosterone's benefits for your heart.

70 years of heart-health benefits

Not one piece of research since the 1930s has shown bio-identical testosterone to worsen any parameter of cardiovascular function—quite the opposite, actually.

All the way back in the 1940s, testosterone was found to be an effective treatment in 91 of 100 cases of angina. Then in the 1970s, research showed it to be effective in improving abnormal electrocardiograms. And in the 1990s, a Chinese study showed improvement in both angina and electrocardiograms in older men using testosterone.

Research continues to confirm that testosterone is good for men's hearts. Two examples taken from very recent studies:

- "Men with proven coronary heart disease had significantly lower levels of total testosterone, free testosterone, free androgen index and estradiol…For the first time in clinical settings it has been demonstrated that low levels of free-testosterone was characteristic for patients with low ejection fraction." Ejection fraction measures the amount of blood pumped from one of the heart's chambers, so low testosterone is associated with less blood being pumped.)

- "Testosterone reduced QT dispersion in [men with] heart failure." Higher QT dispersion, a measurement taken form an electrocardiogram, indicates higher risk of death from cardiac arrhythmia. That means in the above study, testosterone reduced the risk of death from cardiac arrhythmia.

A bone-building boost when you need it most

By the time most men hit 70, they "catch up" with women and have just as much osteoporosis and as many bone fractures as women do. This and many other topics are discussed in detail in the book about testosterone I co-authored with Lane Lenard, Ph.D., Maximize Your Vitality and Potency for Men Over 40. So I'll just quote one bit of more recent research here: "After controlling for age and body mass index, bone mineral density correlated positively with estradiol and testosterone."

Once again, no one has ever reported that normal levels of bio-identical testosterone are in any way bad for men's bones.

The reason you still need those regular check-ups

If your testosterone levels are low, and you decide to take testosterone (that's real, bio-identical testosterone, not a patentable version) make sure to have your PSA level checked before you start, and then check it again in three to four months. If it rises more than a little in that time, you may have uncovered a pre-existing prostate cancer, so check with your doctor or a urologist right away, and stop using testosterone until you've fully investigated the situation.

Remember: Testosterone doesn't cause prostate cancer (if it did, young men would have the highest rates), but it does increase the growth rate of a cancer that's already there.

But don't settle for "plain" PSA measurement; there are more advanced and more accurate measurements. At present I prefer the "cPSA" (complexed PSA) test; your doctor may prefer another.

Even bio-identical hormones can be dangerous in excess. So no matter how great you might feel, don't take more than your tests show you need!

Natural testosterone: Easier to use than ever

The current trend in testosterone replacement therapy is the application of natural testosterone to the skin (transdermal administration). The first of these methods is the scrotal patch (sold under the name Testoderm®) made from a vegetable source. Scrotal patches tend to be rather inconvenient, though, so there have been some other innovations in testosterone replacement.

The "almost anywhere" patch works in much the same fashion as the scrotal patch but can be applied anywhere except the scrotum or bony areas. This type of patch is sold under the names Androderm® and Testoderm TTS®. The use of Androderm resulted in significant improvements in fatigue, mood, and sexual function.

Two more options in natural testosterone replacement are creams and gels, which are usually much cheaper than the patches.

Finally, an oral form of natural testosterone can be formulated by a compounding pharmacist and can essentially function as the most convenient and inexpensive natural testosterone delivery system. (However, I don't usually prescribe the oral form to my patients, having found the other methods to be a bit more effective.)

The quickest, most efficient way to find a knowledgeable, open-minded doctor who will consider prescribing natural testosterone is to locate one who is a member of the American College for Advancement in Medicine (ACAM). Members of this professional organization are skilled and knowledgeable in the prescription and use of natural hormones, as well as various nutritional, herbal, and botanical products. For a list of ACAM doctors near you, contact ACAM by calling (800)532-3688 or via the Internet at www.acam.org.

Once you have a prescription for natural testosterone, you'll need to find a compounding pharmacist. Compounding pharmacies are located all over the country, so you shouldn't have too much trouble finding one. For a list of compounding pharmacies near you, contact the International Academy of Compounding Pharmacists (IACP) by calling (800)927-4227, (281)933-8400, faxing (281)495-0602, or via the Internet at www.iacprx.org.

Chapter 3:

Forget the Proscar propaganda— shrink an enlarged prostate the natural way

Nothing focuses on the differences between the pharmaceutical and natural approaches to health care more sharply than the treatment of an enlarged prostate, or benign prostatic hyperplasia (BPH). Take finasteride (the generic name for Proscar™) for example. Designed by a computer to fit a particular chemical receptor site, finasteride is a chemical laser beam aimed at the metabolic juncture where testosterone turns into DHT—the enzyme 5a-reductase. By inhibiting the action of 5a-reductase, finasteride drastically reduces the amount of DHT formed in the prostate.

This strategy has had its share of clinical success, not to mention commercial success. But it's also helping to propagate the myth that excess DHT is the cause of BPH. If you believe this myth, of course, then Proscar™ is just what the doctor ordered. But the truth is, BPH is a lot more complicated than just "too much DHT binding too many androgen receptors for too long." Effective treatment requires a strategy that approaches the problem from several different angles

The best alternative to Proscar

You've probably heard a lot about saw palmetto over the past few years. It has a well-deserved reputation for reducing and, in many cases, eliminating the symptoms of BPH. In fact, the results of numerous trials on saw palmetto and BPH are so indisputably good that, these days, you can find this supplement in most supermarkets.

Even better, there doesn't appear to be any side effects from using this herbal preparation.

But when it comes to prevention, I'm willing to bet that no man ever got BPH because of a deficiency of saw palmetto or stinging nettle. In my own practice, I've observed that men who try diet and supplemental essential nutrients first almost always experience a big decrease and sometimes even a complete elimination of their BPH symptoms. BPH may actually be a symptom of zinc and/or essential fatty acid (EFA) insufficiency for some men.

Both zinc and essential fatty acids are essential nutrients, saw palmetto isn't. And, it's more than likely that if one body tissue is deficient in an essential nutrient, there are other tissues, glands, and organs that are also deficient (even if they're not apparent). So if the prostate is "hurting" for lack of zinc and essential fatty acids, you need to make sure to get these nutrients first. These supplements will help the rest of your body, too, wherever they're needed. By contrast, taking saw palmetto will help the prostate, but it won't help the possibly hidden need for essential nutrients elsewhere in the body.

In my clinical experience, zinc and essential fatty acids are the most important parts of a supplement program designed to reverse BPH and its symptoms. And sometimes these two essential nutrients (taken together as supplements) are all that many men with BPH need.

Two of the best and most easily accessible dietary sources of zinc and essential fatty acids are unroasted sunflower seeds and pumpkin seeds. Nearly all other unroasted seeds and nuts are also good sources of these two nutrients.

While food sources of zinc and essential fatty acids may be enough to prevent BPH in the first place, they're usually not sufficient to reverse it. Once BPH and its symptoms have occurred, I usually recommend 30 milligrams of zinc (picolinate or citrate) three times daily to start, tapering down slowly as symptoms recede, along with 2 milligrams of copper. I also recommend taking 1 tablespoon of organically grown, carefully processed "high-lignan" flax oil twice daily along with 400 IU of vitamin E.

Granted, there aren't any clinical studies on this approach. So a few years ago, I did one of my own. I kept track of 19 of my BPH patients (I picked 19 just to stay in the same range as other studies on "mainstream" approaches) who were supplementing with zinc and flax oil only. I observed that 18 of the 19 men in this group had significant reductions in both symptoms and gland size.

One note of caution: There has been some recent research linking alpha-linolenic acid (ALA), an essential fatty acid found in flaxseed and flaxseed oil, with increased risk of prostate cancer. According to these studies, too much ALA can suppress 5-alpha-reductase, so if you decide to try this approach for managing your BPH symptoms, you might want to have your 5-alpha reductase enzyme activity measured. This is easily done from a 24-hour urinary steroid test.

A few more botanical tricks up Nature's BPH-relieving sleeve

Of course, saw palmetto shouldn't be ignored completely. It can make a difference if zinc and essential fatty acids don't completely eliminate your symptoms.

Since it's a complex, naturally occurring substance, you might expect saw palmetto to have a few more therapeutic tricks up its sleeve than a one-trick pony like finasteride, and you'd be right. Exactly how saw palmetto works is not certain. What is certain is that unlike finasteride, it appears to have a variety of different actions, any or all of which may be beneficial for prostate health.

The vast majority of trials of saw palmetto extract in men with BPH have shown it to be an effective and exceptionally safe therapeutic option.

Saw palmetto extract is widely available in health food stores and by mail order from nutritional supplement companies. Keep in mind, though, that not all saw palmetto extracts are alike. It's important to make certain that the product label indicates that the saw palmetto extract is 85 to 95 percent fatty acids and sterol. Anything less may not have the potency to do any good. The dose most often found to be safe and effective is 160 milligrams twice daily. No serious side effects of saw palmetto extract, taken in reasonable doses, have ever been reported.

Another helpful botanical in fighting an enlarged prostate is stinging nettle (urtica dioica). Like saw palmetto extract, stinging nettle extract is a complex natural substance, and it probably helps in several effective ways to combat BPH. Studies have shown that the extract binds the protein called sex-hormone-binding globulin (SHBG). SHBG permanently binds testosterone (and other "sex hormones"), and its levels increase with age as testosterone levels decline. To the degree that they bind to SHBG, the components of stinging nettle extract "crowd out" testosterone, which may raise the levels of free testosterone circulating in the body. Elevated free testosterone may have a variety of beneficial effects all over the body. Specifically in terms of the prostate, though, this added free testosterone may help restore the normal estradiol/testosterone ratio, removing an important stimulus to prostate growth.

Stinging nettle extract is also widely available from health food stores and nutritional supplement suppliers. The dose of stinging nettle extract used most often in clinical studies is about 300 milligrams per day. Stinging nettle makes a great soup and a bowl of soup a day should readily achieve this dosage level. (The active components of nettle appear to be water-soluble). No serious adverse effects have been associated with reasonable doses.

In addition to saw palmetto and stinging nettle, other botanical products that appear to have beneficial effects on the aging prostate are Pygeum africanum bark and a flower pollen extract, Graminaceae, usually called by its brand name, Cernilton™. Since each of these substances may have slightly different mechanisms of action, it is common to combine two or more of them to achieve an additive effect.

The best solution might mean more than one "right" answer

So, why not use all of these treatment options? This may actually be the best solution. It's what I often recommend to my patients. But whatever you do, if you have an enlarged prostate along with its symptoms, don't just reach for the saw palmetto or stinging nettle without picking up the zinc and essential fatty acids too. And make sure to talk to a doctor skilled in natural medicine, who can work with you to develop the best regimen for you.

(Of course, any prostate health supplement program should also include selenium, vitamins E and D, and lycopene from tomato products—and I don't mean ketchup!)

There are several widely available prostate supplements that contain all the useful ingredients mentioned above. Check your local natural food or vitamin store for one that best suits your needs. Though it's perfectly fine to take the supplements individually, one of the combinations could save you time and money—not to mention space in your medicine cabinet!

BPH medications aren't helping? Maybe you're treating the wrong problem

Some men may suffer what they think are typical BPH symptoms (frequency, urinary urgency, nocturia, decreased size and force of stream, incomplete bladder emptying, and dribbling) and get treated (unsuccessfully) for BPH, but the symptoms may not be caused by an enlarged prostate at all.

Instead, they may be caused by a condition known as prostatism, which is related to the muscles in the prostate and the neck of the bladder. These smooth muscle cells are under the control of the sympathetic nervous system, and they tense up and contract just like all other muscles. The feelings that occur mimic the symptoms of BPH.

The key to relieving prostatism is adopting a treatment program that includes something that will relax your muscles. I had one patient who could only empty his bladder completely after a night of ballroom dancing. The motion of the dancing and the social atmosphere relaxed him sufficiently enough to regulate bladder function.

I usually recommend that people take a combination of muscle relaxing herbs.

Kava is a good muscle relaxant and may benefit prostatism. I've recommended it to patients who've had successful results. Other relaxation herbs include zizyphus spinosa, skullcap, and cramp bark, often used as a mixture.

You might need to try a few different approaches and dosage amounts before you find relief. For a list of physicians in your area who can help you determine the best program to fit your needs, contact the American Academy of Environmental Medicine at (316)684-5500 or www.aaem.com.

Chapter 4:

Help for a lagging libido and potency problems—beyond Viagra

If Viagra were harmless and inexpensive, I wouldn't emphasize the use of natural therapies so heavily. But Viagra just poses too many risks to be considered the treatment of choice—especially when there are safe, natural options readily available for you to try.

L-arginine: Just say yes to NO

The first step is to make sure your testosterone levels are where they need to be (see Chapter 2 for more on that). From there, you need to increase your body's levels of nitric oxide (NO). It sounds somewhat ominous (like you're pumping yourself full of rocket fuel), but nitric oxide is actually the natural substance primarily responsible for causing and maintaining erections. It is possible to raise NO levels safely and naturally, enabling normal erections, by raising levels of the amino acid L-arginine, which can be rapidly converted to NO when needed in the body. The best food sources of L-arginine are grains, seeds, beans, nuts, and chocolate. You can also take L-arginine supplements, which are available in most natural food stores. L-arginine is generally considered to be very safe, even at the high doses that may be required for sexual enhancement—3 to 6 grams per day or more. However, if you have cancer or any form of herpes, you should consult your physician before supplementing with L-arginine.

The pre-Viagra treatment of choice still holds its own

For the last 70 or 80 years, the most widely accepted treatment in the United States for sexual problems in both men and women wasn't a "magic" little pill from a patent medicine company. Instead, the mainstream relied on something completely uncharacteristic: An all-natural herb called yohimbine. In fact, until Viagra came along, yohimbine was the only medicine approved by the FDA for treating impotence.

But since yohimbine is completely natural, it couldn't be patented, which means no one could make enormous profits from selling it. So the big patent medicine companies didn't rest until they came up with a "solution" to sexual dysfunction that would boost their stock prices, even if it turned out to cause significant side effects—and so, Viagra was born. But yohimbine is still effective and is available over the counter in a variety of formulations and by prescription in 5 mg tablets.

Yohimbine probably works because it prevents noradrenaline from stimulating a2-adrenergic receptor sites, but it is not clear whether it exerts its effect in the brain or in the penile arteries. The doses of yohimbine most commonly reported to be safe and effective range from 18 mg to 100 mg per day, usually divided into three to four doses.

Although they're nowhere near as dangerous as those associated with Viagra, there are several side effects to watch out for when using yohimbine, particularly when recommended quantities are exceeded (can't imagine one of us guys doing something like that, can you, ladies?). The most common ones include anxiety, dizziness, headaches, and insomnia. Men who have high blood pressure are generally advised not to take yohimbine and use of the herb should be discontinued if you experience any increase in your blood pressure.

Better than testosterone

When testosterone levels decrease, sexual dysfunction isn't the only result. The chemical imbalance can lead to symptoms such as depression, fatigue, and muscle weakness. But researchers specializing in male health and sexual function have reported that a combination of two safe natural metabolites—propionyl-L-carnitine and acetyl-L-carnitine—are even more effective than testosterone in treating the depression, fatigue, and sexual dysfunction that can be associated with male aging.

It's not that testosterone doesn't work—in fact, the researchers reported that testosterone worked significantly better than placebo. It's just that the combination of "carnitines" worked even better.

None of the groups experienced significant side effects. And since they're safe and effective alternatives to testosterone, the carnitines offer the perfect solution for men who have had prostate cancer and can't take testosterone.

A safe alternative for men who have (or have had) prostate cancer

Poor sexual function is especially common in men who have had prostate cancer. For them, taking testosterone usually isn't an option because it could potentially stimulate cancer growth. (In fact, many are even given patent medications that reduce testosterone levels to zero or close to zero.) This is really one of the very few instances where Viagra can be helpful. Of course, Viagra does nothing for other symptoms of low or no testosterone, including fatigue, depression, and muscle weakness.

But researchers have found that taking the carnitine combination mentioned above along with Viagra (when needed) provides significantly more improvement in sexual function for men in this situation than taking Viagra alone.

And as a bonus, the combination of acetyl-L-carnitine and propionyl-L-carnitine can improve your mood, alleviate fatigue, and improve muscle strength and function, making up for many of the problems that go with low or absent testosterone (and which Viagra doesn't help at all).

Better sexual function in a single—natural—formula

Although you can purchase the carnitines separately, propionyl-L-carnitine can be hard to find, so I recommend buying them in combination.

The best formula presently available is called PROPeL, which is a combination of acetyl-L-carnitine, propionyl-L-carnitine, and alpha-lipoic acid. (Alpha-lipoic acid has been found to improve erectile function in lab animals.) PROPeL is available in natural food stores and compounding pharmacies carrying Life Enhancement products, the Tahoma Clinic Dispensary, and Life Enhancement, Inc., www.life-enhancement. com, (800)543-3873.

Three more herbal options for a satisfying sex life

My research files are filled with studies proving the libido-enhancing benefits of herbs. Some of the results I've found most impressive refer to muira puama, ginseng, and Ginkgo biloba. Muira puama's origin is as exotic as its name implies. It is derived from a shrub that grows in the Amazon region of Brazil. Studies suggest that supplements of this herb can increase libido and improve erectile dysfunction. And you don't have to travel halfway around the world to get it. You can find this product in many natural food stores.

Various studies have demonstrated that ginseng has increased serum testosterone levels and that it may improve blood flow to the penis. Gingko biloba is also a major aid in improving blood flow, especially through small arteries like the ones in the penis. Both are available in natural food stores, as well as many grocery stores.

This list might seem a little overwhelming, but I doubt you will need to take all of the items mentioned. Usually one or maybe a combination of two to three will do the job. Whichever combination you decide to try, the dosage amounts I generally recommend to my patients are as follows: 1,000 to 1,500 milligrams of muira puama daily; 100 milligrams of ginseng two to three times daily; and/or 40 milligrams of Gingko biloba three times a day.

In addition to these supplements, don't forget diet and exercise: Supplements can help, but they can't fix everything. We're all creatures of habit. Moving from old unhealthy patterns to new, more health-promoting ones isn't always easy and it won't happen overnight. But it definitely is worth the time and trouble: Making sure your body is healthy overall will lead to a more fulfilling sex life for you and your partner.

Chapter 5:

Detect and reduce your prostate cancer risk with these simple steps

O f course, prostate cancer is the worst case scenario of prostate problems. But there's plenty you can do to prevent it from happening to you. You can determine your own risk of prostate cancer by testing yourself for two major risk factors. And if your test results aren't as favorable as you'd like, you can make a few simple diet changes and take certain supplements to lower your risk.

You need to know your 2/16 ratio too

The first step in reducing your prostate cancer risk is actually one of the same steps women can take for breast cancer: The 2/16 ratio test.

Recently, the journal *Cancer Causes and Control* published a study that directly examined the 2/16 ratio/ prostate cancer relationship. Researchers compared 113 men with prostate cancer to 317 men without prostate cancer. They reported that "...elevated 2-hydroxyestrone urine levels suggested a reduced prostate cancer risk...Conversely, elevated 16 alpha-hydroxyestrone levels were associated with an increased risk of prostate cancer...finally, the [2/16] ratio was associated with a reduced risk of prostate cancer."

This wasn't the first clue that the 2/16 ratio might be relevant for prostate cancer. A few years ago, another study showed some intriguing results. Researchers "followed" the diets of several thousand men for several years and found that men who ate at least three 1/2-cup servings of Brassica vegetables per week had a 41 percent reduction in prostate cancer risk. (Brassica vegetables include cabbage, cauliflower, broccoli, Brussels sprouts, bok choy, and others.) Since these vegetables raise the 2/16 ratio, it seemed reasonable to guess that at least some prostate cancer is related to the 2/16 ratio. Now the new study mentioned above confirms that guess.

The good news is, testing your own 2/16 ratio couldn't be easier. You don't even have to leave home to do it. Some changes in the actual testing equipment have made the process a lot easier. In fact, the testing kits can be mailed to you at home, where you'll collect a urine specimen in the container provided. When you've collected your sample, just mail it back to the lab.

Once you send your sample back to the lab, it generally takes about two to three weeks to get your results.

You definitely want more "good" (2) estrogen than "bad" (16) estrogen—substantially more if possible. So when you get your results, check the proportion of these two substances: Any ratio below 1.0 is unfavorable. Although there's no consensus on an ideal ratio number, I recommend 2.0 or greater if possible.

If your 2/16 ratio is less than 1.0, there's a good chance you'll be able to boost it just by eating a few specific foods. Start with Brassica (or mustard family) vegetables. These include cabbage, broccoli, cauliflower, bok choy, Brussels sprouts and many others. One thing to keep in mind: It is possible for Brassicas to cause suppressed thyroid function and even goiter if you eat a lot of them on a daily basis, so three to four servings a week is a good general range.

The natural cancer-fighting substances in these vegetables—isothiocyanates and indoles—help regulate and improve the 2/16 hydroxyestrogen ratio. In essence, a normal 2/16 ratio means less cancer risk.

You might find that you only need to incorporate one of these foods into your diet to raise your 2/16 ratio, but sometimes it takes a combination to make a big difference. In a lot of cases, just eating these foods will bring a low 2/16 ratio to 1.0 or above in just four to six weeks without any other specific supplementation. But if you find you're still not getting sufficient improvement, you can also take di-indolylmethane (DIM) supplements to boost it even further. DIM is actually a substance found in Brassica vegetables, but it's also available in most health food stores in supplement form. If you need some extra help, take 60 milligrams three times daily, and check your 2/16 ratio again in another four to six weeks.

Of course, it's also important to note that the 2/16 ratio is only one risk factor for prostate cancer, and while fixing this problem definitely lowers cancer risk, it doesn't eliminate it. And, unfortunately, once cancer has started, lowering the amount of "bad" estrogen is not likely to cure the cancer—but it is very likely to slow the progression.

Is your testosterone turning into estrogen?

By now you might be wondering why a test that predicts estrogen-related cancer risk also works for evaluating prostate cancer risk. Well, even the manliest men produce some estrogen. In fact, your body actually turns testosterone into estrogen. This process is called aromatization.

If everything is functioning properly, only a small fraction of your total testosterone becomes estrogen. Unfortunately, as men get older, there's a tendency for this process to speed up, turning more and more testosterone into estrogen. (This is called excess aromatization.) With excess aromatization, your body makes more estrogen than is good for your prostate—and it leaves too little testosterone behind. This raises your risk of both prostate enlargement and prostate cancer.

Excess aromatization is rare before age 40 to 45 (although it is possible). So if you're in that age bracket, you might want to have your aromatization checked—especially if there's a history of prostate cancer in your family.

The excess aromatization test involves collecting your urine for 24 hours. You only need to mail a small amount of the total sample to the laboratory for testing, and, if you want, the 2/16 test can be done on the same specimen. If you have trouble getting your doctor to order these test kits for you, contact a physician-member of The American College for Advancement in Medicine (800)532-3688; www.acam.org or The International College of Integrated Medicine (866)464-5226; www.icimed. com, or Meridian Valley Lab (425)271-8689; www.meridianvalleylab. com for help. Meridian Valley is located in Washington state, where, by law, you can order own your lab tests without a doctor's order.

Boost your manhood with a flower?

When your test results arrive in the mail, look at your total estrogen and testosterone levels. If your total estrogen exceeds the "normal" range listed for men, or if your testosterone level is way too low (less than your estrogen level), that indicates excess aromatization.

If your lab results show excess aromatization, chrysin, a flavonoid derived from passionflower, can slow it down to normal again. Take 500 milligrams of chrysin three times daily. (I've observed that the brand of chrysin containing a very small amount of diadzein, an isoflavone, appears to be more effective.) Then take another test in four to six weeks.

In the majority of cases, a follow-up test shows more testosterone and less estrogen, which means that the excess aromatization has been slowed. I definitely recommend trying chrysin first. But if it doesn't seem to work for you, the only alternative available right now is a patent medication called Arimidex. Carefully adjusted fractional doses of Arimidex will effectively slow aromatization. If you end up needing to take Arimidex, please work closely with a physician who can help you take the smallest dose necessary to do the job.

Make a different sort of "date"

There you have it: Two simple tests for figuring out your prostate cancer risk—and a few easy solutions to lower it if it's too high. In fact, since so many of these steps are similar to breast and cervical cancer risk testing, you and your wife may want to consider ordering your test kits at the same time. Then, if you need to take steps to lower your risks, you'll be able to help each other through the process.

You should still continue to take as many other protective measures as you can—including taking 200 to 300 micrograms of selenium, 20 to 30 milligrams of lycopene, and 3 milligrams of boron per day: The more you protect yourself, the better!

Part IX

Anti-Aging, Memory, Hearing and Vision

Chapter 1:

Five ways to avoid that hearing aid

I'll be honest with you: There's not much new to say about hearing loss. Mainstream medicine hasn't "discovered" the cause or cure for hearing loss, so they're usually not interested in spending much time on it. If your doctor has bothered to talk to you about it at all, it was probably just to recommend a hearing aid. But that's certainly not your only option. I first covered the natural way to approach hearing loss several years ago. Since I hear from so many of you that you still struggle with this problem, it probably bears repeating.

Most of the research points to a link between age-related hearing loss and low levels of vitamin B12 and folic acid. In one study published in the *American Journal of Clinical Nutrition*, researchers examined hearing in 55 women.[1] They found that the lower the women's levels of vitamin B12 and folic acid, the worse their hearing. Specifically, women with impaired hearing had 38 percent lower serum vitamin B12 levels and 31 percent lower folate levels than women with normal hearing.

It sounds easy enough to correct: Just take vitamin B12 and folic acid supplements. But these results were found in women already taking B12 and folic acid. It doesn't seem to add up: Low levels of these nutrients are associated with hearing loss, so why didn't their supplements help? My guess is that their stomachs had something to do with it.

It all goes back to your stomach

In my experience, age-related problems like macular degeneration and hearing loss usually trace back to poor stomach function—especially a condition called hypochlorhydria, or low stomach acid. As you age, stomach function slows down and produces less and less acid. If your stomach isn't producing enough acid, it won't digest your food—or your supplements—efficiently. So even if you're taking the right supplements for the job, they won't help as much as they could if your stomach were functioning properly.

With that in mind, your first step should be to have your digestion tested. At the Tahoma Clinic, we usually test this is by radio telemetry using the "Heidelberg capsule."

To take this test, you'll swallow a small, plastic capsule that contains electronic monitoring equipment. As it moves through the stomach and intestines, the capsule can measure the pH of the stomach, small intestine, and large intestine. This information can help your doctor determine whether or not your stomach is producing adequate amounts of acid.

If your test results indicate low levels of stomach acid, it's a good idea to supplement with either betaine hydrochloride-pepsin or glutamic-acid hydrochloride-pepsin before meals. To start, I usually recommend taking one capsule (5, 7 1/2, or 10 grains) before each meal. After two or three days, if there are no problems, take two capsules in the early part of the meal, then increase your dose to three capsules per meal several days later. The dose is gradually increased until it equals 40 to 70 grains per meal.

Hydrochloric acid should never be used anti-inflammatory medications. This method should only be used when testing indicates a need for it and should always be carefully monitored by a physician.

Your step-by-step supplement guide for fighting hearing loss

If you do have hypochlorhydria, even correcting the insufficient levels of acid and pepsin may not be enought to help you absorb vitamin B12.

So in this case, it's a better idea to take this nutrient by injection. I usually recommend injections of 1 cc of vitamin B12 (containing 1,000 micrograms) and 1/2 cc of folic acid (containing 2.5 to 5 milligrams).

Sublingual vitamin B drops are worth a try, but the absorption is variable from person to person. In other words, they may or may not help you.

In addition to vitamin B12 and folic acid, zinc has also been linked to hearing—especially tinnitus, a condition characterized by ringing in the ears. In a study published in February 2003, researchers found that patients with tinnitus had significantly lower levels of zinc than controls.[2] In another study, researchers found improvement in 46 percent of tinnitus patients taking 50 milligrams of zinc per day for two months.[3]

And last, but not least, on the list of nutrients to combat hearing loss is vitamin D. I know this vitamin keeps popping up over and over again, but that just goes to show you how important it is. Several studies have suggested that vitamin D deficiency might play a role in hearing loss.[4,5]

So, as I've mentioned several times over the past few months, make sure you're getting enough vitamin D—2,000 to 3,000 IU is a good general range.

I can't promise that following the steps outlined above will cure or reverse your hearing loss. But all of these recommendations are as good for your overall health as they are for your ears, and if they help keep you from ever needing that "doctor-recommended" hearing aid too, all the better.

Chapter 2:

The mineral breakthrough helping terminal patients defy death: And why you should be taking a little of it too

Between the lack of any media coverage at all about the hundreds of encouraging lithium research papers, and the general impression that lithium is a prescription "drug" used "only" for bi-polar disease, even the most dedicated anti-aging enthusiasts I meet are seldom taking advantage of the brain-protective and brain anti-aging effects of low-dose lithium.

If you're one of the many people not using supplemental low dose lithium yet, you may want to take another look at it—especially since some very recent research reports have added even more weight to the already heavy mountain of evidence in favor of lithium's brain-protective benefits. In fact, a groundbreaking study appeared in the *Proceedings of the National Academy of Sciences* journal showing that lithium may help halt the progression of a degenerative disease even more deadly than Alzheimer's.

But before I tell you about the new lithium breakthrough, let's review a bit.

Just for the record: Lithium is a mineral element in the same "family" as sodium and potassium. It's not a drug, and definitely not patentable, which is very likely why you haven't read or heard much in the media about its enormous potential for protecting and improving brain health, despite truly abundant and all-positive research.

Back in 2004, I gave a presentation about lithium to a group of physicians, and included 38 of the most important research papers published over the previous decade about lithium and the brain. Below are titles of some of those studies, along with descriptions of what each article reported.

More brain power—literally

"Lithium-induced increase in human brain grey matter"[1]

"Lithium stimulates progenitor proliferation in cultured brain neurons"[2]

The first study is the one that led me to start using low-dose lithium myself. Using MRI scans, the researchers in the first study found that lithium actually increases the numbers of brain cells in older individuals. The second headline explains at least part of how lithium does this. This

---

Using lithium safely

In over 30 years of practice, I've never had a patient using low-dose lithium report symptoms of excess. But just to be on the safe side, it's important to know the signs of lithium toxicity, which include hypertension, tremor, and nausea. Luckily, it's very simple to keep any of these things from occurring in the first place: Taking extra quantities of essential fatty acids will prevent any possibility of lithium toxicity.

I always recommend that anyone taking lithium also take a teaspoonful or two of flaxseed oil (or other essential fatty acid) along with 400 IU of vitamin E (as mixed tocopherols) each day.

study found that lithium stimulates "progenitors," which promote the growth of new nerve cells.

Three-pronged protection against the most common brain-destroyers

"Neuroprotective effects of chronic lithium on focal cerebral ischemia in rats"[3]

"Lithium at 50: Have the neuroprotective effects of this unique cation been overlooked?"[4]

"Lithium exerts robust neuroprotective effects *in vitro* and in the CNS in vivo: Therapeutic implications"[5]

These studies explain more about how lithium protects the brain. There are lots of research articles showing that lithium protects against both internally produced molecules toxic to nerve cells (such as glutamate) and external toxins (including aluminum). But the first group of researchers above reported that lithium not only protects brain cells against toxins, but also against lack of blood flow.

The second article explained that one way lithium protects neurons is by increasing levels of a major neuroprotective protein called "bcl-2." Bcl-2 also increases regeneration of neural axons, the "branches" that project out from the main bodies of nerve cells and contact other neurons.

And the third study headline shows just how impressive these results are: "Robust" is a term rarely seen in the titles of research articles. Basically, scientific publications use it as a restrained code word for "Wow! That really works!"

The best—and least used—treatment for Alzheimer's

"Lithium inhibits amyloid secretion in COS7 cells transfected with amyloid precursor protein C100"[6]

"Lithium protects cultured neurons against beta-amyloid-induced neurodegeneration"[7]

Amyloid and beta-amyloid are byproducts of nerve cell metabolism that, in excess, contribute to Alzheimer's disease. These two studies showed that lithium inhibits amyloid production and protects nerve cells against damage from excess beta-amyloid. Other researchers have reported that lithium also prevents the formation of "neurofibrillary tangles," another contributor to Alzheimer's disease.

And here's another encouraging study "headline" that came out very recently:

"Lithium: A novel treatment for Alzheimer's disease?"[8]

This research review from the Indiana University School of Medicine cites some of the evidence noted above and considerably more, and came to the following conclusion: "One intriguing clinical application is in the treatment of Alzheimer's disease."

But after reading all the other research evidence that came before this, I think its potential goes well beyond "just" treatment of Alzheimer's disease. After all, "a milligram of prevention may be worth a kilogram of cure." And since low-dose lithium is so safe, it really should be a part of everyone's supplement program—especially if you have a family history of Alzheimer's disease, senile dementia, Parkinson's disease, any other neurodegenerative disease (or if you just want to "keep all your marbles").

I generally recommend 10 to 20 milligrams of lithium (as aspartate or orotate) daily. Of course, like any other substance, lithium can be dangerous in high doses, so please be sure to read the box on above about using lithium safely.

Battling inner demons with an all-natural weapon

"Lithium in drinking water and the incidence of crimes, suicides, and arrests related to drug addiction"[9]

"Lithium and the treatment of alcoholism: A critical review"[10]

They may seem unrelated to the previous studies listed, but both of these articles show lithium's potential to protect against a different type of disease—addiction. One study also shows that even very low levels of lithium have a measurable effect: In the first study, researchers found that levels of lithium less than 200 parts per million in drinking water are associated with significantly fewer arrests for crimes committed as the result of drug addition: Homicide, robbery, rape, suicide, and drug trafficking.

The second study was a review of lithium treatment for alcoholism. These researchers concluded that lithium significantly improves mood and behavior in alcoholics, and is even associated with fewer repeat hospitalizations for alcohol intoxication.

New hope for a "hopeless" disease

Unfortunately, despite all of these proven benefits, the mainstream still basically ignores lithium. But when the following research paper was published in February, the title alone was so shocking and such a potential breakthrough against an otherwise rapidly fatal disease that I thought for sure—finally—there would be some mention in the "mass media world" of newspapers, radio, and television.

There wasn't!

So unless you've been actively searching "on-line" because you have a loved one dying of this disease, you'll probably be reading the following "headline" for the first time:

"Lithium delays progression of amyotrophic lateral sclerosis"[11]

You may know amyotrophic lateral sclerosis by its more common names, ALS and Lou Gehrig's disease. This "nickname" came after the disease struck home-run-hitting major-league baseball player Lou Gehrig back in 1939. After his diagnosis, Gehrig deteriorated very rapidly: Less than two years after his initial symptoms of weakness and stumbling appeared, he suffered a helpless, totally-paralyzed death. The same has happened to nearly all other ALS victims. So anything at all which "delays progression" of this terrible disease should receive major media attention—even if just a brief notice to "get the word out" to ALS sufferers.

Actually, the term "delays progression" used in the study's title is quite conservative. Lithium treatment definitely did much better than that.

Quoting from the summary: "ALS is a devastating neurodegenerative disorder with no effective treatment…we found that daily doses of lithium…delay disease progression in human patients affected by ALS. None of the patients treated with lithium died during the 15 months of the follow-up, and disease progression was markedly attenuated when compared with age-, disease duration-, and sex-matched control patients treated with riluzole for the same amount of time." Riluzole is one of several patent medications used to "treat" ALS, with practically no effect.

The researchers observed two groups—16 patients who took lithium along with "routine" riluzole treatment, and 32 who took just the riluzole. The patients in the riluzole-only group experienced an average symptom worsening of 50 percent in just the first three months, and 30 percent of the "riluzole-only" patients died within the 15-month study period. In stark contrast, none of the patients who took lithium died within the 15 months. In fact, none of them even got significantly worse.

This is a fantastic breakthrough, and hopefully it will revive interest in clinical trials—and clinical usage—of lithium for nearly <u>any</u> disease in which brain cells and nerve cells are degenerating.

<u>But don't try this for a loved one on your own</u>! The lithium dosages the researchers administered to the ALS patients in the study were considerably larger than the brain anti-aging doses I typically recommend. While they can be safely tolerated by most adults, they definitely require close and careful monitoring by a physician skilled and knowledgeable in nutritional and natural therapy.

Chapter 3:

Forget those needles—erase your wrinkles with a powdered drink mix: Plus two other all-natural age-fighters your skin will thank you for

A few weeks ago, our 31-year-old daughter came home for a visit. She hadn't seen her mother for several weeks, and not long after she arrived, she asked what Holly had been doing "this time" to make her skin look so good. As she put it, Holly's skin looked "healthier than ever." She commented that her skin tone was deeper and more vibrant and that some of the little wrinkles around Holly's eyes were actually gone.

Holly's always taken very good care of herself: Never smoked, doesn't drink alcohol, eats as much "organic" and "free range" as possible, uses absolutely no sugar, refined food or food chemicals, and takes her vitamins, minerals, and botanicals. She's also used bio-identical hormones for over 15 years, and most of that time she has also used a skin cream containing a tiny amount of estriol (more on that a little later).

Of course, I have always considered her beautiful, but she really does appear much younger than her actual age: In fact, from time to time she's asked to show her driver's license to prove that she qualifies for the "over-55" discount offered at certain places.

But she had been doing something extra "this time." I admit that I hadn't noticed a great difference, but, in my defense, it's harder to see changes in someone you're around every day (or perhaps men just aren't as "tuned in" to those sorts of details as women are). But regardless of whether or not I'd noticed, our daughter certainly had.

Holly's improvements had come about as a result of her taking (for the second time—I'll tell you about the first time in just a bit) a combination containing collagen, hyaluronic acid, and other natural ingredients.

Why these anti-aging "miracles" aren't always all they're cracked up to be

You've likely already heard of products containing collagen and hyaluronic acid (HA). They've both been touted for their skin "anti-aging" effects for a while. And using them is logical since collagen is the major extracellular protein responsible for the strength and flexibility of connective tissue, including the skin. In fact, 25 to 30 percent of bodily protein is collagen. And HA is one of the biological hallmarks of youth: Baby skin has the most and content declines with age.

But if it were as easy as it sounds in the commercials advertising products containing collagen and HA, everyone would be using them— and would have younger-looking skin with fewer wrinkles as a result. Since that isn't the case, you've probably gathered that there are a few problems with using many of these products.

"Generally accepted" opinion has been that swallowing collagen and hyaluronic acid won't do that much good, as they'd be completely digested (or nearly so) in the intestines. So emphasis has been placed on injecting them directly into the skin, especially facial skin, to replace the collagen and hyaluronic acid our own skin makes less of as we grow older.

Since all the "approved" forms of collagen and HA are injectable, they all require visits to a doctor—and they're quite costly. But even worse than these drawbacks is that the injectable forms of collagen and HA used in most cases are not exactly the same as the human forms. Collagen shots typically include cow collagen instead of human collagen, and HA injections come from rooster and bacterial sources, so the chances of unwanted "side effects" are higher. To be fair, there is at least one injectable that uses bio-identical hyaluronic acid.

But it wasn't injections of bio-identical HA that had elicited such praise from our daughter about Holly's appearance. In fact, she hadn't been using injections of anything. Even though most sources agree that taking collagen and HA orally won't help the skin, at least one study—not to mention Holly's first-hand experience—has shown that it does.

Say goodbye to sagging, puffy, wrinkled eyes

In this blinded and randomized eight-week research trial, 40 women ages 35 to 60 took 7.5 or 8.5 grams daily of a product called Toki®. Toki is a powdered drink mix that combines collagen, hyaluronic acid, and other natural ingredients and is sweetened with stevia. According to the researchers, the formulation "resulted in a highly statistically significant improvement in peri-orbital [around the eyes] wrinkling, in peri-orbital aging, and peri-orbital over-all facial aging. The investigator's mean global improvement scores of overall facial aging as compared to baseline photographs were also highly significant."[1]

The women participating in the study also did self-evaluations. And each of them also reported significant improvement in sagging, puffiness, and wrinkling around the eyes, as well as noticeable improvement in overall facial aging—the same improvements our daughter noticed in Holly after she started taking Toki.

This research also certainly appears to disprove the idea that injecting collagen is the only way to prevent it from being broken down during digestion: Levels of collagen in the participants' blood were 114 percent higher at the end of the 8 weeks than at the outset of the study. So apparently, at least some of the collagen swallowed in the Toki formula "made it through" without being broken down in the gut.

Of course. that doesn't prove outright that the very same collagen caused the women's significant facial improvements, but there's no question that something in Toki _did_.

Holly's Toki regimen started with 6 grams (one packet) three times a day for two weeks. Then she tapered back to two doses daily for another two weeks. Now she's following the "maintenance" dose of one packet daily.

First time's a charm

As I mentioned earlier (and as our daughter's comment implied), this isn't the first time Holly has tried injection-less anti-aging treatments. Three or four years ago at yet another convention, she was given a small sample bottle of a hyaluronic acid product called Synovoderma®. Knowing that babies' skin has considerably more hyaluronic acid than adult skin, and that dermatologists and plastic surgeons were using non-bio-identical injections of hyaluronic acid to improve their patients' appearance, she decided that a natural form might be worth a try. At the very least, she knew it wouldn't hurt to swallow it, especially since the capsules contained nothing else but rice bran and beeswax (apparently fillers). So she read the label, and took three of the capsules twice daily.

Towards the end of the first week, she was washing her face, and asked me to come take a look. "There's all this dead skin coming off," she pointed out. "I've never had that much dead skin come off at one time, ever!" Her face cloth was definitely covered with shreds of old skin; the only time I've seen that much coming off someone at once has been the "peeling" that sometimes occurs awhile after a sunburn, and Holly definitely hadn't had that.

For the next few days, more dead skin than usual came off each time Holly washed her face, although each day it was a little less, until the exfoliation subsided to normal. She continued to use three capsules twice daily for three weeks, as the product packaging instructed, then cut back to three a day for several weeks. About that time, our daughter (the same one who visited recently) came by, and noticed an improvement in her mother's facial skin then too.

While it's true that Synovoderma® may be more expensive than many other supplements, and Toki® is definitely more expensive than other supplements, the difference either one can make to your complexion may be worth it. Unlike most of the facial injections, both these supplements are all natural, and very unlikely to cause significant "side effects." And if cost is an issue to you, facial injections are way, way more expensive than either Synovoderma® or Toki®—and take considerably more time and trouble. If you've been thinking at all of cosmetic facial injections, it's worth your while to try one or both first.

But in addition to these, there is one more natural anti-aging tool for your facial skin that you may want to consider.

Bio-identical HRT: Good for you inside _and_ out

The other skin treatment Holly has been using for years is a topical cream containing bio-identical estriol. Usually, when I mention this hormone it's in reference to its role in bio-identical hormone replacement therapy, which is typically prescribed for women dealing with the various symptoms associated with menopause (hot flashes, vaginal dryness, etc.). But over 10 years ago, I read about the results of a 1987 study in which 14 post-menopausal women were treated for three weeks with a topical skin application containing estriol (and compared with another six women who received the same topical treatment without estriol).

According to the researchers, after three weeks "The elastic fibers in the [skin] were thickened, better oriented and slightly increased in number in half of these patients but in none of the control patients. The epidermal thickness was slightly increased in four of the patients treated with estriol."[2] And this after only three weeks!

I guessed that a longer period of time would have shown a greater success rate, and even better results. So I asked my compounding pharmacist friends at Key Pharmacy (www.keynutritionrx.com, 1-800-878-1322) to put estriol together with other ingredients into a skin crème.

Since the quantity of estriol in the skin crème was small, and not likely to have a systemic effect, Holly started using it. Since then, she's noticed that she's gotten considerably fewer and less noticeable wrinkles than many of her friends (and the benefits she's gotten from products like Synovoderma and Toki are just "icing on the cake," so to speak).

But Holly's experiences aren't the only support for this approach to skin anti-aging. In 1996, another research group examined the effects of tiny concentrations of bio-identical estrogens applied to the skin. In this study, 59 pre-menopausal women with signs of skin aging applied crèmes containing either 0.01 percent estradiol or 0.3 percent estriol. The researchers also measured the women's blood levels of estradiol and two other hormones, FSH (follicle stimulating hormone, which stimulates estrogen secretion from the ovaries) and prolactin (which, among other things, stimulates milk secretion in nursing mothers). And skin biopsies were also taken for measurements of collagen in 10 of the women.

According to the researchers: "After treatment for six months, elasticity and firmness of the skin had markedly improved and the wrinkle depth and pore sizes had decreased by 61 to 100 percent in both groups. Furthermore, skin moisture had increased and the measurement of wrinkles...revealed significant, or even highly significant, decreases of wrinkle depth in the estradiol and the estriol groups ...significant increases of Type III collagen labeling were combined with increased numbers of collagen fibers at the end of the treatment period."[3]

The researchers also noted that only blood levels of prolactin increased significantly, while estradiol and FSH did not. They pointed out that this indicated there were no systemic effects from these hormones, only the skin changes.

And in 2005, another research group reported on the use of progesterone skin cream in 40 women during and after menopause. The study measured skin elasticity, epidermal hydration (skin water content) and skin surface lipids, along with measurement of blood levels of estrogen, progesterone, FSH, and LH (leutinizing hormone), which stimulates progesterone secretion.

According to these researchers: "The 2 percent progesterone cream yielded consistent superiority over [placebo] in counteracting different signs of ageing in the skin…Clinical monitoring showed a greater reduction in wrinkle counts (29.10 percent vs. 16.50 percent) and wrinkle depth (9.72 percent vs. 7.35 percent) … and a significantly higher…

How you can ensure your own visit to the Fountain of Youth—or postpone it

If you really want to make absolutely certain you'll have a desperate need for Toki, Synovoderma, or even topical bio-identical hormones, here are a few "sure fire" things you can do. First up: Smoke cigarettes and be sure to drink a lot of alcohol. According to published research, you should also eat plenty of sugar, drink sugar-sweetened fruit and "soft" drinks, eat pastries, cakes, potatoes, processed meats, and drink milk.[4] And, by all means, avoid eggs, beans, spinach, eggplant, asparagus, celery, nuts, olives, cherries, melons, prunes, apples, pears, yogurt, tea, and pure water. If you follow these steps, you're certain to wind up with plenty of wrinkles—likely more of them and deeper ones than you'd normally get too.

I'm not being "smart" (as my teachers would occasionally say). The point I'm attempting to get across is that there's little use in trying these supplements if you don't pay attention to your diet and other habits!

After all, the best thing you can do is prevent as many wrinkles as you can by staying as healthy as possible. Then whatever little lines do eventually appear are much more likely to respond to treatments like Toki and Synovoderma.

increase in skin firmness (23.61 percent vs. 13.24 percent) in the treatment group...No serious side-effects of the treatment were observed."

Ladies, it's never too late to consider using topical BHRT. It's safe, and can be monitored for any systemic effect (and adjusted accordingly in the unlikely event that one should occur). If you're interested in trying this "anti-aging" tool, contact a physician skilled and knowledgeable in BHRT. (See "Alternative Health Resources," page 485.)

But before you do, there is just one small note of caution: Two percent of a hormone (progesterone, in the case of the last study mentioned above) in a skin crème doesn't sound like much. However, it did produce a small but significant increase in blood progesterone in the women who used it. On the other hand, the .01 percent estradiol and .3 percent estriol crèmes used in the other studies didn't increase blood levels of these hormones significantly.

Although your body isn't likely to absorb each of these hormones at the same exact rate, it's probably close, so even though they are applied topically and haven't been shown to affect blood levels significantly, you should still undergo regular interval monitoring for systemic absorption of any topical hormones you take (just as you would during "regular" bio-identical hormone replacement). It's also likely best to keep the concentrations of any topical hormones at no more, and possibly less, than the concentrations mentioned in the research articles.

Chapter 4:

Don't go deaf, blind or lose your mind! Natural strategies for keeping your hearing, vision, and thinking sharp well into old age

"Eh? What's that you say? Louder, please. No, don't bother writing it down, can't see very well, either! Oh, never mind…I probably won't remember it, anyway!"

If you chuckled when you read that, it's probably because it sounds familiar—whether it's something you remember your parents or grand-parents saying, or whether you've uttered similar things yourself. And while it sounds funny on the surface, the unfortunate truth underlying phrases like these is that varying degrees of failing hearing, vision, and mental function are still considered to be "normal" with advancing age.

But they need not be "normal" for you! In previous issues of *Nutrition & Healing*, I've covered prevention and treatment of "age-related" hearing, vision, and cognitive function problems. This time, we'll review them all in one place, while you—and I—can still remember how to lower your chances of going deaf, blind, or losing your mind!

The hormone deficiency that could be destroying your hearing

Dennis Trune, Ph.D., of Oregon Health Sciences University, pioneered the research showing that the naturally occurring adrenal steroid hormone aldosterone can often reverse hearing loss in animals.

Based on Dr. Trune's work, I've had aldosterone levels tested in many individuals with hearing loss (most of them "older"), and a significant number turned out to have low or "low normal" measurements. But after taking bio-identical aldosterone in "physiologic" quantities—amounts that would normally be present in adult human bodies—more than half of these individuals have regained a significant proportion of their "lost" hearing.

I've been surprised by two aspects of bio-identical aldosterone treatment for hearing loss. First, when it works, it works relatively rapidly, restoring a significant degree of hearing within the first two months. In fact, a few of the people I've worked with have literally heard improvement within just two to three weeks.

The other thing that surprised me about aldosterone therapy is that it's capable of restoring a significant degree of hearing even years after the hearing loss initially occurred. So far, the longest interval I've witnessed was in an 87-year-old man who'd lost his hearing 13 years prior to regaining a significant degree of it using aldosterone.

None of the people I've worked with have had any adverse effects from aldosterone therapy, likely because the use of bio-identical, physiologic-dose aldosterone restores levels to those that would be found in the body anyway.

I've focused this treatment on individuals with hearing loss and low or low-normal aldosterone levels, but I do know of one individual—an M.D.—who decided to try this approach for his hearing loss even though his aldosterone levels were quite normal. His hearing did improve, but unless you too are an M.D., D.O., or N.D. who can prescribe bio-identical aldosterone and order lab tests for sodium and potassium (sodium and potassium regulation are two of aldosterone's major responsibilities), please don't take aldosterone, bio-identical or not, if your measured levels are perfectly normal!

Beat the top 3 causes of blindness—
without patent medicine or surgery

Glaucoma, macular degeneration, and cataracts are three very common causes of vision loss—if they're left untreated, that is.

But many cases of these three sight-stealing conditions can be treated by natural means, often avoiding patent medicines and/or surgery entirely. Even better, it's also possible to significantly reduce your risk of developing any of these problems in the first place.

The vision-robbing disease that's
actually a symptom in many cases

Let's start with glaucoma. This condition occurs when the pressure inside the eyeball (intra-ocular pressure) rises. If the intra-ocular pressure rises high enough, it can cause blindness. Conventional treatment of glaucoma uses either patent medications (generally called miotics) or surgery to relieve the excess pressure.

But in 1937, Emanuel Josephson, M.D., an ophthalmologist in New York City, published a book titled *Glaucoma and its Medical Treatment with Cortin*. In it, Dr. Josephson reported many cases of individuals whose glaucoma and high intra-ocular pressure improved after treatment with a substance called cortin. Cortin was the 1930s name for entirely natural injectable extracts from animal adrenal cortex—the part of the adrenal glands which make cortisol, cortisone, DHEA, aldosterone, and all other natural adrenal steroid molecules in natural balance with each other. (Later on, Cortin was renamed Adrenal Cortical Extract, or ACE.)

Some of the improvements Dr. Josephson related were quite dramatic, with the patients' intra-ocular pressure dropping over 20 points to within the normal range. Dr. Josephson carefully explained that Cortin produced such impressive results because many cases of glaucoma don't actually originate in the eye, but instead manifest in the eye as a symptom of weak adrenal glands. In other words, Dr. Josephson discovered that, in many cases, glaucoma is a symptom, not an "independent disease."

Injections of Cortin (which was literally "hormone replacement therapy" for weak adrenal glands) would allow the eyes—which apparently depend on normal adrenal function—to normalize themselves in many cases. In fact, Cortin even helped alleviate high intra-ocular pressure in people who hadn't responded to miotics or surgery.

At the time Dr. Josephson was using it in his patients, Cortin was sold by major patent medication companies, including Parke-Davis. While they couldn't patent the extracts themselves (since they were 100 percent natural) patent medicine companies could patent—and make enormous profits from—the extraction process.

Unfortunately, though, in the late 1940s and early 1950s, patent medicine companies discovered ways to make totally unnatural but very powerful and patentable (and therefore much more profitable) versions of cortisone and cortisol. Even though these space-alien versions have an incredible list of adverse effects when used in human bodies—including diabetes, osteoporosis, high blood pressure, cataracts, and stomach ulcers—the patent medicine industry was so successful in blurring the lines between them and bio-identical cortisone and cortisol (which never have these sorts of adverse effects when used in "physiologic" quantities) that they've become the go-to choice for most mainstream physicians. A more recent example of this type of "blurring the lines" is the inability of the FDA, conventional medicine, and patent medicine companies to distinguish between Premarin and other patentable pseudo-estrogens and bio-identical estrogens. And just like the current situation with bio-identical HRT, *los Federales* used this line-blurring to outlaw Cortin/ACE in the 1970s.

They claimed that it should be banned because, unlike the synthetic version, ACE was "unapproved," and therefore potentially "dangerous"— even though it had been sold and in use for decades with no reported side effects. In an accompanying illogical leap of FDA "logic," after terming ACE "dangerous," they also stated it was "ineffective."

But I personally witnessed its tremendous success in normalizing glaucoma. Several individuals had decreases in intra-ocular pressure from well above 20 (normal is under 20) to below 20 following a series of intravenous injections of ACE. (All intra-ocular pressure measurements were done by ophthalmologists, not me.) Many other physicians practicing natural medicine had seen similar results and we all protested to the FDA. Unfortunately, the public didn't get involved, and side-effect-free ACE remains illegal today.

However, individuals with glaucoma can still improve and even normalize their intra-ocular pressure by using more general techniques to improve their adrenal function. The very best place to start is with your diet, eliminating all refined sugar and refined carbs and making sure to get adequate amounts of salt.

There are also a number of supplements that can help boost adrenal function, including the sodium ascorbate form of vitamin C, pantothenic acid, chromium, vitamins A and E, and ginseng. Another relatively subtle but powerful technique for strengthening weak adrenal glands is "cell therapy" using fetal animal adrenal cells with other related fetal endocrine cells. (There's a brief note about cell therapy on page 341.) For even more information on strengthening weak adrenal glands, check your local library for the book Adrenal Fatigue by James Wilson, N.D., Ph.D.

As you've likely guessed, adrenal-strengthening treatment is most likely to be successful treating glaucoma in people who have weak adrenal function. The 24-hour urine test for natural steroids and other hormones discussed on page 339 can help you and your physician make an official diagnosis, but symptoms of weak adrenal function include lower-than-average blood pressure (especially if the "top"—systolic—number is consistently below 110), dizzy spells when standing up rapidly, and being easily tired out. Being underweight for your particular height and difficulty gaining weight are also common with weak adrenal function, but are not always present.

If you have any or all of these symptoms, check with a physician skilled and knowledgeable in natural and nutritional medicine, as well as bio-identical hormone replacement.

If weak adrenals aren't at the root of your glaucoma, there are still a few other nutritional and natural therapies that may be able to help reverse it. Eliminating any food allergies you might have is a good first step. Research has also shown that daily use of fish oil (I recommend 1 tablespoonful daily) and high quantities of vitamin C (10 to 35 grams daily, split into three to four doses) can help reduce high intra-ocular pressure. Thyroid hormone also lowers intra-ocular pressure in some cases.

And both magnesium (250 milligrams daily) and standardized extracts of ginkgo biloba (40 milligrams three times daily) have been found to improve visual field defects for individuals with glaucoma.

The macular degeneration treatment that starts in your stomach

Just as Dr. Josephson found that many cases of glaucoma don't originate in the eye, but elsewhere in the body, in the 1980s I discovered that many—if not most—cases of "dry" macular degeneration are "symptoms" of digestive malfunction, specifically poor digestion and assimilation of nutrients. So if you're starting to have vision problems, I encourage you to have your digestive function tested. If it's not operating up to par, correcting it (naturally, of course) will go a long way in helping you get the most from the nutrients that have vision-improving potential.

The most useful of those nutrients are lutein and zeaxanthin, which are found in highest concentrations in spinach, collard greens, and other deep green leafy vegetables. Other important nutrients include zinc (found in oysters, fish and other animal protein), selenium (two to four Brazil nuts a day are an excellent source), riboflavin (which comes from brewer's yeast, almonds, mushrooms, wheat bran, and dark green leafy vegetables), taurine (found in organ meats, fish, and other animal protein), and quercitin (good sources include onions, apples, kale, cherries, grapes, red cabbage, and green beans are all good sources). Bilberry and ginkgo are the best vision-supporting herbs.

I encourage anyone with macular degeneration to consider using Ocudyne II capsules (formulated by my colleague Alan R. Gaby M.D. and me), which contain all the nutrients noted above.

Clearing up cataracts, naturally

I wrote about one of the most effective, well-researched cataract treatments in the July 2008 issue, so I'll refer you there for the complete discussion of N-acetylcarnosine eyedrops.

Another option for treating cataracts is a combination of Chinese botanicals called "Hachimi-jio-gan," or Ba-wei-wan. This treatment has been used for centuries in China to treat cataracts, and even has a bit of clinical evidence to support it: In a human study of early cataracts conducted in Japan, Hachimi-jio-gan was associated with lessening of cataracts in 60 percent of the volunteers. In the USA, Hachimi-jio-gan is available as a (much easier to pronounce) formula called Clinical Nutrients for the Eyes, which is available from natural food stores, compounding pharmacies, and the Tahoma Clinic Dispensary.

Rounding out the natural treatment options for cataracts is a single, simple nutrient: Vitamin A. Decades ago, an honest ophthalmologist with a sense of humor wrote a letter-to-the-Editor of a medical journal "complaining" that his income from cataract surgery had gone down by over 2/3 since he started recommending vitamin A to all his patients with any degree of cataract at all. I recommend 30,000 IU of vitamin A (not beta-carotene) for anyone who wants to prevent or treat cataracts. In fact, the only people who shouldn't use this amount are very small children (who don't get cataracts anyway) and pregnant women.

And while we're on the topic of cataract prevention, one of the most important things you can do is eliminate all sources of sugar and refined carbohydrates from your diet! Researchers have found that part of the cause of cataracts is the lens of the eye trying to "help" the body lower high blood sugar by "packing it away" within the lens, which gradually obscures the vision. This explains why individuals with type 2 diabetes have a much greater incidence of cataracts than people with normal blood sugar levels. So even though not eating sugar and refined carbohydrates is better for everyone's health, it's especially important for cataract prevention if you have diabetes—type 2 or type 1—in your family. Eliminating all sources of the milk sugar lactose (milk, ice cream, cottage cheese, and many soft cheeses) will reduce your risk of cataracts, too.

In addition to eliminating refined sugar and carbohydrates, you may also want to consider incorporating some cataract-preventing nutrients (other than just vitamin A) into your daily supplement regimen. Riboflavin, vitamin C, quercitin, zinc, and carotenoids have all been associated with cataract risk reduction. And one study found that people with higher serum vitamin E levels had 50 percent less risk of developing cataracts than people with lower levels. (When you're supplementing with vitamin E, remember to use mixed tocopherols, not just alpha-tocopherol.)

As a side note, patent-medicine "cortisone" preparations that are prescribed to suppress symptoms of asthma, severe allergies, rheumatoid arthritis, and other more severe inflammatory conditions always increase cataract risk. So if you're using prescription patent-medicine "cortisone," check with a physician skilled and knowledgeable in nutritional and natural medicine for effective alternatives.

Your guide for beating cognitive decline (a.k.a "keeping your marbles")

According to health authorities, Alzheimer's disease is slated to become the next epidemic. In fact, current estimates state that nearly half of people over the age of 85 have Alzheimer's, whether it's obvious or not. There are non-Alzheimer's forms of dementia, too, most notably "multi-infarct" dementia, which is thought to be caused by a series of small strokes, and mild cognitive decline, which likely has many causes that have yet to be identified.

The best way to combat any and all of these cognitive problems is to prevent them from occurring in the first place. You keep reading about it over and over again, but an excellent diet is truly the most important aspect of preventing most—if not all—health problems, including cognitive decline. In fact, more and more research is being reported linking blood sugar problems (such as diabetes) and potential blood sugar problems (such as metabolic syndrome and insulin resistance) with a higher risk of Alzheimer's disease. So here we go again: Eliminate the sugar and refined carbohydrates! Make sure to eat several non-starchy vegetables and a wide array of colorful vegetables every day, too. (You want a varied palette on your plate because each color signals a different and necessary-to-good-health group of nutrients.)

It's also a good idea to "eat organic" as much as possible, since organically raised foods have significantly more minerals and vitamins than commercially grown varieties, not to mention a much lower risk of being contaminated with pesticides, herbicides, and miscellaneous non-food chemical additives.

When you can, I encourage you to even go beyond organic produce and also opt for organic, free-range meat and poultry as well. The essential fatty acid ratio in free-range protein is anti-inflammatory, while the essential fatty acid ratio found in grain-fed animal protein actually promotes inflammation, and inflammation is also being implicated more and more as raising the risk of Alzheimer's and other cognitive malfunction.

Along these same lines, one of the best "brain foods" you can eat is fish. (Low-mercury fish, that is.) Not only are the omega-3 fatty acids in fish anti-inflammatory, but they're also essential components of the membranes of every brain cell we have. And since our bodies can't make them on their own, it's critical to get enough omega-3s and other essential fatty acids from supplements (like cod liver oil) and foods (like free-range meat and fish).

Phospholipids are another key component of brain cells. While our bodies can make them, as with many other things (co-enzyme Q10 and glutathione are two prominent examples) our bodies make less and less with age. Eggs—specifically the yolks—are excellent sources of phospholipids, as is the lecithin found in soy. Supplemental lecithin—another good source of phospholipids—is available in any natural food store and is an excellent idea for anyone over 40.

Boost your brain—and your sex life

I can't tell you how many men I've seen at the Tahoma Clinic who have the idea that testosterone is mostly for sexual function. I always let them know that its most important job is maintaining cognitive function. The sex part is important, no doubt, but who cares about sex if you can't remember who you're with or what you're doing with her?

Unfortunately, thanks to this misunderstanding word hasn't gotten around that—just like estrogen replacement for women—bio-identical testosterone replacement for men is extremely important for significantly reducing the risk of Alzheimer's disease and cognitive decline. I'll mention just a few of the highlights here:

- Higher serum estrogen levels in women in their 60s are directly correlated with lower incidence of Alzheimer's in those same women decades later. (And the reverse is true too: Lower estrogens equal higher incidence of Alzheimer's in later years.)

- The 15-year Princeton men's study determined that men who had higher serum free testosterone in 1983 had less risk of Alzheimer's disease in 1998. (Once again, the reverse was also true: Lower serum free testosterone corresponded with higher risk of Alzheimer's.)

- Researchers observing neurons found substantially less accumulation of beta-amyloid, neurofibrillary tangle, tau protein, and other "neuronal garbage" associated with Alzheimer's when those neurons were exposed to "physiologic quantities" of either estrogen or testosterone (depending on whether the neuron was from a woman or a man).

- In numerous controlled experiments, elderly men without Alzheimer's disease do better on tests of cognitive function when given testosterone than men given placebo.

- Testosterone for men and estrogen (that's real, bio-identical estrogen —not horse estrogen) for women is very protective for the entire cardiovascular system, including the blood supply to the brain. (Remember that cognitive decline due to repeated small strokes?)

The bottom line is, if you want to "keep your marbles" for as long as you live, consider bio-identical hormone replacement when it's appropriate for you. Just make sure to be working with a physician who is skilled and knowledgeable in all aspects of this therapy. If you're not sure if your doctor is, one way to find out is to ask the physician's office whether they do routine monitoring of therapy with the 24-hour urine steroid determination. This test is the very best way to check not only the levels of the bio-identical hormones being replaced but also their metabolization (the natural transformation of the starting hormones into pro- and anti-carcinogenic metabolites). Blood and/or saliva testing just doesn't cut it when it comes to bio-identical HRT. See *Nutrition & Healing* for December 2007 for a much more detailed discussion of safety monitoring for bio-identical hormone replacement (and, rest assured, if safety monitoring does indicate that there's an imbalance in the "wrong" direction, it's almost always correctable with nutrients or botanicals).

Small dose, big protection

I've written about lithium's brain-protecting benefits before too (see *Nutrition & Healing* for August 2003 and April 2008), and this is getting a bit long (sorry about that) so I'll be brief: No matter what neurotoxin your brain is exposed to, lithium protects against it.

Not only that, but lithium actually promotes the growth of new brain cells, even in individuals past age 50. So far, no other nutrient has been found to do that.

Yes, high-dose prescription lithium can be toxic, but low quantities like the ones used for boosting cognitive function and protecting brain cells (20 milligrams daily and under) are not associated with toxicity. In over 30 years, I've only encountered two or three individuals who reported a possible reaction to low-dose lithium: These people thought that it might have given them a slight tremor (which went away when the lithium was discontinued). But on the flip side of that same coin, I've also encountered dozens of individuals who reported improvement in benign tremors with the use of low dose lithium.

Even though risk of toxicity from low-dose lithium is very small, I always recommend working with a physician skilled and knowledgeable in nutritional and natural medicine if you decide to supplement with lithium. And to be on the extra-cautious side, I always recommend using supplemental essential fatty acids when using even low-quantity lithium supplements. Essential fatty acids are the primary treatment for toxicity caused by high-dose prescription lithium, so using them in conjunction with low-dose treatment helps avoid that possibility altogether.

Spicing up your brain-boosting regimen

There are many, many more supplemental items that can help you maintain cognitive function, but we're quickly running out of space, so I'll just mention two more: Curcumin and Ginkgo.

Although no one is entirely sure how it works, the research on curcumin's ability to protect against Alzheimer's (as well as its many other beneficial effects) has been more than a little exciting. Areas of the world in which the spice turmeric (which has a high concentration of curcumin) is routinely used have very little—if any—Alzheimer's compared with areas that don't. Perhaps the best aspect of curcumin is that you don't need to take yet another pill to get its brain-boosting benefits. Just use turmeric in your cooking, perhaps an average of 1/4 to 1/2 teaspoonful daily. (For those of you who just can't stand the taste of turmeric, it is available in capsules, too. If you're using it for long-term cognitive maintenance, consider taking two 200-milligram capsules a day.)

Send in "cell reinforcements" right where you need them most

I recently received an e-mail from a couple in their 60s who read the March 2005 Nutrition & Healing article describing the therapeutic and rejuvenating effects of cell therapy.

Cell therapy was pioneered by Dr. Paul Niehans of Switzerland in the 1920s and 1930s and has been available in the USA through the Tahoma Clinic and other knowledgeable practitioners since 1994.

"Cell therapy" isn't the same as the highly controversial "stem cell therapy." Stem cell therapy uses human cells, which are capable of turning into nearly any other cell in the human body, strengthening and rejuvenating any organ that might need help.

Cell therapy, on the other hand, comes from fetal animal cells and is more specifically targeted in that the cells being used have already been differentiated into skin cells, heart cells, lung cells—or whatever you and your physician decide would help you most. Although the exact way in which these fetal animal cells help improve the health of human organs isn't known, experts have determined that fetal cells have the highest levels of "cell growth factors" and of course have brand new DNA specific to that type of cell and organ. And using radio-active tracer studies, German researchers found that approximately 75 percent of these cells appear to find their way to their intended target—no matter where they're injected into the body. For example, even if fetal heart cells are injected into the thigh, approximately 75 percent of them make it to the heart.

After reading all of the fascinating research and case reports about this therapy and then thinking it over for a while, the couple I mentioned above decided to use the "overall anti-aging program" (there are also programs specifically targeted to strengthen a weak

(continued on next page...)

organ or organs), and they wrote to say how pleased they were with the results. Not only did they tell me that they feel younger, but in their message, they also described how cell therapy has improved their energy levels, complexions, and even their sex life.

While cell therapy isn't inexpensive ("overall anti-aging" is usually $2,500-$3,500 per person) it's dramatically less expensive than stem cell therapy, and doesn't require travel to another country. And based on my own observations over the past 18 years, it almost always has dramatic—and noticeable—rejuvenating effects.

Ginkgo has been used for the brain for thousands of years, and (like lithium) has been found to be neuroprotective.

We all know that none of us will live forever, but there's no reason not to live as long as our "genetic programs" will allow—and keep all of our faculties while we're here. If you can do all of the things outlined above (or at least come close), you'll have a much better chance of living as long as your oldest known relative, getting to know your great-grandchildren, and hearing, seeing, enjoying, and remembering those years of life so much better!

This chapter refers to several *Nutrition & Healing* articles. To read the full text of any you're interested in, go to www.wrightnewsletter.com, and log on to the Archives with the username and password printed on page 8 of your most recent issue.

Chapter 5:

Seeing is believing: Real help for macular degeneration and cataracts

Macular degeneration is not an incurable disease, no matter what you hear from most doctors or read in mainstream media. I've been treating patients with this condition since 1985 and have found a way to preserve and restore vision in 70 percent of the cases.

I know it's hard to believe, but I first published case studies concerning recovery of vision in patients with macular degeneration in the *Journal of Nutritional Medicine* in 1990. So why isn't this treatment better known and much more widely used? As usual, the answer is that it's unpatentable. Pharmaceutical companies aren't interested, and government grants are made available almost entirely to test mainstream medical theories. So there aren't any controlled trial results to make mainstream medicine happy…and there isn't any money given to natural medicine to do the testing. It's a vicious cycle, with patients getting the short end of the stick.

But despite the absence of controlled research, macular degeneration is an important and prevalent health problem. This disease involves degeneration of the center of the retina, which is called the macula. The macula is the part of the eye capable of our most detailed vision. We use it for reading, driving, recognizing faces, watching television, and all precise work. Macular degeneration is the leading cause of legal blindness in people over 55 and affects 9 percent of us over 70 (according to one prominent eye journal).

After working with many patients who suffer from age-related macular degeneration (ARMD), I've discovered that it isn't only a problem with our eyes, it's actually a digestive problem too.

I first uncovered this link in 1984 when treating a patient. From there, I began noticing that my other patients with macular degeneration almost always had low levels of hydrochloric acid and lacked enough pepsin to digest their food properly. (In fact, a lot of them don't make any hydrochloric acid at all.) Without it, protein isn't broken down into amino acids effectively, and minerals aren't separated from the foods as well as they could be. This is why, as much as we all hate needles, many people respond so much better to treatment with intravenous injection of nutrients rather than just swallowing supplements.

Since the mid-1980s, I've started everyone with macular degeneration on IV treatments, simply because more people get better—and sooner, too. If all the digestion tests come back normal (which is unusual) then I consider going to an all-oral treatment. We usually start as soon as tests are done, which can be in a day or two.

The most important minerals for macular degeneration healing— zinc and selenium—are central to the IV treatment. In fact, those are the only two I used for much of the 1980s. Since then, I've expanded the list to include all known essential minerals, as well as vitamin B12 and the other B-complex vitamins. That improved results a little further, and costs only very slightly more.

It doesn't work every time; but halting or reversing the problem about 70 percent of the time certainly isn't bad.

Most people see improvement with this treatment in as little as four to six weeks. If you don't have any results at all after eight weeks, the treatment probably won't help.

If you don't want to try the intravenous therapy or can't find access to it, you can take oral supplements. They don't usually work as quickly or dramatically, but they can still help. But if you decide to go this route, your first step is to have your digestion tested and corrected if problems exist (one common symptom of poor digestive function is cracking, peeling, and chipping fingernails).

Improving the stomach's digestive function with the "digestive replacement therapy" of betaine hydrochloride-pepsin or glutamic-acid hydrochloride-pepsin will help improve many health problems by improving the available supply of essential nutrients.

If hydrochloric acid treatment is recommended for you, start by taking one capsule (5, 7 1/2, or 10 grains) of either betaine hydrochloride-pepsin or glutamic-acid hydrochloride just before each meal. After two or three days, if you don't have any problems, take two capsules before meals, then three capsules another two or three days later. Gradually increase your dose in this stepwise fashion until you get to 40 to 90 grains per meal.

Treatment with hydrochloric acid can be dangerous and should only be used when testing indicates a need. If this is the case for you, the treatment process should be carefully monitored by a physician.

Once your digestion has improved, you will be able to absorb the following nutrients and herbs much more efficiently. So at that point, you can begin the following daily supplement regimen: 30 milligrams of zinc picolinate or zinc citrate, twice daily; 4 milligrams of copper, preferably copper sebacate, taken at a different time of day than the zinc; 1,000 milligrams of taurine taken in between meals; 800 units of vitamin E; 300 micrograms of selenium; and 80 milligrams of bilberry, twice daily.

Don't give up if you don't improve immediately. Keep in mind that it takes several months or even longer for the herbs and nutrients to "build up" in your system and begin making a difference.

Obviously, convincing your Medicare or HMO physician that your ARMD is being caused by your lack of stomach acid would probably be pretty close to impossible. You really need to see a physician who can treat your eyes as part of your whole body. If you are too far away to travel to the Tahoma Clinic, the American College for Advancement in Medicine (800)532-3688; www.acam.org) can usually offer a recommendation closer to home.

And, of course, no discussion of eyesight is complete without mentioning cataracts too. Over two decades ago, I read an article by an ophthalmologist who wrote that his income from cataract surgery had declined by 2/3 since he started recommending vitamin A to individuals with early cataracts. He noted that few cataracts actually disappeared, but that progression of most of them did slow drastically, and often stopped where it was. I was impressed that this ophthalmologist cared more for his patients than for his bank account and have passed his recommendation along ever since.

So my first recommendation is to add 40,000 IU of vitamin A (not beta-carotene) to your program each day. Use the liquid "micellized" form, which absorbs more reliably.

N-acetyl-carnosine (NAC) eyedrops are one of the most promising new treatments. In the latest double-blind, placebo-controlled trial, 90 percent of NAC-treated eyes showed improvement in corrected visual acuity and 88.9 percent showed an improvement in glare sensitivity after just six months.

N-acetyl-carnosine is available as a product called CAN-C, from a few online sources, a few compounding pharmacies and natural food stores, and the Tahoma Clinic Dispensary.

Another research report involved a group of Chinese herbs, collectively called Hachimi-jio-gan (or just "Clinical Nutrients for the Eyes," which is much easier to pronounce). Patients in early stages of cataracts were treated with Hachimi-jio-gan. Sixty percent had some regression, and 20 percent didn't progress any further. If you want to try Clinical Nutrients for the Eyes, take 150 milligrams twice daily.

In another study, bilberry stopped the progression of cataracts in 48 out of 50 of the participants. If you try bilberry, take 80 to 160 milligrams three times a day. And be sure to use a product with a 25 percent standardized anthocyanidin content.

These treatments are all safe, and if they don't work for you, the worst that can happen is that you'll eventually decide to proceed with cataract surgery. But even if you do ultimately need surgery, these approaches will most likely make that necessity come much later than it would otherwise.

Chapter 6:

Stay sharp into your 90s with these all-natural brain boosters

Years ago, I had a patient named Vincent who came to me worried about his memory.

"My wife thinks I'm losing it," he told me. "I was just passing it off, but now I think she's right. Last week, I drove off and left the boat at the launch for the second time in a month, with the dog in it too! Had to drive all the way back to get the boat and the dog."

After an examination and interview, Vincent's description of his symptoms formed a fairly typical pattern. He described a stretch of heartburn that subsided after treatment with antacids, as well as increasing gas—both of these symptoms indicate progressive stomach failure.

Vincent's tests disclosed weak digestive functioning and low levels of amino acids and DHEA. With the help of the appropriate amino acids, vitamin B12 injections (along with other B vitamins), DHEA supplementation, and digestive correction, Vincent's memory was much improved within eight months.

You'll need a doctor's help with testing and determining an individual supplement program. For a list of doctors in your area who are skilled in nutritional medicine, contact the American College for Advancement in Medicine at (800)532-3688 or www.acam.org.

Brain-stimulating herbal supplements are also gaining more and more media attention and popularity. One such herb, Bacopa, was shown to significantly reduce anxiety and improve mental performance in an uncontrolled trial involving 35 patients who underwent treatment for one month. (The daily dose was equivalent to 12 grams of dried herb.) In addition to promoting mental function, Bacopa has the ability to raise the general resistance of the body to stress and to improve visual and motor perception.

Check your local natural food store for Bacopa supplements. If they don't carry them, contact the Tahoma Clinic Dispensary (425-264-0059; www.tahomadispensary.com) for more information on the product Memoractiv, which contains Bacopa.

Chapter 7:

The secret to halting hearing loss: Start with your stomach

Evidence is accumulating that, like macular degeneration, age-related hearing loss is related to suboptimal digestion and assimilation. In a recent study, 55 women with inefficient hearing were shown to have low levels of vitamin B12 and folic acid. Based on this research, it is possible to say that improved levels of all micronutrients may well prevent age-related hearing loss. And the best way to do that is to improve your digestive function. (One common symptom of poor digestive function is cracking, peeling, and chipping fingernails.)

First, have your digestion tested. A doctor from the American College for Advancement in Medicine can help you with that. If problems exist, improving the stomach's digestive function with the "digestive replacement therapy" of betaine hydrochloride-pepsin or glutamic-acid hydrochloride-pepsin will help many health problems by improving the available supply of essential nutrients.

If hydrochloric acid treatment is recommended for you, start by taking one capsule (5, 7 1/2, or 10 grains) of either betaine hydrochloride-pepsin or glutamic-acid hydrochloride just before each meal. After two or three days, if you don't have any problems, take two capsules before meals, then three capsules another two or three days later. Gradually increase your dose in this stepwise fashion until you get to 40 to 90 grains per meal.

Treatment with hydrochloric acid can be dangerous and should only be used when testing indicates a need. If this is the case for you, the treatment process should be carefully monitored by a physician.

Once your digestion has improved, you'll be able to absorb vitamin B12 and folic acid much more efficiently. Take 800 micrograms of each per day.

Chapter 8:

Alzheimer's disease:
New hope for a "hopeless" situation

As you know, there's very little available for Alzheimer's patients (and their families) that can offer even partial relief from the turmoil this disease causes. So when new treatments are developed or discovered, it's usually big news—a ray of hope for people stuck in a seemingly hopeless situation. One of these newly developed treatments, called Memantine, was recently approved in Europe. Apparently, it "works" by protecting brain cells against damage caused by a major excitotoxin, glutamate. But protecting against glutamate-induced nerve cell damage is also one of the well-known actions of lithium. So if it's true that this newly approved patent medication slows the progress of Alzheimer's disease in this way, then lithium should slow Alzheimer's disease progression, too. Of course, lithium treatment, which isn't patentable and doesn't have nearly the profit potential of patented Alzheimer's medications, hasn't made any headlines. But that doesn't mean it isn't a promising option for patients struggling with Alzheimer's disease.

There are many other research findings that also strongly suggest that lithium will protect against potential Alzheimer's disease and slow the progression of existing cases. Researchers have reported that lithium inhibits beta-amyloid secretion, and also prevents damage caused by beta-amyloid protein once it's been formed. Beta-amyloid peptide is a signature protein involved in Alzheimer's disease: The more beta-amyloid protein, the worse the Alzheimer's becomes.

Over-activation of a brain cell protein, called tau protein, also contributes to neuronal degeneration in Alzheimer's disease, as does the formation of neurofibrillary tangles. Lithium inhibits both of these nerve cell damaging problems.

And you've likely read that individuals with Alzheimer's disease usually have excess aluminum accumulation in brain cells. While it's not yet known whether this excess aluminum is a cause, an effect, or just coincidental, most health-conscious individuals take precautions to avoid ingesting aluminum. Unfortunately, it's impossible to completely avoid all aluminum, since it's naturally present in nearly all foods. But lithium can help protect your brain against aluminum by helping to "chelate" it so that it can be more easily removed from the body.

Although Alzheimer's disease and senile dementia aren't technically the same, they do share many of the same degenerative features so there's every reason to expect that lithium will help prevent or slow the progression of senile dementia, too.

For general brain anti-aging, I recommend taking 10 to 20 milligrams of lithium (from lithium aspartate or lithium orotate) daily. I've actually been recommending these amounts since the 1970s. At first I was exceptionally cautious and asked all of my patients taking lithium to have regular "lithium level" blood tests and thyroid function tests. After a year or so, I quit asking for the lithium level blood tests, since 100 percent of them came back very low. Another year after that, I stopped requesting routine thyroid function tests, too, only doing one when I was suspicious of a potential problem. In the 30 years since, I've rarely found one.

In cases of Alzheimer's, though, you might need higher doses of lithium. High-dose lithium (capsules containing approximately 30 milligrams of lithium from lithium carbonate) is available only by prescription. But low-dose lithium (capsules or tablets containing 5 milligrams of lithium from lithium aspartate or lithium orotate) is available from a few natural food stores and compounding pharmacies, as well as from the Tahoma Clinic Dispensary.

To be on the safe side, I always recommend that anyone taking lithium also take a teaspoonful or two of flaxseed oil (or other essential fatty acid), along with 400 IU vitamin E each day.

When you hear the word homocysteine, chances are you immediately think of heart disease. While too much of this substance does contribute to cardiovascular disease, elevated levels also increase your risk of Alzheimer's disease. However, it's not clear whether homocysteine has a direct effect on brain cells or whether the extra Alzheimer's risk is due to homocysteine's effect on blood vessels that serve the brain.

But even though no one knows for sure whether added folate helps prevent Alzheimer's by directly helping maintain brain cells or by reducing blood vessel damage, the net effect is the same: Adequate folate can help reduce your risk of Alzheimer's disease.

This brain-protecting effect extends to everyday cognitive function too. The term "cognitive function" includes not only memory, but also many other measures of abstract thought, including verbal and mathematical reasoning, test performance, and general alertness. Many research groups have reported associations between folate insufficiency and poor cognitive performance. So getting enough folate will help keep you thinking clear well into your golden years.

So how much folate should you take? As much as you need! I'm not trying to be elusive or "smart." I've seen folate requirements vary from none at all in people who get a sufficient supply from their food to 20-30 milligrams daily. Fortunately, there's a simple, inexpensive, and highly accurate test you can take to determine just how much you need.

Instead of blood or urine screens, I prefer measuring folate levels using something called a functional test, which is individualized to you. This type of test measures a function that depends on a certain nutrient. Your specific numerical reading or level of that nutrient doesn't really matter. What does matter is whether you personally have enough of that nutrient to keep the chosen parameter functioning optimally.

Along with the cells that line your intestinal tract, blood cells are the most rapidly dividing cells in your body, constantly duplicating DNA to make brand-new cells. So this is the function that I find works best to measure folate adequacy. Specifically, I look at neutrophils, which are a certain type of white blood cell. The "neutrophilic hypersegmentation index" tells us what percentage of neutrophils had too little folic acid to properly duplicate their DNA. Obviously, 0 percent is best, since you want all of your rapidly dividing cells to be supplied with enough folic acid to properly duplicate.

Just about any laboratory with a microscope and an educated technician should be able to do this test. But, oddly enough, many labs don't. It requires a very small amount of blood smeared on a glass slide under a cover slip. The technician examines the slide for neutrophils, and reports what percentage of them are "hypersegmented" (lacking sufficient folate during the final stages of their development). The price should be $25 to $30.

If you can't get your doctor to order this test, remember that you can actually order your own in many states. Washington state is one of those, so if your local lab doesn't do the neutrophilic hypersegmentation index, have them draw the blood and send it to Meridian Valley Labs (425-271-8689, www.meridianvalleylab.com), where I'm the medical director.

If your test result is 0 percent, congratulate yourself! You've been eating enough folate in your food and/or taking enough to make sure that even your most rapidly dividing cells have all they need.

If you're close to 0, say 1-5 percent, you're still in pretty good shape. With just a little more folate-containing food or perhaps a little more folic acid supplement, you'll usually get to 0 percent quite easily.

If you're over 5 percent, it's time to make some changes. Don't fool yourself that 95 percent normal neutrophils is pretty darn good just because 95 percent got you an "A" in school. Think about what the number means in this context: 5 percent of your rapidly dividing cells don't have enough folate available. (Remember, it takes only one rapidly dividing cell that wasn't able to properly repair its own DNA to result in cancer. And even though an abnormal test result doesn't mean you have cancer, it does mean you have a slightly higher risk, as well as higher risk of dementia and Alzheimer's disease, not to mention all the other conditions folate helps to prevent.) So getting serious and reducing your risk is a very good idea, especially if your test result is 5 percent or greater.

Take a look at the list of folate-rich foods: Anything green, beans, nuts, wheat germ, liver (organically raised, of course), other organ meats, oysters, salmon, and brewer's yeast. There must be at least one or more of these you can add to your menu more often.

If your test result is above 5 percent, you should also take a folic acid supplement—5 milligrams daily—until a repeat test shows a 0 percent result. Keep in mind that you'll need to be very patient: Since this test relies on examination of neutrophils, which have a life span of six to eight months each, the lab might not see much change until that long after you start supplementing.

If your test is 15-20 percent or above, and especially if you're over 55, it's a good idea to increase your folic acid supplement to 5 milligrams, two to three times daily, once again until your test drops to 0 percent.

If your test doesn't improve at all, or even gets worse after six to eight months, you may have run into a folate absorption problem that you'll need a physician's help to overcome. Nearly every other nutrient is absorbed better if your body needs it; improved iron absorption during iron deficiency is one of the best-known examples. But folate absorption is the opposite; there's a "threshold" level of folate deficiency beyond which folate is less and less well absorbed until it's hardly absorbed at all—sometimes even in huge oral quantities. This threshold varies from person to person, so the only way to know if you've crossed the "no folate absorption threshold" is to try to improve your results, and see if they actually do get better over time.

If they don't, you have two options: Those "huge" oral doses—100 milligrams daily or more—or injections. Even though folic acid injections are very safe, you still need a prescription, not only for the folic acid, but, in many states, for the needles and syringes as well. (And if you don't already know how, you'll need to learn self-injection.) If you go the injection route, you should use 2.5 to 5 milligrams of folic acid twice weekly for six to eight months.

If you're going to take the trouble to inject folic acid, talk to your doctor about adding vitamin B12—1,000 micrograms daily—to the injection, since folic acid and vitamin B12 are almost always found together in biochemical reactions in your body.

If you opt to try large oral quantities of folic acid, be sure to also take at least 30 milligrams of zinc (preferably zinc picolinate or zinc citrate, with 2 milligrams of copper) at a different time of day. There's some suspicion that taking large oral quantities of folic acid over a long time might cause a zinc deficiency.

One other precaution: If you are on any type of anti-seizure medication at all, don't take more than 1 milligram of folic acid daily—even if your test shows you're deficient-unless you're working with a physician skilled and knowledgeable in nutritional and natural medicine!

You've likely gathered that I'm not a fan of the usual 400- or 800-microgram daily doses of folic acid. All too frequently, they don't work, leaving the test results just as bad as ever after six to eight months of supplementation. Yet folic acid supplements in quantities of greater than 800 micrograms are hard to find due to FDA guidelines.

Check your natural food store, compounding pharmacy, or the Tahoma

Clinic Dispensary for 5- and 20-milligram capsules, or bottles of folic acid liquid, which contain 2 milligrams per drop. These will help put you on the right track much faster than "regular" folic acid supplements.

Part X
Essential
Health Secrets

Chapter 1:

Vitamin K: What's it good for?

Have you ever seen a bottle of vitamin K supplements in your natural food store, pharmacy, or grocery store? Even though vitamin K is essential to life and quite safe in its natural forms, supplements of it are very hard to find. That's probably because the vast majority of us have only a vague idea about what the vitamin can do—so there's very little demand.

Most of us have heard that vitamin K has "something to do with blood clotting." In fact, Drs. Henrik C.P. Dam (Denmark) and Edward A. Doisy (United States) were awarded the Nobel Prize in Medicine in 1943 for original research uncovering vitamin K's functions in blood clotting. Since then, however, research has shown numerous other benefits, ranging from tooth decay to anti-aging; you should consider what vitamin K can do for you.

Detecting a deficiency—signs are few

Each of us probably received just one deliberate "dosing" with vitamin K in our lifetimes, and that was shortly after birth to prevent "hemorrhagic disease" of the newborn. Since then, we've absorbed small amounts of vitamin K from our diets and elsewhere, but accumulating research says that for many of us, relying on dietary sources may not be enough.

Severe vitamin K deficiency causes uncontrollable bleeding, but mild to moderate degrees of such a deficiency don't ordinarily cause obvious problems. There are two physical signs that indicate you might need vitamin K supplementation.

The first is easy bruising. While this can also be due to a lack of flavonoids (which help keep small blood vessels strong), it's definitely safe and worth a try to use supplemental vitamin K (5 to 10 milligrams daily) to try to stop the problem. After six to eight weeks, it should be possible to tell whether vitamin K is helpful or not.

The second physical sign concerns women only. Many women have told me over the years that supplemental vitamin K totally eliminates menstrual clots, whether the clots are large and painful or only small and negligible. I've heard this so often that (unless proven otherwise) I'm assuming that any degree of menstrual clotting means insufficient vitamin K. Usually 5 to 15 milligrams daily will be enough to eliminate this clotting within two to three monthly cycles.

Although I'm aware of only these few physical signs of vitamin K deficiency, it's quite possible that one or more of the conditions that follow are (at least in part) also signs of insufficiency for the individuals involved.

Fight tooth decay naturally

In 1948, Leonard Fosdick, Ph.D., of the Northwestern University School of Dentistry published research demonstrating that Vitamin K could prevent tooth decay.[1] He had prepared chewing gum with and without vitamin K and asked an experimental group to chew the vitamin K gum after each meal. A carefully selected control group chewed gum without vitamin K. Dr. Fosdick reported: "It was found that the experimental group produced 60 percent to 90 percent fewer carious lesions than did similar control patients."

Dr. Fosdick's report was the eighth in a series starting in 1936. This series of publications carefully traced one major cause of dental caries to decalcification of tooth enamel and dentine by acid. He found that the decalcifying acids were produced by anaerobic metabolism (fermentation) of simple sugars and, to a small degree, starches.

In a 1942 publication, Dr. Fosdick pointed out that the enzymes involved in this acid production could be inhibited by silver nitrate, fluoride, and vitamin K.[2] (If the acid-producing enzymes could be inhibited, he claimed, the reduction in acid production would be accompanied by less caries, as his subsequent 1948 research paper demonstrated.) Dr. Fosdick comments on these three methods:

- **Silver nitrate**: "The application of silver nitrate by dentists is another good example of the use of an enzyme poison. The main difficulty with this procedure is that it discolors the teeth. Nevertheless, there is widespread use of this method with more or less favorable results."

- **Fluoride**: "Fluorides were one of the first-known inhibitors of the enzyme system necessary for acid production. In all probability, the application of this method of caries control may be quite successful. *However, it is extremely hazardous to contaminate the drinking water of a large portion of our population without having more complete information concerning the toxic and obscure effects of long-continued ingestion of the fluoride ion.*" [Editorial emphasis added for obvious reasons.]

- **Vitamin K**: "Another substance that interferes with the [acid-forming] enzyme system is 2-methyl-1,4-napthoquinone [menadione, or vitamin K3], with certain derivatives. These substances seem to interfere with the enzyme system at one of the initial stages of the series of chemical reactions involved in the formation of acids. *On this basis, it would be equal to or superior to the fluoride ion. Furthermore, preliminary experiments indicate that this material has a toxicity far less than that of the fluoride ion and may be ingested over long periods of time with no untoward result.*" [Emphasis again added for the same obvious reasons.]

Although at present Dr. Fosdick's vitamin K chewing gum is not available, Donal Carter, Ph.D., and I have formulated a dental spray containing vitamin K3 called DentaMist, which is available through Tahoma Clinic dispensary, (888)893-6878, www.tahoma-clinic.com, and Life Enhancement Products, (800)543-3873, www.life-enhancement.com.

Nausea and vomiting during pregnancy

Vitamin K (5 milligrams) and vitamin C (500 milligrams) taken simultaneously are a very effective but little-known treatment for nausea and vomiting during pregnancy. Though I'm not an obstetrician, I've observed success with this combination dozens of times.

As reported by Richard J. Merkel, M.D., 64 of 70 women (91 percent) who experienced nausea and vomiting during pregnancy were completely relieved of all symptoms within three days by simultaneous administration of vitamin K and vitamin C.[3] (Dr. Merkel actually used only 25 milligrams of vitamin C with 5 milligrams of vitamin K, but these small doses are no longer available.) Three of Dr. Merkel's patients were relieved of vomiting but not nausea, and only three (4.5 percent) were not helped at all. In "an advanced case of hyperemesis gravidarum (hyper-vomiting of pregnancy) in the second trimester and a case of pseudocyesis (pseudo-pregnancy), this medication appeared to be dramatically beneficial when other means of treatment had failed." Dr. Merkel carefully noted that "in all cases the prothrombin time (a standard measure of vitamin K deficiency) and bleeding time were normal before and after medication." He found that using vitamin K or vitamin C alone failed to give relief.

In his research, Dr. Merkel used menadione, the synthetic water-soluble form of vitamin K, which is safe in small doses. This water-soluble form doesn't require any digestive aid. I've found that phylloquinone works nearly as well, especially if taken with a high-lipase digestive enzyme containing just a small amount of bile salts (often found in the pill with the enzyme). Phylloquinone and vitamin C are also available for (simultaneous) injection and work well that way. (For more information, see "Where to start and what to look for" on page 369.)

Chronic pain

In 1955, researchers in Sarajevo reported on the effects of vitamin K injections on pain.[4] They first determined that (in mice) vitamin K was more effective than morphine in its *thermoanalgesic* properties (relief of pain from burns). Then, they gave vitamin K injections to 115 individuals with chronic pain (due to terminal cancer) controllable only with morphine. Ninety-five of the 115 were able to eliminate morphine and rely on the vitamin K injections for pain relief.

At Tahoma Clinic, Davis Lamson, N.D., and I tried this treatment and found it nearly as effective as did the original researchers. Unfortunately, the type of vitamin K used in the original research was discontinued by its manufacturer, so we were forced to switch to other types. We found the other available types effective in only 40-50 percent of the individuals who tried them. (However, when working with chronic pain, 40-50 percent is still a worthwhile number.)

Currently, we work with a preparation containing 30 milligrams of vitamin K (phytonadione form) per cc. Individuals learn to self-inject 20 to 30 milligrams intramuscularly each day for a two-week trial period. If it's effective within that time, we have each individual adjust the dose and frequency according to what it takes to control pain adequately. (For example, a woman with severe rheumatoid-arthritis pain found that 30 milligrams (1 cc) every three to four days was just the right amount for her.) If it's not effective within those two weeks, we discontinue.

Reversing soft bones and hard arteries

It's been known for years that Vitamin K is important to healthy bones. It is essential to the final step in the activation of *osteocalcin*, a protein essential to normally calcifying bones. Women with fractured hips have been shown to have significantly lower vitamin K levels than women without fractures.[5] A study of 16 individuals with osteoporosis found that serum vitamin K levels were only 35 percent of vitamin K levels in a non-osteoporotic group of the same age.[6]

I've observed decreases in urinary calcium loss (as well as decreases in bone peptide loss) in women after they started taking vitamin K; lessening of urinary calcium excretion in women after menopause has also been reported by researchers.[7,8] The vitamin is also of major importance in healing fractures;[9] I've seen supposedly non-healing fractures recover completely once vitamin K treatment was started.

But isn't it interesting that while vitamin K can help put calcium back where it belongs, into bones, it may simultaneously prevent calcium from depositing in arteries where it *doesn't* belong? Japanese researchers reported that vitamin K2 had exactly this effect in studies involving experimental animals.[10] Dutch researchers found that a group of 113 postmenopausal women with calcification of the aorta had reduced vitamin K levels. In a follow-up study, the same researchers reported that postmenopausal women with aortic calcification also had a significantly lower bone mass.[11]

Although this evidence can't be called at all conclusive, it certainly suggests the possibility that a major function (perhaps the main function) of vitamin K may be to keep calcium "in all the right places" and at the same time to prevent it from getting into the "wrong" ones. Vitamin K is *the* vitamin necessary to attach gamma-carboxyglutamic acid (an amino acid) to proteins. This attachment enables proteins to "grab, hold, and manipulate" calcium. Without vitamin K, this process doesn't work optimally.

Is vitamin K an anti-aging vitamin?

It's relatively well-known that as part of the aging process, calcium "leaks" from the bloodstream through cell membranes into the interior of cells, where (in excess) it interferes with the optimal functioning of intracellular metabolism. If vitamin K could somehow help reverse this process, by keeping calcium from leaking into the wrong places, it would be a major anti-aging nutrient. Terri Mitchell, a contributor to *Life Extension* magazine, has just written an excellent general review of vitamin K in which the anti-aging question is addressed.[12] Much more research is needed in this area.

Where to start and what to look for

As with most supplements, the first place to supplement with vitamin K is in our daily diet. The best sources of dietary vitamin K are green vegetables, especially kale (817 ppm, or parts per million); spinach (400 ppm); endive (231 ppm); broccoli (205 ppm); Brussels sprouts (177 ppm); cabbage (147 ppm); and lettuce (122 ppm). Soybean oil and canola oil (193 and 141 ppm) contain the largest amounts *not* found in green vegetables, with olive oil a distant third (49 ppm). Whole soybeans contain 47 ppm and avocados 40 ppm, but in general, grains, meats, fish, fruits, nuts, seeds, oils, and non-green vegetables (corn, beets, carrots, potatoes, tomatoes, etc.) contain very little vitamin K.

The natural, plant-synthesized dietary source of vitamin K is called *phylloquinone*, though it's still frequently referred to as vitamin K1. Intestinal bacteria (including normal E. coli and Bacteroides species) also synthesize various forms of vitamin K, previously termed (as a group) vitamin K2 but now generally called menaquinones. Menadione, an entirely synthetic molecule with vitamin K activity, was developed in the 1940s and called (at the time) vitamin K3.

There's usually much more of the menaquinones (vitamin K2) than phylloquinone (vitamin K1) found in our livers. Despite this, phylloquinone is the major active form of vitamin K used by our bodies—the menaquinones are not used as effectively. Menadione, being a synthetic molecule, is not normally found in our bodies except when deliberately supplemented.

Both phylloquinone and the menaquinones are fat-soluble and absorbed along with other dietary fats. Menadione (vitamin K3) is water-soluble. Phylloquinone has no known toxic effect; high doses of menadione, however, on rare occasions has caused hemolytic anemia (easily breaking blood cells) and liver toxicity. For this reason, menadione is not usually used when treating small children.

At present, supplemental sources of vitamin K are a bit hard to find. For many years, Standard Process Laboratories has made available *Chlorophyll Complex,* an all-natural plant concentrate containing a useful amount (1.1 milligrams) of vitamin K per capsule. *Vitamin K Drops* (2 milligrams per drop) are available from Scientific Botanicals. Both of these products are also available at the Tahoma Clinic dispensary (888)893-6878, www.tahoma-clinic.com, with which I am, of course, affiliated. Very recently, the Life Extension Foundation (800)544-4440, www.lef.org, has made available *Super K* (10 milligrams per softgel).

Knowing what to take

Do we really need to take a vitamin K supplement? If there's a family history of osteoporosis, definitely. There's also enough preliminary evidence to say that if there's a family history of arteriosclerosis ("hardening of the arteries"), you probably should. And of course, there are the other applications that we discussed.

How much supplemental vitamin K should you take? Fortunately, vitamins K1 and K2 are very safe; only K3 (as noted above) in enormous doses has caused problems. Except in special circumstances, 5 to 15 milligrams daily appears to be sufficient.

Caution: Vitamin K can "interfere" with the function of the drug Coumadin (an anticoagulant). (Actually, the drug Coumadin seriously interferes with the function of vitamin K, thus preventing normal blood clotting…and may cause any or all vitamin K deficiency problems, both short- and long-term…but that's a topic for another time.) **If you're taking Coumadin, DON'T take vitamin K!** It's wiser to check with a physician skilled and knowledgeable in nutritional and natural medicine to discuss alternatives to Coumadin first.

Chapter 2:

Beat unrelenting fatigue with a natural adrenal tune-up

For too many people, fatigue and weakness are constant parts of daily life. Middle-aged workers grow steadily, inexplicably worn out. Young, active, hyper-responsible (and overly stressed) individuals suddenly burn out. And, many times, they don't find the cure they need by visiting their doctor. Often, the symptoms aren't caused by the things most doctors instinctively look for, such as a malfunctioning thyroid, so the individual is left tired, weak, and lacking effective treatment.

In many cases, the mysterious cause of their fatigue lies in the adrenal gland.

We've know about hypoadrenalism since the 1800s, and successful treatment has been available since the 1930s. Yet weak adrenal gland function continues to be one of the most prevalent undiagnosed conditions. The adrenals are the primary stress-response glands in the body. If they aren't operating efficiently, severe exhaustion and other problems can result.

Many people, mostly women, suffer from this debilitating condition for literally decades without a proper diagnosis. The problem is often ignored by conventional medicine, or diagnosed incorrectly since the main symptoms—weakness, fatigue, and exercise intolerance—mirror those of many other conditions. Other symptoms of hypoadrenalism include dizziness upon standing, heart palpitations, low blood pressure, and (usually) low weight for the person's height.

The good news is that, once they have been diagnosed properly, patients suffering from hypoadrenalism can be treated with natural therapies that often lead to a full recovery. Effective treatment often involves a long list of necessary items but is usually worth the effort, as it can help individuals with weak adrenals feel considerably better in just a short time.

The following is a case history of one woman's struggle with weak adrenals and her return to a normal, energy-filled life.

Running on empty: Kathy's story

Kathy C. looked tired. Her walk was slower than most others in their 30s and even sitting down seemed to take extra effort.

"I just don't have any energy," she said. "As long as I'm careful and don't do anything extra, I can get by OK. But if I try to do a little more, there's just nothing there. Used to be if I'd get out and exercise, I'd feel better, but now I just feel worse the next day."

Kathy explained that she had battled fatigue for several years. One doctor diagnosed her with chronic fatigue syndrome, but nothing she tried seemed to help—not rest, not dietary changes, not even vitamins. Recently, Kathy began losing weight without really trying.

"I'm back to my high school weight," she said. "No matter how much I eat, I don't gain anything."

In addition to the weight loss, Kathy was also having heart palpitations and dizzy spells when she stood up quickly. She visited a cardiologist who administered an EKG, a treadmill test, and an echocardiogram, then dismissed her, saying her palpitations would pass.

After noting that Kathy's blood pressure was on the low side—98/60—I recommended that she undergo an adrenal function test. The adrenals are the body's No. 1 stress-response glands. Much like the treadmill test Kathy did to measure her heart's response to stress, an adrenal function test measures how our adrenal glands respond to a standardized stress.

The most accurate adrenal function test involves a 24-hour urine collection followed by an injection of ACTH, the hormone that stimulates the adrenal glands to respond to stress. After the ACTH injection, there is another 24-hour urine collection. The two urine collections are measured for over a dozen natural adrenal steroids and are then compared.

Combatting adrenal reserve failure

Three weeks later, Kathy was back. She looked disappointed. "I got copies of my adrenal function test results in the mail, and they both look normal. In fact, they both look pretty much the same; maybe the first one's a little bit better than the second, but they're both in the normal ranges. I guess weak adrenals aren't a problem for me after all?"

I explained that, actually, her tests fit the definition of "adrenal reserve failure" exactly. Since the adrenals are stress-response glands, they should make considerably more of each steroid hormone when stressed. Our hearts don't beat at the same rate or even a little slower after exercise than before, and our adrenals—if they are functioning properly—don't make the same amount of hormone after stress as before.

Kathy's adrenals actually made <u>less</u> hormone after the ACTH injection. At this point, weakness is a serious problem. Her adrenal glands were operating at *maximum* capacity and "going all out" just to keep her walking around. When they were called on to do more—from exercise, hard work, or the ACTH injection—they just couldn't. It was as if Kathy had her car's accelerator all the way to the floor just to maintain 35 miles an hour.

I recommended that Kathy begin immediate treatment with low-dose natural cortisol, DHEA, and salt.

An adrenal boost in your salt shaker

She looked surprised, apprehensive, and amused all at once. "Cortisol sounds a little scary, but you said salt? Just plain old salt? I thought salt is bad for us; everything I read says, 'Cut back on salt, don't eat salt.' Won't it raise my blood pressure too much?"

I smiled. "If your blood pressure were normal or a little high to begin with, it might. But starting where you are, a five- to 10-point rise in your blood pressure would be good for you and you'd likely feel better."

She admitted that she and her family had cut way back on salt about three years ago, when her husband's doctor warned him that his blood pressure was creeping up. Unfortunately, in joining her husband in salt reduction, Kathy might have worsened her own problem without knowing it. I advised her to reinstate salt as a normal part of her diet, using the maximum amount that tasted good to her.

Clearing up cortisol concerns

Next on Kathy's list was cortisol. She was somewhat concerned about this recommendation, since cortisol is a form of cortisone, and she had heard that cortisone was dangerous. Actually, cortisol is a natural substance produced by our adrenal glands and is necessary for handling stress. It can be dangerous if we take too much or if our adrenal glands make too much (though this is very rare). But Kathy's adrenal glands weren't making *enough*, and this was contributing to her exhaustion.

Adrenal help from natural hormones

From there, we moved on to DHEA. DHEA is very safe when used in amounts no greater than what our bodies ordinarily make. For women, 15 milligrams is a good place to start—so I asked Kathy to begin taking that amount each day.

Speed up the healing process with vitamins and herbs

Extra salt, cortisol, and DHEA all help to partially rest the adrenal glands so they have more energy to repair themselves. But we can help the repairs go faster with nutrients, herbs, and other supplemental items. Watching diet is important, too. Without basic good nutrition, supplements don't help nearly as much.

Kathy was one step ahead of the game in this respect: She was already following a diet consisting almost entirely of whole, unprocessed foods and very little sugar or chemicals.

She was also already taking a basic multiple vitamin, which took care of her need for vitamins A, E, and B-complex. But I recommended that she also take 1 gram of pantothenic acid twice a day and additional vitamin C, in the form of sodium ascorbate—at least 1 gram three times a day (although 2 or 3 grams three times daily is even better if it doesn't cause loose bowels or excess gas). Adrenal glands actually have the highest vitamin C content of any organ in the body, but weak adrenals need extra help.

Kathy began to look a little nervous about all the supplements she would need to take. But I told her the next item on the list might even be fun: Licorice. Licorice contains substances that slow the liver's breakdown of steroid hormones. It's like putting a dam in a river; the water builds up behind it. Kathy's own adrenal hormones would build up so that, in times of stress, they would not be depleted so quickly. Kathy was advised to look for licorice with no added artificial color or sugar and to eat six or more pieces daily.

The final items on Kathy's list were Adren-Plus, a combination of botanicals that have been shown to improve adrenal health in laboratory animals, and an adrenal glandular composed of whole dehydrated animal adrenal cortex. (The best ones come from animals raised in New Zealand without hormones, antibiotics, or any known exposure to mad cow disease.) Adrenal glandulars contain all the raw materials needed for our own adrenal cells to repair themselves. Adren-Plus and adrenal glandulars are available through the Tahoma Clinic Dispensary. Kathy was advised to take one capsule of each three times daily.

Learning to let go of hyper-responsibility

Before Kathy left, we also talked briefly about stress reduction and about learning how to deal with unavoidable stress. Many individuals I work with who have weak adrenals have done some of the damage to themselves by being "hyper-responsible," taking too much of the world's burden on themselves. The most important thing they can learn is not to impose stress on themselves.

Meditation is one technique proven to help reduce stress and improve adrenal health and many other body functions. Some people prefer that; for others, pastoral counseling or regular prayer can be very good. Kathy decided to give meditation a try.

Kathy came back in three months. She looked much better. "My old energy's back," she said. "I've been chomping at the bit to do everything I haven't been able to do, but I'm learning not to do it all at once. It is both a 'body and mind' thing, isn't it?"

Good health always is.

Chapter 3:

Test yourself for hidden food allergies just by checking your pulse and weight

One of the recommendations I make on a regular basis to Tahoma Clinic patients and to *Nutrition & Healing* readers is to have thorough allergy testing done. Over the years, I've found that hidden food allergies and sensitivities often play a major role in a person's overall health—determining them and eliminating or desensitizing to the trigger foods almost always results in a significant improvement. But I know the idea of allergy testing puts unpleasant visions of being poked and prodded for hours on end into many people's minds—not exactly an experience anyone would really be eager to have. If you've been hesitant to have clinical allergy screening done and want to be sure you really need it before you make an appointment, I have some good news: You might be able to do that just by taking your pulse.

Years ago, Dr. Arthur Coca popularized the "pulse test" for food allergy. He found that some (but definitely not all) allergic individuals have a significant increase in their resting pulse after eating a particular food allergen. Others have observed that eating certain trigger foods causes them to retain fluids, which manifests as a significant weight gain that doesn't disappear by the next morning (like most water-weight gain).

These are observations you can make on your own, right at home. To get started, get yourself a notebook that you can use to record each day's measurements, and make sure you have an accurate bathroom scale. Weigh yourself each morning and evening for several days (a week if possible) and record those numbers in the notebook. During that same week, take your resting pulse just before—and again one hour after—your largest meal of the day (and if possible before and one hour after other meals too).

At the end of the week, take a look at your measurements: A person's pulse might increase as much as eight to 20 beats or more per minute after certain meals; it's also not unusual to see 2 to 6 pound (or more) weight gain in one day. And the added "weight" can persist for two or more days. If you notice that either situation occurred in your observations, it means that you do indeed have some form of food allergy. Once you've determined that you do have food allergies, then you should go ahead and make an appointment to have complete clinical testing done to determine what specific foods are causing problems for you. The American Academy for Environmental Medicine (AAEM) is a good resource for finding a doctor in your area who can help you with testing and even desensitization to your allergens (AAEM contact information appears on page 485).

Two cautions: While either a "positive" pulse or water weight test (or both) almost always signals food allergies, "negative" tests do not necessarily mean that you don't have them. Any body system can react to food allergy: Some allergies may affect your pulse or weight, while other allergies don't affect pulse or weight at all. Also, if you just happen not to eat any of the things to which you're allergic, your self-observation will be "negative." So if you have persistent health issues that don't seem to get better no matter what you do, you should still consider having thorough screening done even if you get a negative result on your self-test.

Chapter 4:

One program, two months, lasting relief from almost any symptoms: And the older you are the better it works

There's a program we use at the Tahoma Clinic that helps a lot of the patients we see—usually in just about two months, and no matter what their symptoms are. And unlike many other treatment programs, which work better if you're younger, the percentage helped with this program increases with age: The older you are, the more likely it is to help. It's nothing flashy or high-tech. In fact, you might consider it a little boring—at least until you learn what it can do for you and your health.

This "miracle" program is nothing more than supplemental nutrients: Replacing the ones your body is missing and boosting levels of the ones it's not getting enough of.

I talk about vitamin and mineral supplements every month in *Nutrition & Healing*, but, in this case, there is a "catch": The program we use with such great success at the Tahoma Clinic uses an intravenous (IV) drip to provide these essential nutrients.

Every time I recommend IV treatments, I have some needle-shy readers and patients ask me why they can't just take oral supplements. There are a few very specific reasons why oral supplements aren't always the best option, but before we get into those, let me share how this therapy has helped my patients suffering from conditions ranging from hypertension and osteoporosis to depression and insomnia.

Quench your body's nutrient needs with the 22-ingredient "cocktail"

On her first visit, Paula D. told me that she was mildly hypertensive and had been diagnosed with hypoglycemia and insulin resistance.

To deal with this, she had previously put herself on a high-protein, low-carbohydrate diet. But in order to lose weight she'd had to eliminate all fruits and even most vegetables, which left her feeling like she wasn't getting all the nutrition she needed.

She was right: We tested Paula's blood for amino acids, her hair for minerals, and her stomach for acid production and found some unsettling—but common—results. Her stomach function was very low, and probably had been that way for several years. Her amino acid test disclosed abnormally low levels of five of the eight essential amino acids. And her hair mineral analysis showed a "malabsorption pattern." The majority of the nutrient minerals were below median—many of them quite far below.

Based on these results, I recommended the "rapid IV nutrient replacement" program to Paula. And since her gastric analysis showed that she had practically no stomach acid, which is an essential part of digesting protein as well as minerals from other foods, I recommended she take hydrochloric acid with pepsin capsules with meals from then on. I also advised her to continue taking the multiple vitamin and mineral supplement she'd been taking before, along with extra calcium and magnesium, since most people need more calcium than a once-a-week IV can accommodate.

So every week, Paula had two IV drips: One containing 14 different minerals, and another containing all eight essential amino acids. She also received intramuscular injections of vitamin B12, folic acid, and adenosine monophosphate (AMP), the immediate precursor of adenosine triphosphate (ATP), the principal "energy molecule" for every cell in our bodies.

After two months on this program, Paula came back to discuss her situation. Right away, I noticed that she looked considerably better, and she said she felt much better too.

Her blood pressure was significantly lower, her hypoglycemic symptoms were gone, she'd cut the thyroid supplement she'd taken for years from 90 to 60 milligrams daily, and she'd lost 18 pounds. She also told me she'd been able to add back in many more non-starchy vegetables and still lose weight.

"I have *much* more energy. My head's clear, and I feel more grounded. My memory's improved, I'm more focused, and I can concentrate better. Even my reading comprehension's better. I've been able to get back to walking three miles every day. I need less sleep. I'm even growing less facial hair!"

Another patient, Betty M., came to the Tahoma Clinic with problems of osteoporosis, fatigue, intermittent abdominal bloating, and lack of energy. Like Paula, Betty had hypertension, but she also had high cholesterol, high triglycerides, and a slight elevation of "hemoglobin A1C," a blood test which indicates either mild diabetes or recurrent episodes of high blood sugar preceding actual diabetes.

After her initial screenings, we discovered that Betty also had very little remaining stomach acid, and multiple low levels of essential amino acids and nutrient minerals. I recommended the rapid IV nutrient replacement program to her, along with a high-quality multiple vitamin-mineral, calcium and magnesium, and, in her case, extra strontium because of osteoporosis. I also recommended hydrochloric acid-pepsin capsules with meals.

Like Paula, Betty was considerably improved after just two months. Her energy was restored, she was sleeping better, and she reported she'd regained interest in many of the activities she'd "just stopped doing." Her blood pressure was significantly lower, and her hemoglobin A1C was now well within normal.

IV nutrients bypass your body's roadblocks

If Betty and Paula had been decidedly against needles or IV treatment, I <u>would</u> have recommended oral amino acid and mineral supplementation, along with other nutrients. An entirely oral program would definitely have helped them feel better—but progress would have been much slower. To achieve solid improvement without intravenous or injectable nutrients would most likely have taken them up to a year, or even longer. There are several reasons why:

- Even when digestion is optimal, as it usually is in a young person, no nutrient is 100 percent digested and then assimilated. The "food" your body assimilates most efficiently is, unfortunately, the worst one for you—refined sugar. But most nutrients, especially minerals, are assimilated at less than 40-50 percent efficiency. Quite often, you only assimilate 20 percent or less of the essential nutrients from what you eat. And this is if your digestion is operating completely up to par.

- In most cases, digestion <u>isn't</u> optimal, which further compounds the problem of absorbing or assimilating nutrients from your food. As we all get older, the efficiency of digestion and assimilation almost always declines, as does our vision, hearing, strength, and many other functions. This happens even when there aren't any specific digestive or absorptive defects, and, of course, it's aggravated by specific conditions such as low stomach acid (hypochlorhydria), weak pancreatic digestive function, low or absent (because of surgery) gallbladder function, and other digestive/absorptive defects.

- Not only is your own stomach working against you, but the foods you're putting in it probably aren't helping much either. Even if you avoid packaged, processed foods, the things you do eat may not be as nutritious as they should be. Unless most of your diet is organically grown, the nutrient content of nearly any food you eat is considerably less than it was for the same food a century or more ago. For example, in the 1960s, the United States Department of Agriculture (USDA) published a map showing that in 37 of the 50 (U.S.) states, agricultural soils were deficient in zinc. This is still the case for the large majority of all minerals. It takes years—even de-cades—of organic farming to restore both the quantity and avail-ability of the entire range of nutrient minerals to optimal levels.

- And on top of all that, hidden food allergies, sensitivities, and intolerances, estimated to affect over half of us, also interfere with nutrient assimilation to variable degrees.[1]

So all of these factors are standing in the way of you absorbing—ei-ther from foods or supplements—all the nutrients your body needs to be healthy and disease-free. But when nutrients are injected intravenously or intramuscularly, they bypass those roadblocks and go straight into your blood stream where they can be delivered immediately to the areas that need them. While it's true that some of them are promptly excreted again by the kidneys and liver, your body knows what it's doing, so if it really needs one or several of the supplemental nutrients, it will "hang on" to a larger proportion.

An example: Years ago, Dr. Mildred Seelig, a foremost expert on magnesium, found that magnesium-deficient individuals would rou-tinely retain more of a standard dose of magnesium given intravenously than individuals not deficient in magnesium. And it's well known that minerals of all sorts are stored away in our bones, where they can stay for literally decades, to be used as needed.

Other factors to consider when digestion isn't the issue

The majority of people who respond to rapid IV nutrient replace-ment have developed low levels of multiple essential amino acids and minerals because of poor stomach function. But there are other causes of nutrient maldigestion and malbsorption, too.

For example, Jim K. came to the Tahoma Clinic with fatigue, anxiety, digestive upset, and depression. He'd seen several mainstream physicians over the prior few years, and the last one had given him a prescription for a patented antidepressant. Although the antidepressant had lessened his depression, he also experienced some of its adverse effects, including decreased libido.

As I mentioned a few months ago in the May issue, most individuals who "respond" to patented antidepressants actually have low levels of essential amino acids, so I recommended that Jim have his levels measured, along with a hair mineral analysis and gastric analysis.

Seven of the eight essential amino acids were low, along with the large majority of his minerals, so I expected that his gastric analysis would be abnormal, too. To my surprise, it was almost normal. We discussed Jim's personal history and family history further, and based on our conversation we decided he should have a blood test done for gluten/gliadin (two sub-fractions of grain protein) intolerance. This test came back quite positive.

I recommended that Jim see the Tahoma Clinic nutritionist to help with planning a totally gluten- and gliadin-free diet program. But since his amino acid and mineral tests had been so poor, I also recommended the rapid IV nutrient replacement program. As with Paula and Betty, I also recommended he continue taking a multiple vitamin and mineral, along with a fish oil high in EPA and DHA, which would help target his symptoms of depression (supplements of these essential fatty acids have been linked to lessening depression in many studies).

Three weeks after eliminating all gluten and gliadin and following the injectable nutrient program, Jim observed a definite improvement in his digestive symptoms, along with a significant lessening of fatigue and anxiety. He said he thought his depression was less, too. At our consultation following the completion of the two-month program, he reported "plenty of energy," and no anxiety. He was eager to start tapering off his patent medicine antidepressant, which he did successfully (working with his doctor, of course) over the next few weeks.

So individual problems or factors like Jim's gluten intolerance can also play a major role in your body's ability to absorb nutrients. Diet and lifestyle choices can also impact your nutrient levels, as I encountered when Leslie N. came to the Tahoma Clinic.

Leslie said she'd felt poorly for many years: Her energy was very low, she had chronic insomnia, and she "just felt out of sorts." Because of her insomnia, I recommended she have the blood test done for essential amino acids. The test returned with all eight essential amino acids below normal.

I suspected that I knew the reason: Like a small percentage of individuals I work with, Leslie was a strict vegan (eating no animal products of any kind). We checked her minerals with the hair test and also extended the testing to other nutrients. Leslie's results were consistent with what I've observed in other vegans: In addition to low amino acids, she was low in iron, zinc, vitamin B12, and other nutrients found in higher quantities in animal proteins, which, as a vegan, Leslie had completely eliminated from her diet.

I have a great deal of respect for those who choose this diet option; it usually reflects a great deal of thought given to the meaning of life and our role in it. But when it results in clearly sub-optimal health, I have an obligation to discuss it with the affected individual.

So I presented Leslie with two options: She could continue as a vegan and supplement with all the nutrients she wasn't getting enough of, or she could consider including small amounts of animal protein not derived from killing animals, such as unfertilized eggs. She said she would need time to think it over, so in the meantime, I recommended the rapid IV nutrient replacement program, which is not derived from animal sources. I also recommended she take a "vegan-friendly" high potency vitamin-mineral supplement.

After the two-month program, she reported she "felt like a new person." Her energy was back, insomnia gone, and she was doing things she'd postponed doing for years.

Can you afford to do it?
Can you afford not to?

The combination of amino acids is available through routine IV material suppliers and compounding pharmacies as "Freamine," as are vitamin B12, folic acid, and AMP, which I gave to Paula as part of her program. A caution about adenosine monophosphate (AMP): It should *not* be given intravenously except in very special circumstances, and this program is no exception. It should only be given intramuscularly under a physician's supervision.

The 14-mineral combination (called a "comprehensive re-mineralization IV") is one I've worked with at Tahoma Clinic for over 20 years. It's available to your physician through McGuff Compounding Pharmacy Services in Santa Ana, California (800-854-7220; www.mcguffpharmacy.com).

The major drawback to the rapid IV replacement program is cost. Including their administration, the intravenous amino acids and minerals add up to over $1,900, and the injectable vitamin B12, folic acid, and adenosine monophosphate add up to a little less than $100 for the two-month program. There's also the time involved with intravenous administration; usually it's one or two trips to a clinic a week for two months.

However, there's no arguing with the results. With oral supplements alone, it routinely takes considerably longer, often over a year, to achieve results. But with the IV program, improvement is almost always substantial and quick, occurring in just two months.

And as long as you correct or compensate for any other factors (hypochlorhydria or gluten intolerance, for example), the results are usually permanent. Occasionally, someone does have to come back in for more IV sessions if, for some reason, he or she hasn't been able to stick to the recommended follow-up program. The need for follow-up or additional

IV treatments is more likely in the 75-80+ age group, but it can happen.

Maintenance generally involves taking more than just a multi-vitamin/mineral, since most folks do come in with specific problems that require support from an individualized group of supplements. Plus, we often work with patients to tailor a program of numerous "anti-aging" supplements too. But once the two-month IV program is completed, these and any other necessary supplements can just be taken orally.

If you want to explore rapid intravenous nutrient replacement with your doctor, make sure that she or he is skilled and knowledgeable in nutritional and other natural therapies. If you need a list of natural medicine physicians in your area, contact one of the organizations listed in the "Alternative Health Resources" section on page 485.

Chapter 5:

Send even the most stubborn infections—cold sores, toenail fungus, and more— into hiding for good

No matter what type it is or where it's located on your body, there's one thing that you can count on with any skin infection: It's not going to be pleasant—or pretty. These sorts of infections can leave you with itchy, pus-filled blisters, painful, scabby lesions, and thick, yellowed nails. And those are some of the more basic symptoms. Unfortunately, left untreated, it can get even worse.

But as is the case with eczema, skin infections are another instance where topical use of herbs—four in particular—can be a godsend, offering relief just as effective as any patented drug, and in some cases, even faster.

From the Outback to your toenails

Let's start with one you may have heard of already: Tea tree oil. It's made from a plant native to Australia (in fact, we can thank the aborigines for its contribution to herbal medicine), and in recent years it has become more well known as an addition to various cosmetics. But tea tree oil also has powerful antifungal and antimicrobial properties.

Numerous studies have shown that local application of tea tree oil can be very effective against fungal infections of both the nails and skin. In one double-blind, randomized, controlled trial, 117 patients with toe-nail fungus used either tea tree oil or a solution containing 1 percent of the antifungal drug clotrimazole twice a day for six months. At the end of the trial the tea-tree-oil group experienced relief just as significant as the clotrimazole group.[1]

In another double-blind, randomized, placebo-controlled trial, 104 patients with a fungal infection of the foot called tinea pedis used either a solution containing 10-percent tea tree oil, one containing 1 percent of the antifungal medication tolnaftate, or a placebo cream. Unlike the drug group, tea-tree-oil-treated patients didn't experience complete eradication of the fungus at the end of therapy. However, both the tea-tree-oil group and the tolnaftate group showed clinical improvement in symptoms such as scaling, inflammation, itching, and burning compared to participants in the control group. So the tea tree oil appeared to improve the symptoms but not remove the fungal cause.[2] There were no adverse reactions reported.

I would venture to guess that the tea tree oil cream used in this trial was too weak, because another placebo-controlled trial found that a cream using a stronger concentration of tea tree oil _was_, in fact, able to cure tinea. In this particular study, a 50-percent solution produced the best healing effect, although about 8 percent of the subjects using it did encounter a mild rash from the high concentration of oil.[3] So for tea tree oil, the stronger the solution or cream the more effective it is at killing infections, but also the higher the risk of an adverse skin reaction.

Tea tree oil also works for a condition that all too many women battle on a regular basis: Yeast infections. In one study, 28 with chronic vaginal infections due to a strain of yeast called *Candida albicans* received vaginal capsules containing 0.02g tea tree oil in gelatin for daily use over 90 days. After one month, 75 percent of the patients were completely healed, and only one patient experienced any side effects (in this case, vaginal burning).[4]

Other studies have shown that the results from tea tree oil are as good as those from the standard drug suppositories sold in pharmacies for yeast infections, without causing irritation, burning, or other side effects.[5]

What you can do when life gives you lemons— and cold sores

The next herbal infection fighter on our list is one that's a little less well-known: Lemon balm. But creams containing it can be very effective for relieving the cold sores brought on by the oral form of the herpes simplex virus (Type 1). In fact, one study found an improved healing rate for 75 percent of patients using lemon balm, as well as an increased time between outbreaks in 50 percent of cases. Compared to conventional treatments the average healing time of lesions was halved to about five days and the time between outbreaks was approximately doubled.[6]

In another multicenter study on 115 patients, 87 percent of the participants using lemon balm were completely healed within 6 days of treatment. And 69 percent of these patients had an extended time between outbreaks that was a full month longer than those using conventional drug treatment.[7]

In a more recent clinical trial, 66 patients with recurrent herpes-related cold sore outbreaks were treated with either the lemon balm cream or a placebo. The cream was applied to the affected area four times a day for five days. Compared to the placebo, symptoms were significantly reduced by the second day, which is important because this is around the time when symptoms are typically at their worst.[8]

Since these studies found that lemon balm cream effectively lengthened the time between outbreaks, it's reasonable to assume that it might also be able to prevent outbreaks altogether—or at least increase the time between breakouts even more—if it's applied regularly to cold-sore-prone areas.

Lemon balm cream can also be used to treat herpes simplex Type II infection, and probably other similar viral skin infections including shingles. (A technical note: If you decide to try this approach, the creams used in the studies contained 1 percent of a concentrated 70:1 extract of lemon balm.)

Two "garden-variety" herbs take on big-name herpes medication

Rounding out our list are two herbs, rhubarb root and sage, that have been pitted head-to-head against one of the most recognized herpes medications—Zovirax (acyclovir).

In a double-blind, controlled trial involving 49 patients using creams containing either 2.3 percent sage, 2.3 percent sage and 2.3 percent rhubarb, or Zovirax, the average time for the herpes sores to fully heal was 7.6 days with the sage cream, 6.7 days with the rhubarb-sage cream and 6.5 days for acyclovir.[9]

So while Zovirax had a slight advantage over the sage cream, the herbal combination worked just as well—without the side effects associated with the drug.

Chapter 6:

Harnessing the healing power of light

Part I: What you need to know about UV rays—beyond sunburn

Despite what the sun-screen industry would like us to believe, the drastic increase in use of these lotions and potions over the past several decades hasn't made a big impact in skin cancer rates. But what it *has* done is made people afraid of ultraviolet (UV) light. While it's true too much radiation from the sun can result in skin damage (not to mention a painful sunburn), those harmful effects are hardly the extent of what UV radiation is capable of—and its potential benefits far outweigh the risks.

As you've read in these pages numerous times, UV rays from the sun are the best source of the vitamin D your body needs to ward off cancer and dozens of other health problems. But that's just the beginning of what ultraviolet light can do.

Not only is it an extremely effective disinfectant with the ability to kill bacteria, viruses, and fungi in the air and on surfaces,[1-3] but UV light also has the potential to prevent—and even cure—infections and diseases that other treatments are powerless against.

A strong history leads to an even more promising future

Using ultraviolet light as a medical treatment may sound like a new technology, but the medical use of ultraviolet light for the prevention and treatment of disease is not at all a new area of research. This form of therapy has been studied since the late 19th century, when researchers first experimented with UV light in patients with lupus and sepsis. In fact, back in 1903, a Danish physician named Niels Ryberg Finsen won a Nobel prize for his work with UV light and the treatment of disease.

There are even a few forms of ultraviolet light therapy that "mainstream" medicine uses. Ultraviolet radiation can eliminate or reduce pathogens floating in the air. This process is called air ultraviolet germicidal irradiation, or UVGI. UVGI is an important technology in many hospitals, research centers, and laboratories where contamination with bacteria and fungal spores poses a serious health risk.[4,5] One recent study evaluated the infection rate in an operating room in which total joint replacements had been performed over a 19-year period. Infection rates were three times higher when only regular (laminar) airflow was used as compared to an ultraviolet light plus laminar airflow system. The UV lowered the number of bacteria in the entire environment, thereby reducing the infection rate, rather than just reducing the number of infectious organisms present at the surgical site.[6] The researchers concluded that UV light is a very effective means of lowering the rate of infection during total joint replacement therapy.

The most common form of UV light therapy used by the mainstream for treatment purposes is probably for psoriasis. UV radiation works well for this condition because it penetrates the skin and slows the abnormal rate of skin cell growth.[7,8] It's also commonly used to treat acute tissue rejection in patients who have had heart transplants.[9] And in 1988, the FDA even "approved" UV light therapy for the treatment of a form of non-Hodgkin lymphoma called cutaneous T-cell lymphoma.[10]

But despite these mainstream uses, UV light therapy is still considered "experimental" and "investigational" (or even "quackery") for many of the healthcare problems affecting people all over the globe. The application that seems to be the most controversial is ultraviolet blood irradiation.

Blood irradiation was developed in the 1920s, when a piece of equipment called the "ultraviolet blood irradiation (UVBI) device" was created to irradiate blood "extracorporeally" or outside of the body. UVBI was developed for medical use by an engineer, Emmet K. Knott and Virgil Hancock, M.D., and was used early in the 20th century to treat many types of diseases, including a wide variety of infections, many of them otherwise fatal. When antibiotics and vaccines were developed in the late 1940s and early 1950s, UVBI was almost completely set aside, even though a number of diseases, including hepatitis, streptococcal toxemia, and viral pneumonia, actually responded better to UVBI therapy than to antibiotics and vaccines, and even though UVBI was repeatedly described as quite safe in multiple publications.

With the rise in antibiotic resistant strains of bacteria and the growing interest in therapies that are less toxic, there is a reviving interest in UVBI as a therapy against infection. Even though it's vastly underutilized, UVBI is still available here in these United States, and has remained a very important treatment modality in Russia and other countries, where many "modern" studies of its effectiveness have been conducted. So this month, we'll cover the "modern" research, almost all reported since 1990, demonstrating that UV is "still" effective treatment for many problems.

Help your body create its own, internal vaccine

UVBI also goes by the terms light therapy, phototherapy, photophoresis, and photoluminescence. It uses UV light of varying wavelengths to destroy blood-borne pathogens, as well as to treat diseases not clearly linked to specific pathogens, and to improve general health. During a session, a small amount of blood, ranging from 60-250 cc, is withdrawn from a patient and sent through a chamber where it is irradiated with specific frequencies of UV light (since certain frequencies have different effects), and is then reintroduced into the body. This creates a kind of self-generated vaccine that can have many beneficial effects.

UVBI treatments sometimes include the addition of other compounds, either before or after irradiation. This combination therapy has been termed "photodynamic antimicrobial chemo-therapy, or PACT. PACT is used along with UV light to inhibit pathogens in blood products.[11] Conventional medicine has even embraced one form of PACT that involves exposing blood with-drawn from a patient's body to UV radiation and a substance called 8-methoxypsoralen (8-MOP). This is the form of UV therapy used to treat cutaneous T-cell lymphoma, as well as systemic sclerosis and several other inflammatory conditions.[12,13]

But "alternative" physicians, especially those who've read the older research, often accompany or follow UVBI therapy with hydrogen peroxide, which acts as a "synergist" to increase the effectiveness of UVBI.

While not all the mechanisms of action of UVBI are understood (some aren't even guessed at yet), research has found that it increases the oxygenation of the blood,[14] increases important blood markers that indicate healing, and inactivates viral, fungal, and bacterial toxins, including botulism and diphtheria toxins. It also improves chemical balances and cell permeability. And what makes UVBI even more impressive is that it not only begins working after just one treatment, but the effects are cumulative and persist for some time after each treatment session.

Several animal studies have demonstrated these quick, long-lasting effects. For example, when a group of horses that had been exposed to the anthrax virus had their blood treated, investigators noted increased hemoglobin content as well as red and white blood cell counts. An important measurement of inflammation, the erythrocyte sedimentation rate (ESR), increased after the first hour and remained elevated until the fourth day, and returned to normal after six days—but none of the horses "came down" with anthrax. The UVBI apparently stimulated the destruction of the infectious organisms.[15]

Light as air: UVBI offers major benefits for chronic lung disorders

One of the most important uses for UVBI in humans is in the treatment of lung diseases, including asthma, COPD, and bronchitis. In one study of chronic bronchitis, patients who were given UVBI treatments every two to three days experienced significantly more improvement than the control group that received only conventional therapy.[16]

UV blood irradiation even has positive effects in patients with chronic forms of tuberculosis, which are notoriously difficult to treat.[17] But following UVBI therapy, patients experienced reductions in their clinical symptoms, and increases in one of the standard measurements of breathing capacity called forced expiratory volume (FEV). They also had decreased levels of the bacterial pathogen, Mycobacteria tuberculosis, and improved markers of overall blood health (hematological indices).[18]

Studies have also shown that UVBI helps alleviate the inflammation of the trachea and bronchial tubes ("tracheobronchitis") that often occurs after tracheostomy surgery (the creation of a new opening for air entry into the trachea at the base of the neck).[19]

No job too big

High blood pressure is still one of many people's primary concerns. You may be surprised to learn that UVBI can help bring blood pressure levels back to normal ranges. In one study, arterial blood pressure in hypertensive patients who underwent five to seven sessions of UVBI dropped an average of 24 percent from initial levels. The general health of patients also improved and the clinical effect persisted for four to eight months, on average. Blood pressure isn't the only aspect of cardiovascular health of which to be aware, and UVBI certainly isn't the only natural treatment that can help alleviate hypertension, but researchers suggest that it may be a beneficial addition to other therapeutic measures for the treatment of cardiovascular disease.[20]

While UVBI is a good addition to the other effective natural treat-

Breathe easier without the blood

If you have asthma or other breathing difficulties but the thought of blood irradiation leaves you a bit squeamish, less-invasive forms of UV light therapy may still help. One animal study evaluated the ability of UV-B rays to induce airway immunity. A group of mice were exposed to enough of a dose of UV-B radiation to cause skin redness. Several days later, the researchers induced airway allergies in the mice. The results of the study demonstrated that UV-B radiation effectively reduced airway hyper-responsiveness to the allergens, suggesting it as a possible therapy for asthma and other inflammatory diseases of the respiratory system.[21]

Another recent study involving a small group of mold-sensitized asthmatic children looked at the effectiveness of UV irradiation units installed in their homes' central heating and cooling systems. The UV irradiation of home air was found to be effective in reducing airway hyper-responsiveness and other clinical symptoms, and is a promising therapy for the treatment of allergic asthma.[22]

ments for hypertension, there are very few treatments—natural or otherwise—that are effective for terminal kidney (renal) failure. But in one study in which patients with chronic renal failure were treated with UVBI, immune function was stimulated, a low white blood cell count was corrected, and patients demonstrated overall improvement.[23]

Making cancer treatments safer

As I mentioned earlier, UV light therapy has been used successfully as a treatment for cutaneous T-cell lymphoma, a type of cancer that is generally very resistant to chemo-therapy and radiation. But this isn't the only cancer application for UVBI. It also helps combat some of the negative effects of traditional chemotherapy and some of the hazards associated with cancer surgery.

In one study, patients undergoing chemotherapy which had caused a significant drop in their red blood cell counts had 200 ml of blood removed, then irradiated, and immediately returned to them. The red blood cell counts returned to normal.[24]

During surgery, patients of course lose blood, and surgeons try to recover some of it to give back before the surgery is over. This process is called "intra-operative blood salvage." But during cancer surgery, the lost blood could be contaminated by cancer cells, so surgeons are hesitant to salvage it. In one study (done "*in vitro*," not on a living patient) using a number of cancer cell lines and tumor preparations, researchers irradiated salvaged blood to see if the process could eliminate the potential for cancer cells to spread. Following irradiation of tumor-cell-contaminated blood, even though cancer cells were still present, there were no signs of them spreading. The authors of this study concluded that there was a clinical basis for using UVBI during surgery as a means of salvaging useable blood.[25] A later study using intra-operative blood salvaged by using UVBI confirmed these results and concluded that UVBI is an important way to save blood resources while avoiding cancer cell spread and the necessity for transfusion, which carries its own set of risks.[26]

And speaking of risks associated with blood transfusions, results of a recent study showed that UV light combined with amotosalen (a synthetic but relatively safe version of naturally occurring plant com-pounds called "psoralens" found in figs, celery, parsley, and other plants) could inactivate parvovirus B19, a virus that may be transmitted through blood transfusions but, until now, evaded attempts to disable it.[27]

Germ-killing with UV

In addition to all the benefits we've gone over so far, ultraviolet light is also particularly effective in killing antibiotic resistant strains of bacteria, which are a serious and increasing problem in many hospitals and other healthcare facilities these days.[28,29] And like the asthma treatments mentioned in the sidebar on the previous page, UV light therapies for these forms of potentially deadly bacteria are done without withdrawing blood from patients. In one study patients with chronic body-surface ulcers were treated using a lamp that emitted ultraviolet C (UV-C) light, held about an inch away from the wound site. After just one 180-second treatment, there were significant reductions in all types of bacteria, most notably *Pseudomonas aeruginosa*, as well as *methicillin-resistant S. aureus* (MRSA), which has been making headlines worldwide recently. A second study of the effects of UV light treatment on antibiotic-resistant strains of *S. aureus* and *Enterococcus faecalis* showed similar results with exposures as little as 5 seconds.[30] These results confirm other studies showing that UV-C can kill many types of bacteria present in superficial, chronic wounds.

When UV light is applied at the site of an infection it inactivates pathogens by creating something I'm normally warning you to avoid: Free radicals. But, in this case, free radicals are a good thing, since they're causing oxidative damage to the invading organisms, not to your internal organs.[31]

As you've seen, all of this modern research has shown UV light and UVBI to be a safe and effective (not to mention inexpensive) treatment with rapid clinical response for a wide variety of acute and chronic conditions. But conventional medicine still hasn't gotten around to employing it as often as it should, as was done with great success (and reported in many, many peer-reviewed professional journals) in the 1920s through the 1950s. In 2008, UVBI therapy is done almost entirely by physicians—including Tahoma Clinic physicians—skilled in natural and nutritional medicine, as well as intravenous (IV) therapies (see "Alternative Health Resources," page 485.) But with the ever-increasing spread of antibiotic-resistant micro-organisms, it's well past time "conventional" medicine goes "back to the future" and starts using this long-ago-proven therapy. The UV-treated conditions we covered in this chapter—all but one reported in the past two decades and the majority since the year 2000—are just the tip of the proverbial iceberg when it comes to UVBI's healing potential.

In Part II, I'll tell you about those research reports published right here in these United States from the 1920s through the 1950s documenting the use and effectiveness of UV light and UVBI to safely and effectively treat tens of thousands of humans with infections, including viral pneumonia, staphylococcal septicemia (serious, often fatal systemic staph infection), polio, erysipelas (streptococcal skin infection), puerperal sepsis (an often fatal infection also termed "childbirth fever"), staphylococcal skin infection (furunculosis), paralytic ileus (paralysis of the bowel after surgery), and thrombophlebitis (vein inflammation followed by blood clot). You'll also read about UV light's benefits for more common conditions like rheumatoid arthritis, herpes, psoriasis, and diabetes.

Thanks to Lauren Russel N.D. for her organization and summary of the data I collected for this chapter.

Part II: Time-tested strategies for beating superbugs and more of today's deadliest health threats

In Part I you read about the benefits of ultraviolet light—and not just the vitamin-D-producing effects we generally associate with the sun's rays. While vitamin D production is certainly one of its critical functions, ultraviolet (UV) radiation goes way beyond that.

Let's take a step back and look at the beginnings of this time-tested therapy and how—despite what mainstream naysayers would like you to believe—it has remained a highly effective tool for fighting a vast array of health problems, from everyday ailments like asthma and arthritis to deadly infections like pneumonia and cancer.

The makings of a modern-day miracle

Niels Ryberg Finsen, a Danish physician and scientist, is considered to be the founder of modern "phototherapy," the technical term for treating disease using ultraviolet light. When his own health started to fail, Finsen became interested in the bacteria-destroying effects of sunlight. This led him to develop ultraviolet treatment for a form of tuberculosis that affects the skin, known as lupus vulgaris. Finsen's UV therapy for lupus vulgaris had a 98 percent success rate[1] and in 1903, he was awarded the Nobel Prize in Medicine and Physiology "in recognition of his contribution to the treatment of diseases, especially lupus vulgaris, with concentrated light radiation, whereby he has opened a new avenue for medical science."[2] His work created a basis for the ultraviolet sterilization techniques still used today in bacteriological research and radiation therapy.

Building on Finsen's work with lupus vulgaris, one of the earliest areas of research into UV therapy was its effects on skin infections. One of the earliest pioneers of UV therapy was Dr. Walter H. Ude, who successfully treated a potentially serious streptococcal skin infection called erysipelas. In nearly 100 cases, he reported a 100-percent cure rate using ultraviolet irradiation.[3]

Research into the use of external irradiation continued, focusing on mumps, which was very common among school-age children at the time. But UV light prevented the most severe complications associated with mumps. And, like many of the other applications we'll go over, mumps patients often responded after just one treatment.

Although it wasn't the first time UV radiation had been used internally, the most successful transition from external use of ultraviolet light to blood irradiation was made by a Seattle-area physicist named Emmett K. Knott, who developed and patented a treatment he called "photoluminescence." This form of treatment took advantage of the bacteria-killing properties of ultraviolet radiation by directly irradiating the blood stream to kill microorganisms. In 1928, Knott used photoluminescence to treat his first patient, who was suffering from a severe systemic infection (septicemia) following an abortion. (For centuries, "childbirth fever"—the same sort of systemic infection but following childbirth—was a major cause of death for young women.) By the time she received UV therapy, the woman's condition had deteriorated to the point where she was considered beyond the help of medicine. But after her blood was irradiated and re-introduced into her body, she made a full recovery. Later on, she was able to have a healthy child, despite nearly dying of septicemia.[4]

Knott and another Seattle-area doctor, obstetrician Dr. Virgil K. Hancock, went on to publish their accounts of UV therapy in 1934. It was the first article on the efficacy of what eventually came to be known by the term we use today, ultraviolet blood irradiation (UVBI) for treating infection.[5]

By 1942, Hancock and Knott had successfully treated 6,520 patients using UVBI without any harmful effects whatsoever. Their pioneering work was pivotal to fostering understanding of how this method could be used to treat bloodstream infections and cure many patients thought incurable by conventional medicine.

What happens during UVBI?

But besides providing the basis for today's research and understanding of UV therapy, Knott and Hancock also created a very simple process for conducting their UVBI treatment. Using a syringe, a small amount of blood (approximately 300ccs, 10 to 11 ounces) was drawn from the vein of a patient, a natural anti-clotting agent was added, and the blood was then passed through a machine that irradiated it using ultraviolet light at a specific frequency for about 10 seconds. The flow of blood was then reversed with the syringe and re-injected into the patient. Treatments ranged from one single irradiation to a series of treatments if necessary, but usually no more than two were performed per patient in any given day.

Acute conditions, like colds, pneumonia, toxic conditions, and viral diseases generally responded to treatment within a few hours and usually required only one or two treatments. Chronic conditions were treated once or twice a day for up to three times a week, except for two conditions—atopic dermatitis and porphyria. Hydrogen peroxide is typically administered at the end of each treatment to improve the effectiveness of

---

Even more weapons in Mother Nature's arsenal against infectious bacteria, viruses, and fungi

While UVBI is the best researched and reported, it's only one of our defenses against "supergerms." There's also considerable research on the effectiveness of silver as a germ-killer, and—like UVBI—silver kills bacteria, viruses, and fungi without inducing resistance. Then there's intravenous ozone, also a "non-discriminate" germicide. And these are only three of many more potential tools.

So when the news reports proclaim the arrival of the Grim Reaper in the form of antibiotic-resistant bacteria, rest assured that Mother Nature can—and will—come to the rescue for those of us smart enough to turn to her for help.

UVBI.[6,7] (A more detailed account of that protocol can be found in the book *Into the Light*, by William Campbell Douglass, M.D.)

Like Emmett Knott, Dr. E.W. Rebbeck used UVBI for patients experiencing septicemia (systemic infection) following childbirth and abortion. While many of his patients were near death when they came to him at Shadyside hospital in Pennsylvania, all of them recovered following UVBI treatment. And in over 4,000 treatments he administered, he observed no adverse effects at all.[8]

Dr. Rebbeck's results were so outstanding that Shadyside Hospital established UVBI as a standard *preventive* treatment, rather than using it just to treat already septic cases.[9]

While polio is rare these days, it was a major health threat when this early research into UVBI was going on. Another physician, Dr. George Miley, and his colleague Dr. Christensen reported that in the 58 cases of polio they treated with UVBI, they only lost one patient. All other patients, ranging from those with mild to severe disease, improved significantly within 24-48 hours.[10]

Dr. Miley also demonstrated that UVBI was an extremely effective therapy for viral pneumonia. His patients experienced improvement within 24-76 hours, elimination of cough in one week or less, and complete clearing of the lungs (confirmed by chest x-rays) within 24-96 hours. And all of this resulted from only one UVBI treatment.[11]

Ironically, in 2008, "mainstream medicine" still has no reliably effective treatment for viral pneumonia, but continues to criticize UVBI as "quackery."

Arthritis, asthma, shingles, and more: UVBI shows promise against "everyday" problems too

Early research into the applications and benefits of UVBI suggested that it might be useful in the treatment of many common health conditions too. Clinical studies following up on these claims have shown promising results in the treatment of several autoimmune disorders, including scleroderema, rheumatoid arthritis, and organ rejection.[12-14] Other studies have been conducted into its effectiveness in the treatment of type 1 diabetes and multiple sclerosis.[15,16]

Dr. Miley, who pioneered the use of UVBI for pneumonia, also used UV therapy to treat cases of asthma that showed no improvement despite elimination and desensitization of all possible allergens and only temporary relief (or none at all} following the injection or inhalation of adrenaline (cases like this are technically referred to as "intractable" asthma). Of the 56 intractable asthma patients he treated with UVBI, 45—that's 80 percent—showed definite improvement, and they maintained the improvement for up to a year.[17,18]

In Into the Light, Dr. Douglass reports his experience with UVBI treatment of asthma. He points out that individuals with severe asthma are likely to have an asthma attack after the first UVBI treatment, but after the second or third treatment there is often marked decrease in the frequency and severity of attacks. But aside from the initial worsening, he reports (like all the other researchers) a complete absence of any toxic effects of UVBI.[19,20]

In the 1930s and 1940s, Dr. Miley also treated 11 patients with very resistant boils caused by a bacteria that's still causing problems for many people today, *Staphlyococcus aureus*. But after two to four treatments, most of Dr. Miley's patients experienced a reduction in the number and rate of recurrence of boils.[21]

He also reported that UVBI worked well for patients struggling with cases of shingles that conventional methods had been unable to alleviate.[22]

Poison control goes back to basics

Many of the early researchers focused their attention on the ability of sunlight and UV radiation to detoxify certain poisonous substances like the toxins produced in botulism, tetanus, and even snake venom.

In one notable case, Dr. Miley reported that a patient dying from the effects of botulism and unable to see or swallow recovered within 48 hours after treatment. She was able to leave the hospital within two weeks after a single UVBI treatment.[23]

Miley also observed that UVBI-treated patients with peritonitis, an infection and inflammation of the intestinal lining, showed signs of recovery within less than 35 hours, and complete recovery within 82 hours following treatment. And he reported that patients suffering from appendicitis recovered completely in less than two days.[24]

The amazing thing about these reports is that most of the results were achieved after only one treatment. Among those patients treated by Miley at Hahnemann Hospital in Philadelphia was another patient with serious blood poisoning following abortion that antibiotic therapy had failed to control.[25] Prior to treatment with UVBI, the patient was near death. Within 48 hours of treatment, however, she was no longer in a morbid state.[26] She subsequently made a complete recovery.

Miley also treated another patient who was in a state of systemic infection and profound shock, including irregular heartbeat, following removal of a gangrenous appendix. Within *minutes* after the patient's UVBI-treated blood was returned to his body, he improved significantly and all signs of shock—including the irregular heartbeat—were substantially diminished. By the next day, the patient was able to sit up in bed and function normally. Although he needed two more UVBI treatments to eliminate all toxic symptoms, he also made a complete recovery.[27]

In yet another amazing case, a patient with pelvic abscess and steady decline despite antibiotic therapy was detoxified within 72 hours of receiving blood irradiation therapy. She was given a UVBI treatment prior to undergoing surgery to remove the pelvic infection and recovered without any side effects.[28]

Making UV light even more effective against cancer

In previous issues of *Nutrition & Healing*, you read about combining

UV radiation with other substances. These compounds are called photosensitizers. While this concept has been understood and applied since the 1800s, the most recent example is the combination using UV radiation along with a compound called 8-methoxyopsoralen (8-MOP) that comes from a plant that grows along the Nile to treat T-cell lymphoma.[29]

While photosensitizers aren't necessary to achieve good results from UVBI treatment, they do improve its effectiveness.[30] The use of photosensitizers in the treatment of cancer, for example, can improve treatment outcome since the rapidly dividing cancer cells absorb more of the photosensitizer compound. Then, when the blood is irradiated, more of the cancer cells will contain the photosensitized compound and be killed by the light.

One of the first researchers to investigate UVBI for treating cancer was Dr. Robert C. Olney. In five cases of cancer treated with UVBI using the UV-A light, he reported a 100-percent recovery rate.[31]

Since Dr. Olney's early work, UVBI has been used to treat early and advanced lung cancer, advanced esophageal cancer, early and advanced head and neck cancers, and ocular cancers.[32-34]

Exactly how UVBI works is a mystery, but the results are real

UVBI appears to work by stimulating the body's immune defenses, but exactly how it does this still hasn't been identified. Some researchers have theorized that perhaps humans may be susceptible to an "ultraviolet light deficiency." And based on the cancer- and infection-fighting effects it has, it does seem possible that UVBI could correct an underlying vitamin D deficiency (which increases the risk of a vast array of health problems). Of course, it's likely that UV light has many more effects in addition to stimulating vitamin D synthesis, but this aspect could play a role in its success.

But regardless of knowing exactly how UVBI works, all of the research done since the 1920s shows that it does work. In case after case of serious and life-threatening acute infections treated with UVBI therapy at Hahnemann and other hospitals, Dr. Miley reported that his patients all recovered without ill effects.[35-40]

The same is true of the subsequent research as well: Most physicians using UVBI have noted that, within 12-24 hours after treatment, patients usually experienced a reduction in headache, nausea, chills, fever and other symptoms of toxicity. And most go on to full recovery following as little as one treatment.

Whatever happened to UVBI?

As you've seen from all these case studies, UVBI had two decades (late 1930s through early 1950s) of proven effectiveness in the treatment of serious infection, often relieving symptoms within hours of treatment. Success after success was reported in dozens of medical journals, both "major" and "minor," by responsible investigators and practicing physicians. UVBI was in use in hospitals and clinics alike, and no harmful effects were observed in tens of thousands of treatments. The overwhelming majority of bacterial infections were eliminated, and viruses yielded to UVBI too. Even fungal disease was improved.

So why did a treatment with such an outstanding record of success just "disappear"? Whatever happened to UVBI?

Antibiotics are what happened. Antibiotics "got off the ground" during World War II (1941-1945 for these United States) and did indeed save the lives of many soldiers and airmen suffering from infections that occurred after being injured. Although many antibiotics (like penicillin) were actually derived from Nature (penicillin from a mold), the average bacteria had never seen them before in such quantity and with such frequency. Bacteria had no defenses against this never-before-seen antibiotic onslaught, and anti- biotics became "lethal weapons" against bacteria: One infection after another gave up and died. Not only that, but it was undeniably much easier to swallow tablets or capsules than to have an intravenous procedure, however effective it might be. The "golden age" of successful bacteria fighting was proclaimed and UVBI was "obsolete," (not to mention that it was no longer covered by patents from the 1920s and 30s).

But bacteria are living things, and living things don't like being killed. Living things usually find a way to survive, even when their numbers are greatly reduced at first. When they're forced to learn new ways by affliction and hardship, surviving living things frequently emerge much stronger than they've ever been, more ready than ever to do battle, and this time, more likely to win.

That is exactly what has happened with bacteria and antibiotics in the 21st century. By now, everyone has heard of—and many are very afraid of—"supergerms," bacteria resistant to nearly all types of antibiotics. Medical "authorities," *los Federales*, and the media all tell us that we have almost no defenses against these supergerms.

But we do! Regardless of main-stream skepticism, UVBI is still one of our best defenses against super-germs. And even though they've "fallen out of fashion," so to speak, UVBI treatments have continued to be done by many alternative medical practitioners. Unfortunately, present-day "conventional" practitioners now view UVBI as "quackery." In fact, back in 2006, our old "friend," the Washington State Medical "Quality" Assurance Commission (M"Q"AC) launched an investigation of the Tahoma Clinic just for mentioning of UVBI on Clinic's website. (Ironically, this investigation took place in the home state of Emmet K. Knott and Dr. Virgil K. Hancock, the Seattle-area residents who presented some of the most successful, life-saving UVBI-treated cases to a meeting of the King County Washington Medical Society—in 1934!)

But it's well past time for the mainstream health authorities to give up their skepticism about this time-tested therapy and to realize that there are many treatment possibilities for illness besides patent medications, un-natural radiation, and surgery. The list of health problems improved by UVBI is a long one, and includes diabetes, asthma, COPD, hypertension, chronic renal failure, some cancers, rheumatoid arthritis, psoriasis, paralytic ileus, thrombophlebitis, and irritable bowel syndrome. It's time to re-open the medical journals of the past, read all about these (and many more) successes of UVBI, and start applying them to today's health problems.

I am grateful to Lauren Russel N.D. for her excellent job in organizing the voluminous information collected for this chapter. I am also very grateful to William Campbell Douglass M.D. for the largest collection of data ever assembled concerning clinical applications of UVBI.

Chapter 7:

The two vitamins that could save your life in the ICU—and why many hospitals won't give them to you

I've been called a cynic on more than one occasion, particularly when it comes to mainstream medicine. There are a number of general reasons why—things like the patent medicine industry's greed and *los Federales*' collusion with them. But there are also some very specific reasons—things that I've experienced first-hand—that have contributed to my continued mistrust of the medical system in this country. One of the worst examples occurred several years ago, back in 2002, when one of the local hospitals here in the Seattle area refused to implement a treatment protocol that would save more lives and cost less money simply because the treatment involved using vitamins.

This was actually one of my first experiences as one of the members of the Board of Trustees for the regional "Level 1" trauma center hospital, located in Seattle, but serving Washington, Alaska, Idaho, and Montana. Fortunately for me, a well-respected naturopathic physician had been appointed to the Board two years or so before, so the very intense and public opposition from "conventional" medical doctors and their allies that greeted her was considerably muted in my case. Nonetheless, when it came time to choose a subcommittee to serve on, I deliberately steered clear of the one with "health care" in its title, figuring that my background in naturally oriented health care wouldn't earn me a very friendly reception. Instead, I joined the "finance" subcommittee, which I thought might not seem as threatening to the administration or some of the staff.

The same year I was appointed to the Board, a team of physicians based at the very same hospital published the results of a randomized, prospective trial of 595 critically injured individuals admitted to the intensive care unit (ICU). The research concluded that early, preventive administration of anti-oxidant vitamins E and C significantly reduced the incidence of multiple organ failure, decreased pulmonary complications and the need for mechanical ventilation, and shortened the length of time spent in the ICU, with no side effects attributable to the antioxidants.

It occurred to me that this use of antioxidants might save the hospital considerable money, too. So I asked the hospital's chief financial officer to analyze this aspect. The answer I received was that the total hospital charge for each patient receiving antioxidants was $88,897 compared with $93,874 for those who did not, a difference of about $5,000 per patient.

When I did the math and applied that $5,000 savings to each of the 595 patients in the study I found that the hospital could have saved $2,975,000 if the entire group had been treated with the antioxidant therapy. I also learned that the hospital treated approximately 2,500 patients for similar injuries each year. If all of those patients were treated with antioxidants it was possible the hospital could save up to $15 million per year.

Potentially saving almost $15 million dollars per year certainly seemed like a financially worthwhile matter to me, so I proposed to the finance subcommittee that this research—done at our own hospital, with no reported side effects—be applied in the future to all ICU patients admitted under the same circumstances.

My suggestion was referred to a committee of the medical staff. After six months of "study," the finance subcommittee was told that my suggestion would not be implemented, as the antioxidant vitamins E and C given "might not be safe." When I pointed out that the physicians at our very own hospital who conducted the study had found no adverse effects, I was told that it was a "medical matter," and none of the finance subcommittee's (or the entire Board of Trustees') business.

So much for the Hippocratic oath. Here the hospital's own physicians had discovered a side-effect-free treatment that could potentially save the hospital up to $15 million yearly—not to mention potentially decreasing multiple organ failure in critically injured human beings—and they refused to use it for the singular reason that it involved nutrients! It's enough to bring out the cynic in even the most optimistic of people.

But in the five years since this scene transpired, whenever time allowed, I've looked for evidence proving the safety and effectiveness of vitamins E, C, and other antioxidants for treating critically injured individuals.

I've found quite a bit of research that supports this treatment protocol for all sorts of very serious injuries. And while I doubt it will change any policies at our "Level 1" regional trauma center, the information below could very well save your life or the life of someone you love.

So if any of your loved ones are severely injured, *give the rest of this chapter to the doctors involved!* I just hope they're more open-minded to "evidence-based medicine" (even if the evidence supports nutritionally based therapies) than the committee that reviewed the study done at our own hospital in 2002.

When fighting free radicals becomes a matter of life or death

Even when you're healthy, normal metabolic processes generate free radicals. Normally, though, most of these free radicals get eliminated by the antioxidants you get from your diet and supplements. But when you're critically ill or have undergone severe trauma, your body experiences a variety of physiologic stressors above and beyond those caused by the illness or trauma itself. Inflammatory processes are much worse and the body's normal methods of coping with oxidative stress are interrupted, which causes an imbalance between the formation of free radicals and the ability to remove them.[1,2] This leads to an excess of free radicals circulating in the bloodstream and tissues. And all those excess free radicals wreak havoc throughout the body, breaking down cell membranes, damaging DNA, and even killing cells. Recent research shows a link between oxidative stress and dysfunction in organ systems.[3,4]

In fact, most deaths that occur in intensive care units (ICU) result from the cascade of events that follow severe oxidative stress—things like multiple organ failure, septic shock, and acute respiratory distress syndrome (also known as ARDS).[5-7]

This is where antioxidant therapy comes in. First, let's go over some additional details from the study done at the Level 1 regional trauma center where I serve on the board.

More vitamins, fewer deaths

In this particular study, researchers enrolled 595 individuals between the ages of 16 and 74 who were either general surgery or trauma patients and had come to the hospital within 24 hours of injury.[8] Patients were randomized to receive 1,000 IU of vitamin E via the intestines and 1,000 mg of vitamin C intravenously every 8 hours for the duration of their stay in the ICU.

The researchers chose these particular vitamins not only for their general health-promoting and immune-boosting benefits, but also because a number of studies have demonstrated their ability to work together to improve antioxidant defenses.[9-12] Vitamin E prevents damage to cell membranes by squelching free radicals. And when it's used in combination with vitamin C, which has its own free-radical-scavenging abilities, the nutrients work together to dramatically decrease oxidative stress and all the complications that come along with it.

Among the group receiving the antioxidants, there was a 19 percent reduction in deaths from pulmonary causes (ARDS and pneumonia) and a 57 percent reduction in the incidence of multiple organ failure. The anti-oxidant group also had a decreased need for mechanical ventilation, which resulted in a shorter time spent in the ICU. And as I mentioned earlier, on top of all these benefits, there were no adverse effects.

Another randomized, double-blind, placebo-controlled study on the same vitamins showed similar results. The researchers examined the effects of oxidative stress in 216 critically ill patients.[13] Roughly half (105) of the patients received a combination of 500 milligrams of vitamin C and 400 IU of vitamin E via feeding tube for 10 days. The other 111 patients received a placebo mixture.

The researchers found that antioxidant supplementation not only reduced oxidative stress but it also reduced overall mortality over the course of 28 days.

Reduce burn complications by 45 percent

But there are even more specific studies supporting the potential of antioxidants to help severely injured patients get on the road to recovery more smoothly. For example, the oxidative stress that occurs after burn injuries often results in the release of excess histamine. Excess histamine increases the production of the enzyme xanthine oxidase, which generates hydrogen peroxide and superoxide, two potent free radicals that cause additional tissue damage.[14,15] Another critical aspect of burn injuries is the significant loss of body fluids caused by the burn. To combat this, patients receive what are known as "resuscitation fluids."

So in a prospective, randomized study in a Japanese trauma center, researchers examined whether high-dose vitamin C could prevent some of these complications in burn patients.

The Japanese study enrolled 37 patients who were burned over more than 30 percent of their total body surface area and who were treated within 2 hours of injury. Patients were randomly divided into a group to be given IV vitamin C or a control group. The researchers found that the vitamin C reduced resuscitation fluid requirements by 45.5 percent, decreased wound swelling, and reduced the risk of respiratory dysfunction.[16]

While this study was small, other studies have also shown that high-dose vitamin C can reduce the tissue damage following burns as well as decrease the need for resuscitation fluids.[17,18]

The "other" antioxidant you need in urgent situations

While vitamins C and E have produced some amazing results, they're not the only antioxidants worth taking in critical situations. It's always best to cover as many bases as possible, and adding selenium to the mix can help you do that.

Selenium is another antioxidant that supports the immune system, protects the body from tissue damage, and helps maintain thyroid function. And research shows that, like vitamins C and E, it may also decrease rates of infection, promote healing, and increase survival in critically ill patients.

It certainly can't hurt, considering that in a study of 60 critically ill patients in an ICU, plasma selenium concentrations were found to be well below minimum values.[19] Decreased levels of plasma selenium have been associated with increased amounts of tissue damage, infection, mortality, and organ failure. Most of the clinical trials that have been done used daily doses of selenium ranging from 200 to 1,000 mcg and showed significant reductions in infection and time spent in the ICU.[20]

Of course, despite the fact that these studies on selenium have been very promising, the "experts" claim that "more research is needed." But after reviewing the existing evidence for the past five years, I can firmly say that the only thing that we really need more of is a willingness on the part of mainstream, conventional medicine to use these safe, effective nutrients to save the lives of people who need urgent, critical care.

Chapter 8:

Killer appliances?
9 ways to protect yourself from the new pollution more deadly than lead poisoning

Many historians actually attribute the decline of Rome—at least in part—to lead poisoning from Roman water pipes. Of course, the Romans had no clue: They couldn't see, smell, or taste the lead that leached from the pipes. But the fact that it was invisible and silent didn't mean that it wasn't deadly. In fact, countless Romans developed chronic illness and even died from lead poisoning, without ever realizing what had happened to them.

And if you're wondering why I'm bringing up such "ancient" history, it's because, today, in the 21st century, we may be just as clueless. Our technology has exposed us all to an invisible, untouchable pollutant with strong possibilities of doing far worse to us than lead did to the ancient Romans.

But the good news is we're not entirely defenseless against all this invisible pollution. In this chapter, I'll cover some things you can do to defend your health against at least some of it. First, though, it's important for you to fully understand what you're up against.

Everyone's at risk

This new invisible pollutant is our overwhelming 24/7 exposure to hundreds if not thousands of electromagnetic frequencies and wavelengths never before experienced by humans or any other life on Earth.

Of course, exposure to some electromagnetic radiation isn't a new phenomenon. Humans have always co-existed with minimal exposure to very low frequency electromagnetic fields (EMFs) that occur naturally from the sun and natural energy fields generated by the Earth, the human body, and other living things. But with the development of electricity, manmade sources of EMF exposure—from very high to very low frequencies—have increased dramatically over the last 120 years. And these exposures are everywhere: Nearly every habitable area of our planet has some degree of artificial electrical electromagnetic field.

EMFs are made up of two things—electric fields and magnetic fields. These fields radiate power, which is often referred to as energy "waves." Electrical engineers and scientists often compare EMFs in wires to water flowing through a hose. Electromagnetic energy isn't restricted to flowing in wires anymore, though: Energy waves get transmitted through the air to all kinds of receivers—antennas, cell phones, laptop computers, etc.

There are two types of EMF exposure. The first type is generated by electrical appliances and power lines and is known as "extremely low frequency electromagnetic fields" or ELF. The second type is radiofrequency radiation (RF). RF is most commonly generated by equipment used to transmit wireless signals, such as cellular towers and antennas, broadcast transmission towers, and the equipment receiving these signals, such as cell and cordless phones.

The number of repetitions of each electromagnetic wave—called cycles per second—is termed "Hertz" (Hz), named after a pioneer 19th century researcher. Although most electrical current is generated at around

60 Hz, poor power quality caused by high-frequency voltage changes often contaminates the 60-Hz transmission frequency.[1] This "dirty" electricity exposes us all to high-frequency radiation (much higher than 60 Hz) through the wiring, electrical outlets, and electronic devices we've come to depend on every day. To put all these frequencies into perspective, consider that an electric train has a frequency of 20 Hz, whereas wireless communication commonly operates at 1 billion Hz (1 GHz).[2]

Health concerns about EMF exposure, particularly magnetic field exposures, have been cropping up since 1979, when two researchers discovered a relationship between childhood leukemia risk and "exposure to EMF radiation from electricity transmission lines."[3]

Since then, the safety of EMF has been the subject of quite a bit of debate and speculation. The research has continued too, and the fact is, electrical hypersensitivity, or overexposure to radio-frequency radiation, also known as "radio-wave sickness," is growing at an alarming rate. In fact, up to 50 percent of the population may be hypersensitive.

Cancer, Alzheimer's, diabetes, and more: The many faces of radio-wave sickness

I was made aware of this problem by a mother who told me that her 13-year-old son had been having abrupt and very noticeable behavior worsening multiple times daily for years. The episodes occurred at the exact same times every day when he was at home, but he didn't have these problems at all when he and his mother were out of the area. After months of painstaking research, she discovered his behavior changes were "triggered" by the rotating radar beam from the local Naval Air Station that "swept over" their home at exactly those times. They tried nutritional, biochemical, and acupuncture treatments, but nothing worked, so they moved to another area well away from the radar beam. The abrupt behavior changes completely disappeared.

Unfortunately, the problems associated with EMF go far beyond the behavioral experiences this young boy experienced. Studies conducted over the last two decades suggest that EMF is both neurotoxic and carcinogenic.[4]

Since that first study back in 1979, EMF has been implicated numerous times as a risk factor in childhood leukemia, in some cases even at very low exposure levels.[5-7]

A number of studies have examined the occupational risk of exposure to EMF and have found that electrical workers are at significantly increased risk for brain tumors and acoustic neuromas (a type of brain tumor that affects hearing).[8,9] Experts say that the risk is similar to that for lung cancer from second-hand smoke.[10,11]

But it's not just on-the-job exposure that's dangerous.

Although still one of the most controversial areas of research, more than a dozen studies suggest an increased risk of brain tumors (gliomas) and acoustic neuromas from the use of cell phones. Risk may be increased in people who have used cell phones for more than 10 years, particularly if that use is only on one side of the head.[12-14]

RF exposure may disrupt cellular communication, cell membrane function and metabolism, and trigger the activation of proto-oncogenes (genes which pre-dispose to cancer) and stress hormones. Other effects attributed to RF exposure include DNA breakage and chromosomal aberrations, cell death, increased production of free radicals, and changes in brain function.

Exposure risk has also been studied for other adult cancers.15 EMF exposure has been indicated as a possible risk factor in the development of breast cancer because of its effects on melatonin levels (declining levels of melatonin have been associated with breast cancer risk).[16,17] According to one researcher, "Collectively, the data are consistent with the idea that exposures to EMF, as defined, are associated with some increase in breast cancer risks..."[18]

Beyond cancer, EMF has been associated with exacerbating or contributing to many illnesses ranging from diabetes[19] and multiple sclerosis, to asthma, fibromyalgia and attention-deficit disorder.[20]

And studies have also found a relationship between exposure to EMF and neurological conditions like Alzheimer's disease and amyotrophic lateral sclerosis (ALS). In fact, in some cases, there's been a doubling and even tripling of the risk for developing ALS.[21,22]

Current "protection" doesn't measure up

One of the biggest problems we face is that all of this EMF and RF technology was invented and put to use without thinking about the potential health risks. And the current regulatory standards just aren't offering enough protection. Despite all the studies showing that EMF and RF exposure are risk factors for numerous—and serious—health problems, the FCC hasn't done an adequate job defining safe exposure standards. In fact, exposure standards for RF are based on the weight and height of a 6-foot-tall male, which leaves out a vast majority of the population.[23]

A consortium of international scientists and public health professionals put together a BioInitiative Report outlining the problem and insisting existing public safety limits for ELF and RF are inadequate.[24] The report calls for more research to establish standards and guidelines that protect people from health risk, which isn't exactly an easy thing to do.

Not only is EMF technology everywhere these days, but studying EMF is complicated by many factors, such as the effects of different and over-lapping frequencies, amount of exposure, distance from source of exposure, and amplification of signals.

In the meantime, the only thing you can do to protect yourself from high-frequency radiation is to reduce your exposure to it.

What your transistor radio can tell you about your home

A few years ago, Holly and I bought an abnormal frequency detector (a "Stetzerizer" microsurge meter) through www.stetzerelectric.com.

We weren't surprised to find that our home had abnormal readings in nearly every room. But you may not even need a special device to test your own home.

You can check for electrical pollution by taking a small, hand-held radio and tuning it to 500 AM, usually the lowest possible frequency on the dial. Turn up the volume and you'll hear a noise. Then, bring the radio close to electrical equipment, like dimmer switches, fax machines, computers, microwave ovens, telephones, and compact fluorescent bulbs. When you bring the radio close to a source of electrical energy, the noise coming from the radio will likely increase, which indicates electrical pollution.[25,26]

When Holly and I discovered the electrical pollution in our house, we installed Graham/Stetzer filters everywhere necessary. The Graham/Stetzer filter, or "Stetzerizer," is a capacitor (a filter of abnormal frequencies) that plugs into any 110-volt electrical outlet (the universal household plug-in) and eliminates high-frequency electrical waves generated between 4 to 100 kHz.[27,28] It usually takes about 20 Graham/Stetzer filters to protect a typical home from electrical pollution coming from televisions, lamps, toasters, and other electronic equipment.

Studies have shown that these filters improve health, often quite dramatically, and reduce the effects of EMF in homes and offices.[29]

In many case studies, patients have reported significant improvement in their health within a few hours to a few days. Sometimes the improvement in health is immediate. These positive health effects include a decreased number and severity of headaches, increased energy, better balance in patients with MS, decreased blood sugar levels in patients with diabetes, and increased wellbeing.[30]

In one particular study, Graham/Stetzer filters were installed in a school in Wisconsin that had been classified previously as a "sick" building. Previous attempts to fix the problem by removing mold had had no effect on symptoms.[31] But after the Graham/Stetzer filters were installed, there was a dramatic decline in the number of headaches experienced by teachers and students, reduced symptoms of asthma among students, and improvements in memory, concentration and energy, and general wellbeing.[32]

Similar effects were noted in another study, this one conducted in a school in Canada, where 50 Graham/ Stetzer filters were installed. After six weeks, the teachers, who were unaware of the study, reported that they had fewer headaches and body aches and were less frustrated, irritable, and tired. They also had a general sense of improved health and mood. Although the results weren't as conclusive for students, teachers reported that they were less disruptive.[33,34]

And speaking from personal experience, I have been sleeping noticeably better ever since we installed ours. (And just to allay any concerns, I am not and have not been associated with the sale of these products in any way.)

Simple ways to protect yourself starting today

Some other things you can do to reduce or eliminate your exposure to high-frequency radiation:

1. Have dimmer switches replaced with regular switches and replace halogen lamps with regular light bulbs.

2. Remove or bypass variable speed drives on heating and cooling systems.

3. Replace "touch lamps," wireless plug-in jacks, compact fluorescent lights (CFLs), and fluorescent bulbs with electronic ballasts.

4. Don't buy a plasma TV. If you already have one—sorry about that—stay as far away from it as you can while still being able to see the on-screen picture. And don't buy another one!

5. Make sure that any new electronics you buy already have harmonic noise filters installed.

6. Position electrical equipment on outside walls so that radiation isn't projected into other rooms of your home or office. It's particularly important to avoid electronics in areas around beds. If possible, keep electronic equipment, including your digital alarm clock, at least six feet from your bed.

7. Unplug electrical appliances when they're not in use and use power strips that you can turn off.

8. Don't hold your cell phone against your head, especially if you use it a lot. Switch sides to reduce exposure on any one side. Or, even better, use a plug-in device which keeps the cell phone away from your head. Wireless devices, like Bluetooth technology, can also increase EMF exposure, so it's better to use speakers or a headset.[35,36]

For more suggestions on limiting your exposure to this potentially deadly pollution, you can refer to the website www.electricalpollution.com, and click Electrical Pollution Solutions. Also check www.stetzerelectric.com.

Thanks to Lauren Russel N.D. for her research and other contributions to this chapter.

Chapter 9:

Nature's equal opportunity libido booster

Just because all of the attention has been focused on men doesn't mean that women don't struggle with their sexual function as they get older. In fact, lagging libido may very well be even more common in women than erectile dysfunction is in men. But there's one natural solution to both problems —and it has nothing to do with a "little blue pill."

In the early 1980s, I worked with a 50-something year old woman whose DHEA levels were below the limits of laboratory detection on repeated tests. Effectively, she had zero DHEA. She started using supplemental DHEA at physiologic levels—the amounts needed to achieve the usual level in human bodies. At a visit nearly a year later, here's what she told me:

She'd been seeing a psychiatrist for years for mild depression. "Nothing really bad," she said, but with one somewhat unusual aspect—she thought that something was the matter with "everyone out there" because they were all obsessed with sex!

She couldn't understand why "sex was everywhere," since it "just wasn't that big a deal" to her. She said she considered many, many other

428 • Treasury of Natural Cures

things more pleasurable and fun. And she told me that she'd felt that way all her adult life.

But a few weeks after starting DHEA, she'd absent-mindedly stroked her arm lightly, and shocked herself by getting "turned on." That had never happened "in all my years, even when a man who other women told me was attractive was doing the stroking!"

About the same time, she noticed that some men were becoming attractive to her now, and her psychiatrist pointed out she didn't seem depressed any more, even mildly. She (the psychiatrist) encouraged her to consider acting on her new-found attraction. She did, and told the psychiatrist (and later me) that she'd finally discovered that nothing at all had been the matter with "everyone out there."

"It was me!" she said. (As you might have guessed, she continued her DHEA.)

Another intelligent and observant woman had a similar experience. At one of her first visits, we reviewed her fairly extensive supplement list, which she'd mostly studied and started on her own. When we got to her DHEA—which was 50 milligrams daily, taken orally in a capsule—I pointed out that taking DHEA orally isn't actually the most efficient method.

Finding the path of least resistance

If you think about it for a moment, you'll see what I mean: Your body doesn't naturally put DHEA into your intestines, like food. DHEA is made in your adrenal glands, then released into the veins that drain your adrenal glands and kidneys. From there it goes straight to the heart, which pumps the unchanged DHEA molecules to every cell in your body. So every cell that can use DHEA gets its supply of these as-yet-unmetabolized DHEA molecules, and then uses them for whatever purpose Nature intended.

Contrast this with what happens with "oral" DHEA, the kind in capsules which many people are still swallowing every day. That DHEA goes into your intestines, and from there it's taken directly to your liver, just like food or anything else you swallow. Your liver's job with food is to break it down and transform it into forms useful to build and restore our bodies. But your liver's job with internally secreted hormones—including DHEA—is mostly to get rid of them. It just makes sense: Ovaries and testicles start making much, much more estrogen and testosterone at puberty; if much of it wasn't disposed of by our livers every day, we'd be so jam-packed full of these hormones for the next 30 years that the term "sex-crazed" might truly apply!

So when you swallow DHEA, your body is getting rid of most of it before all your cells get a chance to use it. As usual, the better option is to copy Nature!

Like testosterone, estrogen, and progesterone, DHEA should be used as a transmucosal, topical cream, rubbed into the mucous membrane of the inner labia or vagina (for women) or the anal mucosa—the area "just outside" (for men). That way, it's most effectively absorbed and most closely copies the way that Nature routes each hormone around your body. (Transdermal DHEA creams—which are rubbed into the skin—are OK initially, but too often lose their effectiveness over time.)

When I explained this all to the woman who'd been taking oral DHEA supplements, she agreed that it made sense to switch. So I wrote her a prescription for the same amount of DHEA to be rubbed in transmucosally.

At her next visit, she told me she'd had to cut back her use of DHEA dramatically, from 50 milligrams taken orally daily to 15 milligrams rubbed in transdermally "most days" since even taking it every day was sometimes too much. I asked her why. She smiled, and said she'd started using DHEA in her late 30s after experiencing a notable drop in her libido and finding low blood levels on tests. (DHEA levels "peak" in both sexes usually between ages 25 and 30, and decline—sometimes rapidly, sometimes more slowly—after that.) She said "it helped my libido and I just generally felt better."

But after switching to trans-mucosal DHEA at the same 50 milligram dose she told me, candidly, "I got so darn horny it was too distracting! My husband was happy, of course, but I also have a job, so we agreed I'd use that much on appropriate occasions, and cut back to a more reasonable amount the rest of the time, especially during the week, so I could get my job done!"

Of course, these are just two anecdotes. I've heard many others, not as dramatic, but similar. And don't forget that even though testosterone is "stronger," DHEA works for men struggling with erectile dysfunction too. Working with 53 men ages 21-68 with chronic prostatitis (a common problem for men), Russian researchers found a significant correlation between lower serum levels of DHEA sulfate (one measurement of DHEA) and erectile function, regardless of the man's age.[1] (For those of you who want "real science" to prove that Nature and Creation were right about the trans-mucosal/trans-dermal "route of administration" for DHEA and other hormones, please refer to the following study: Labrie F, et al. "Bioavailability and metabolism of oral and percutaneous dehydroepian-drosterone [DHEA] in post-menopausal women." *Journal of Steroid Biochemistry and Molecular Biology* 2007; 107:57-69.)

You almost always need a prescription for DHEA cream, but you also need a physician skilled and knowledgeable in bio-identical hormone replacement to help you with measuring and balancing all of your hormones, so if you're interested in trying DHEA, it's really better to work with such a physician for over-all health improvement and maintenance.

See the Alternative Health Resources section on page 485 for a list of organizations that can help you find a natural medicine physician near you.

Chapter 10:

New secrets for reading your body like a book

When's the last time you read a mystery novel? Whether you prefer Sherlock Holmes, Miss Marple, or Charlie Chan, all these great detectives have one thing in common. They use common sense and hard facts to uncover the most obvious signs in order to solve the mystery. But what does a mystery novel have to do with you? Everything.

Imagine if you could read your own body just like a book...Well, you can. By looking at the right signs, you can solve the mystery of whatever's ailing you. Page by page, you will uncover clues for conquering illness and disease. By the end of your quest, you will have found the true path toward optimum health.

Here's how it works.

There are warning signs written all over your body that point directly to a larger problem with your health. But all too often we shrug off changes to our skin, hair, fingernails, and other parts of our bodies as a natural part of growing older.

And, in the age of the 10-minute routine checkup, your doctor probably doesn't take the time to look for hidden warning signs pointing to larger problems like heart disease, diabetes, food allergies, and nutritional deficiencies. Too often, your doctor takes your weight, measures your blood pressure, and sends you on your way.

The good news, however, is that the signs can be written all over your body and they are simple for you to spot. And once you know what to look for, you can take the steps needed to prevent or even cure many serious illnesses.

With this special report, you'll learn exactly how to read your body like a book. You'll begin to look more closely at your skin, hair, eyes, tongue, and other parts of your body to find vital clues for lurking illnesses.

Before you read the next few pages, I recommend you take out a pen and look into the mirror. Using the box on the next page, place a check next to each symptom you see on your body today. You might be surprised by how many signs you'll find.

Then, read the following report to discover what your body is trying to tell you. In most cases, you'll find there are natural, inexpensive, and non-prescription remedies for your most worrisome problems. Sometimes, it's even just a matter of making slight changes to your diet.

However, you'll notice that in many instances, I don't give direct dosage advice. When you're making self-observations like these, it's always a good idea to compile a complete list of the things you notice and meet with a doctor skilled in nutritional medicine before making any changes or additions to your supplement program. Your specific combination of symptoms might require a different nutrient and dosage combination than someone else, and your doctor can help you tailor a program specifically suited to your own needs.

For a list of naturally oriented physicians in your area, please contact the American College for Advancement in Medicine (800)532-3688; www.acam.org; the American Association of Naturopathic Physicians (866)538-2267; www. naturopathic.org; or the American Academy of Environmental Medicine (316)684-5500; www.aaem.com.

COMPLETE BODY CHECKLIST

- ❏ Rosy cheeks
- ❏ Yellowish skin
- ❏ Teenage acne
- ❏ Adult acne
- ❏ Psoriasis
- ❏ Eczema
- ❏ Skin tags
- ❏ Dry skin
- ❏ Raised dry spots
- ❏ Forehead wrinkles
- ❏ Varicose veins
- ❏ Easy bruising
- ❏ Cracked, callused feet
- ❏ Earlobe creases
- ❏ Cracked ear skin
- ❏ Dry, flaky scalp
- ❏ Sensitive scalp

- ❏ Premature gray hair
- ❏ Thinning body hair
- ❏ Pale tongue
- ❏ Scalloped tongue
- ❏ Bumpy tongue
- ❏ Bleeding gums
- ❏ Canker sores
- ❏ Cracked lips
- ❏ Cold sores
- ❏ Dark circles under the eyes
- ❏ Cloudy eyes
- ❏ Red, watery eyes
- ❏ Eye hemorrhages
- ❏ Cracked nails
- ❏ White spots on fingernails
- ❏ Neck or back pain

CLUE # 1: Skin

Your skin is your body's largest organ. Don't miss the obvious signs of illness.

Problems throughout the body very often surface first on the skin. Even dry skin can point to a more serious problem. Look hard in the mirror and read the signs.

❏ Rosy cheeks

Your dermatologist probably doesn't talk about it…but many skin ailments are directly related to problems in your stomach.

Do you have rosy cheeks and/or broken capillaries on your nose? Do you find that many people assume you're a heavy drinker? What most of us don't realize is there's often a strong correlation between red faces and low stomach acid production. And Father Time is the culprit.

As we get older, our stomachs stop producing adequate levels of hydrochloric acid and pepsin. By taking supplements of these elements, you can often correct this simple digestive problem. You'll feel and look a whole lot better!

Is your face generally red all over? Is it most noticeable on your forehead and cheeks? Maybe you even suffer from medium to large acne-type bumps. Your dermatologist has probably diagnosed it as acne rosacea and put you on some type of prescribed medication. But did you know this, too, almost always signals low stomach acidity? Taking supplemental hydrochloric acid and pepsin will not only help aid your digestion but also, in all likelihood, help combat your acne rosacea.

Here's what you can do. Take one capsule (5, 7-1/2, or 10 grains) of either betaine hydrochloride-pepsin or glutamic-acid hydrochloride-pepsin just before meals. If there are no problems, then gradually increase the dosage over several days to the recommended amount (40 to 90 grains per meal). This kind of treatment should always be carefully monitored by a physician. Also, hydrochloric acid should never be used in combination with aspirin, Butazolidin, Inodicin, Motrin, or any other anti-inflammatory medications. These medications can cause stomach bleeding and ulcers, so using hydrochloric acid with them increases the risk.

❏ Yellowish skin

Many people over 50 have a slightly yellow tone to the facial skin. Most of us just chalk this up to getting older. But there is something you can do to get back the rosy glow of your youth. Vitamin B12 injections have been found to help restore the healthy pink-red tones to the face and even support the health of the nervous system. A lack of B12 frequently is due to an older stomach that also isn't making the amounts of hydrochloric acid and pepsin that it once did.

Don't shrug off a brownish-yellow discoloration of the skin on the front of your legs either. This is very often an early warning sign for insulin problems and diabetes.

A slightly yellow tone to the skin all over your body often points to a larger problem. Your thyroid might be under functioning. You must be persistent in discussions with your doctor, because a slight hypothyroidism often doesn't show up in a blood test.

You should also watch out for the other telling signs of an under functioning thyroid, such as persistently low body temperature, dry skin, poor hair, and weak nails.

❏ Teenage acne

Teenagers everywhere suffer from chronic acne and are taken to the dermatologist for a quick fix. But most often, by eliminating refined sugar from their diets, teenagers can stop spending hours in front of the mirror trying to cover up the problem. Eating more foods with zinc and essential fatty acids, like unroasted sunflower seeds and pumpkin seeds, is also very helpful. For very serious cases, however, supplements can be most effective. Also, if the teenager's acne is very severe, it's likely he or she probably has some type of food allergy.

***Note:* Sixty percent of all undiagnosed ailments involve some type of food sensitivity. There are many ways to identify food allergies and sensitivities. Physicians and other health-care practitioners have found that elimination diets, certain types of skin tests, blood tests, muscle testing, electrodermal testing, and radionics are all helpful in the identification of food sensitivity.

Many teenagers also suffer from rough, bumpy skin on the backs of their arms. This often points to a deficiency in vitamin A. Eating lots of carrots, sweet potatoes, yams, and squash can be very helpful. Sometimes, this also points to a lack of essential fatty acids and B-vitamins.

❑ Adult acne

If you're over 25 and still suffer from acne, you undoubtedly have some type of food allergy. For complete acne relief, these allergies need to be identified and dealt with. However, topical application of "creams" containing niacinamide, azelaic acid, tea-tree oil, and pantothenic acid can reduce acne for teens and adults alike.

❑ Psoriasis

If you have psoriasis, you know all too well what those silvery scales or red, raised patches on your hands, arms, and face look and feel like. The elements nickel and bromide in very small quantities can help cure this chronic skin problem.

❑ Eczema

If you have red, cracking skin on your hands and other parts of your body and have been diagnosed with eczema, food allergies are part of the problem. Eggs, dairy and peanuts are the foods most likely to trigger allergies. Also, supplemental zinc and essential fatty acids are very necessary for children and others with eczema.

❑ Skin tags

As we get older, many people develop seemingly harmless skin "tags" under the arms, behind the neck, and in the groin area. But they're definitely not something to ignore…and are more than just a cosmetic problem.

Even though skin tags are thought to be viral in origin, these skin growths can be a distant warning sign for type 2 (maturity-onset) diabetes. You should definitely ask your doctor for a glucose-insulin tolerance test. (This test is used to determine "insulin resistance." The ordinary glucose-tolerance test will not find insulin resistance, which is a precursor to type 2 diabetes.) Even if diabetes doesn't run in your family, skin tags sometimes indicate a higher risk for you!

❑ Dry skin

Do you apply a moisturizer after shaving or taking a shower? Cosmetic companies have made millions of dollars marketing their special creams to women and men who suffer from dry skin. But dry skin points to a nutritional deficiency of essential fatty acids. If you increase fish, nuts, and salad oils in your diet, your dry skin won't come back even in the harshest of winters!

❑ Raised dry spots

Many older women suffer from small, slightly raised dry spots, called "actinic keratosis," on their hands and forearms. Rubbing Retin-A, a natural acidic form of vitamin A, into these patches often helps reduce the size or take them away entirely if used persistently. A prescription is required, so check with your doctor.

❑ Forehead wrinkles

Most of us have them. Wrinkles are a part of getting older, right? But if your wrinkles run vertically on your forehead and are accompanied by abdominal pain, there's a good chance you have a duodenal ulcer. I recommend taking a test for Helicobacter pylori. If the test turns out positive, try a natural substance called mastic. Talk to your doctor about using 500 milligrams three times daily for four to six weeks.

❏ Varicose veins

Most women accept varicose veins as a part of motherhood and growing older. And, yes, they do run in certain families. But so does a higher requirement for flavonoids, which strengthen veins and prevent varicose veins in the first place.

Flavonoids are found in citrus fruits, blueberries, and all other red, blue, and purple fruits and vegetables, as well as a long list of botanical supplements, including hawthorn, bilberry, ginkgo, horse chestnut, pycnogenols, and many others. Vitamin E and magnesium are helpful too. A diet high in fiber decreases the pressure inside the abdomen, allowing the blood to return from the legs to the heart more easily with less "back pressure."

❏ Easy bruising

Let's set the record straight. Easy bruising doesn't mean you're a weakling. It actually points to a potentially serious nutritional deficiency that can lead to uncontrolled internal bleeding.

Easy bruising is often due to a vitamin K deficiency or a lack of flavonoids (which help keep small blood vessels strong) in your diet. Try supplementing with vitamin K (5 to 10 milligrams daily). (You may have a bit of difficulty finding an adequate-dose vitamin K supplement, but keep trying.) If insufficient vitamin K is the problem, you should see a difference after six to eight weeks. If vitamin K isn't sufficiently helpful, use a supplement of one of the sources of flavonoids listed above.

❏ Cracked, callused feet

It's true. Most men, and many women, don't pay much attention to their feet. But we all should...rough skin on our feet can signal serious nutritional deficiencies. If you have cracked feet and heels, your body lacks the essential fatty acids it needs. Flaxseed oil, 1 tablespoonful daily, is one of the best-balanced sources. Be persistent: Ten to 12 weeks may pass before the cracks disappear. In some cases, it may be necessary to add supplemental zinc too.

Calluses along the edge of your heel mark a deficiency in vitamin A (not beta-carotene). Again, it may take 10 to 12 weeks of supplemental vitamin A (not beta-carotene) to lessen the calluses. A dosage of 40,000 IU daily is safe for adults.

❏ Earlobe creases

Do you have diagonal creases across your earlobes? If so, it might mean you're at higher risk of developing cardiovascular disease. If you're eating right, getting regular exercise, and taking vitamin E, it's probably nothing to worry about. But you may want to have your cholesterol, tri-glyceride, homocysteine, and C-reactive protein levels checked.

❏ Cracked ear skin

If you have cracked skin behind your ears, your body isn't getting all the nutrients it needs. Add more zinc and essential fatty acids to your diet through pumpkin seeds, sunflower seeds, and fish oil supplements until it's healed.

CLUE # 2: Hair

There's no such thing as care-free hair.

Some women and men spend hundreds of dollars a year at the hair salon in search of shiny, healthy, and care-free hair. But frequent trips to your stylist and high-priced shampoos can't change what a good look in the mirror should tell you.

Whether you have got a dry and sensitive scalp or thinning and dull hair, your diet, not your shampoo, is often the cause of the problem.

❑ Dry, flaky scalp

A dry, flaky scalp at any age reflects a diet too high in refined sugars and lacking in fatty acids. Dull, lifeless hair points to the same serious problem, not a buildup of shampoo.

Eliminate those refined sugars! Add dietary sources of essential fatty acids, such as fish, unroasted nuts and seeds, and salad oils. (Roasting nuts and seeds destroys much of the fatty-acid content). In addition, supplementing with at least 1 tablespoonful of flaxseed oil daily plus B-complex vitamins is usually necessary for a minimum of three to four months to restore a normal sheen to hair and eliminate that dry, flaky scalp.

❑ Sensitive scalp

If your scalp is always tender to the touch, or if pulling on your hair hurts, try taking cod-liver oil (this works especially well for children), or for adults, try vitamin-D supplements. But be careful; it's possible to take too much vitamin D!

❑ Premature gray hair

There might be a natural way to prevent premature graying. Try adding some extra PABA (paraaminobenzoic acid, a B vitamin) to your supplement program. Some people have also found success using the Chinese herbal "ho-shou-wu" or "fo-ti."

❑ Thinning body hair

By the time they reach middle age, many women begin losing hair on their heads. Hair loss on a woman's head (except in women who are pregnant, have recently been pregnant, or are taking estrogen) is probably caused by low stomach acid, also known as hypochlorhydria.

As we age, our stomachs stop producing adequate levels of stomach acid and pepsin. This leads to poor digestion of essential proteins and impedes the growth of new hair. By supplementing your diet with hydrochloric acid-pepsin capsules, you'll begin to digest and absorb protein properly and your hair loss should stop.

Hair loss on your lower legs and especially an abnormal loss of underarm or pubic hair frequently indicates that you have seriously low androgenic-hormone (DHEA and testosterone) levels in your body. And when you have low hormone levels, your immune system can't function properly. See Part VII: Women's Health for important information about hormone-replacement therapy.

CLUE # 3: Mouth, Tongue, and Lips

In a routine exam, your doctor usually looks into your mouth at your throat. And, yes, dentists look closely at your teeth and gums. But who takes notice of your tongue?

You should! The tongue is a very important health indicator in the body, and you should learn how to read the changes to it and other parts of the mouth.

❏ Pale tongue

A healthy tongue looks rosy red. Does your tongue look pale in the mirror? It might mean that you're anemic and need more iron in your diet. Liver from organically raised animals is the best source. Also, be careful to look for hidden gastrointestinal bleeding as a cause of anemia.

❏ Scalloped tongue

If your tongue looks a little swollen and "scalloped" around the edges, don't assume that the condition is caused by pressure from your teeth. It's most likely due to food allergies. Have yourself tested right away.

❏ Geographic tongue

Does your tongue look like a geographic map, with smooth areas, raised rough areas, cracks, grooves, and contours? In fact, it's called a "geographic tongue." You're missing folate, vitamin B12, and zinc in your diet. Once again, liver from organically raised animals is a good source for all three. Fresh green, leafy vegetables are good sources of folate; chlorella from the natural food store has both folate and B12.

Very rarely, "geographic tongue" is a genetic and unchangeable condition; however, almost always, it reflects a lack of these nutrients in your body.

❑ Bleeding gums

Periodontal disease can be corrected in many cases by supplementing with coenzyme Q10 and folate. A folate "mouthwash" can be especially helpful in reducing the bleeding.

❑ Canker sores

Do you have canker sores that keep coming back? These are very likely related to food allergies. Watch out for things that trigger the sores and eliminate them from your diet. Lactobacillus acidophilus will also help lessen recurrences. Also, avoid toothpaste with "sodium lauryl sulfate."

❑ Cracked lips

If you have persistent cracks at the corners of your mouth and no amount of moisturizer gets rid of them, look to your diet once again! Your body is probably lacking riboflavin, vitamin B2, and other B vitamins.

❑ Cold sores

We know cold sores are associated with the viral infection herpes. To get rid of these tiny, yellow blisters, you should add more selenium to your diet. Selenium is found in garlic and onions. You may also need to take a regular selenium supplement to control unwanted recurrences.

CLUE # 4: Eyes

❏ Dark circles under the eyes

Your mom's not always right. Dark circles under the eyes don't always mean you're not getting enough sleep. They might point to a more serious problem…especially in children.

Dark circles and horizontal creases on the lower eyelids (called "Dennie's lines") often indicate serious food allergies that can affect behavior patterns in children and adults alike. For example, nearly all children diagnosed as "hyperactive" have allergies and sensitivities, especially food allergies. Try eliminating dairy and refined sugars from your diet and observe the results.

❏ Cloudy eyes/cataracts

If you have cloudy patches in the lenses of your eyes and have been diagnosed with cataracts, you may be suffering from abnormal sugar-insulin metabolism. You should immediately eliminate all refined sugar from your diet. Here's how it works: The lenses of our eyes respond to high blood sugar levels by "helping" to remove some of the excess. Unfortunately, the lenses have nowhere to store this excess sugar, so, over time, it literally "condenses" into cataracts.

There's also a possibility that lactose in cow's milk and other dairy products might have contributed to your condition. There is some evidence that vitamins B2, A, and C, along with zinc and selenium, can slow down vision loss. There's also one exciting study showing that bilberry can stop and even reverse cataracts if it's taken when the problem is at a very early stage.

❏ Red, watery eyes

If you have chronic red, watery eyes, try eye drops with vitamins A and C to control the symptoms and strengthen the surface of the eyes.

This will also clear up any viral infections in your eyes. You'll likely need to visit a nutritionally knowledgeable physician or a compounding pharmacist to obtain these drops.

❑ Eye hemorrhages

When the normally white part of the eye turns bright red with blood, you've had a scleral hemorrhage. This could be an early warning sign for hypertension. Be sure to check your blood pressure. You'll also want to think about ways to strengthen your blood vessels with foods containing flavonoids and vitamin C, as well as deep green vegetables for their vitamin K.

CLUE # 5: Fingernails

Like your skin and hair, your nails replenish themselves regularly. Because of this, they're often very visual outward signs of what's going on inside your body.

❑ Cracked nails

Maybe you've always felt that your nails just don't grow. They're thin and weak. They bend, chip, and crack easily. Like most problems with your hair and skin, this points to a problem in your stomach involving low acid and pepsin production. Again, not enough protein and nutrients are being digested and absorbed into your body; as a result, the fingernails can't grow properly. Weak fingernails can also indicate an intolerance for refined sugars and in more serious cases point to a weak thyroid.

❑ White spots on fingernails

White spots on the fingernails almost always point to a zinc deficiency in the body. The problem is that zinc isn't found in large quantities in many foods. You'll probably need to supplement with zinc capsules. For some people, white spots can mean low levels of pancreatic enzymes or gluten-gliadin intolerance, both of which contribute to zinc malabsorption.

CLUE # 6: Bones and Joints

❑ Swollen joints

As we get older, many of our joints begin to ache and perhaps swell a little. Your doctor might call it osteoarthritis and recommend an anti-inflammatory drug that can cause stomach damage.

I recommend taking glucosamine and chondroitin to naturally repair the damaged joint cartilage and prevent swelling. Niacinamide is an essential supplement as well. Many people have also found that by eliminating "nightshade" vegetables such as tomatoes, potatoes, pepper, eggplant, and tobacco from their diets for several months results in a dramatic improvement.

During and following menopause, many women develop tender little lumps at the end joints of their fingers. Hormone-replacement therapy can help, but keep it natural. Extra vitamin B6 and niacinamide can also prove effective.

❑ Neck and back alignment

If you have neck or back pain, it's an obvious sign that you should see a chiropractor. But you shouldn't wait until you're laid up in bed before getting an adjustment.

Here are a few simple tests to determine if your alignment is correct:

1. Try rotating your head as far as possible to the left and right. If rotating is limited on either side, you should head to your chiropractor or osteopath for a neck adjustment.

2. Press firmly on the vertebral spines (those little bony bumps) on the back of your neck. Do you feel any tenderness?

* * * * *

It's important when diagnosing and treating yourself that you know exactly what to look for. What are the signs that show you are likely to develop certain diseases...and what are the natural options available? You need to learn how to read your body like a book...and then figure out how to heal it.

And, of course, always consult your physician before making any changes to your current treatment program.

Chapter 11:

The miracle mineral: Clearing up everything from acne to arteriosclerosis

Can you imagine drinking dirty, contaminated water right from a river? In most cases, you'd have a lot more to worry about than a case of infamous "Montezuma's revenge." Depending on what part of the world the water is in, it could be infested with all sorts of disease-triggering bacteria (cholera comes to mind, but that's just one example). But despite all this danger, I have a friend, a retired Indian physician, who likely drank contaminated water for 30 years while he traveled from village to village in Africa—and he never got sick once. All he did was add a few drops of a common solution (after straining the sediment and debris through a cheesecloth, of course) two or three minutes before he drank it.

It sounds preposterous, I know. But it wasn't some "magic potion" brewed up by an exotic shaman that he used to disinfect his water—it was plain old iodine. Fortunately, the water available in the places most of us travel to is considerably cleaner, but, to be on the safe side, when my wife Holly and I travel, we always carry a small bottle of potassium iodide, a form of iodine combined with molecules of potassium and usually referred to by its abbreviation—SSKI. We put one or two drops into any water we're not absolutely sure about.

You probably remember iodine as the orange liquid your mother put on any cuts or scrapes you came home wearing like a badge of honor as a child. But as you're probably already guessing, iodine's potential goes far beyond being a simple disinfectant. There are literally dozens of uses for iodine and SSKI—and most of them are ones you'd never expect.

Iodine, iodide, SSKI, what's the difference?

Before we get into SSKI's other healing benefits, I thought I should take a minute to clarify what exactly this substance is, and how it's different from plain, old iodine. Iodine is a basic element, like calcium, zinc, oxygen, etc. The word "iodine" usually refers to two iodine molecules chemically "stuck together" (I2), just as the word "oxygen" usually refers to two oxygen molecules "stuck together" (O2). Since pure iodine is more reactive to other elements, it's more likely to cause problems, so iodine is usually used as "iodide," a word that refers to one iodine molecule combined with another molecule—often potassium (KI). So, even though they're not technically the same, for simplicity's sake, I've used the terms iodine and SSKI interchangeably in this chapter of the report (though always meaning SSKI unless noted otherwise).

The "SS" in "SSKI" refers to "saturated solution of potassium iodide." If you've read or heard anything at all about potassium iodide, it's probably been in association with terrorist attacks or nuclear power plant disasters. Potassium iodide (usually taken in tablet form) is recommended by public health authorities to protect the thyroid gland against accumulation of radioactive iodine that would be released by an atomic bomb or by a nuclear power plant meltdown. But in reality, potassium iodide is very effective for lots of less drastic scenarios and is a home remedy with literally dozens of uses.

The germ-killing travel companion
no one should be without

Holly and I have cut back considerably on airline travel this year because of the thoroughly disagreeable "airport Gestapo" experience. But even without all that, there are plenty of other unpleasant realities that go along with air travel. For example, when you sit in the cabin of an airplane for several hours (or more), you're breathing recycled, germ-laden air. That's why it's not uncommon to come down with a respiratory infection ("airline sinusitis") following a flight. So when we're forced to travel by air, Holly and I drink a few ounces of water with 10 drops of SSKI. The SSKI rapidly accumulates in any and all body secretions, including in the sinuses, where it inhibits or kills bacteria, viruses, and fungi before they can cause an infection.

There have also been times when we've gotten to our destination— usually a conference somewhere—and one of the women in attendance comes to me with the embarrassing and uncomfortable symptoms of a bladder infection. Certainly not the sort of infection you want to catch when you're far away from home (and your doctor). Luckily, I always carry a small "backup" bottle of SSKI, which I give to her with instructions to take 10 to 15 drops in water or juice every three to four hours (while awake) until the infection is gone.

SSKI is close to 100 percent effective in eliminating bladder infections, but the amount needed is a relatively high dose, so it's important to use it with caution. Make sure to read the sidebar "Using SSKI safely" on page 454.

So far, I've been telling you about SSKI's ability to kill germs in one place or another. We'll return to this important home remedy use for SSKI, but for now let me tell you about some of its other uses.

End years of suffering with painful breast and
ovarian cysts in as little as three months

Many women develop "fibrocystic breast disease," which is characterized by painful cysts in the breasts. In the 1970s, I learned from Dr. John Myers (one of the pioneering researchers in the use of trace elements) that iodine can minimize and possibly eliminate even the most severe cases of fibrocystic breast disease. In minor to moderate cases, 6 to 8 drops of SSKI taken daily in a few ounces of water will frequently reduce fibrocystic breast disease to insignificance within three to six months.

I've seen remarkable results even in patients with very severe fibrocystic breast disease—sometimes there's improvement in as little as an hour or two. In these very severe cases, I use a form of iodine called Lugol's solution, which is applied to the vaginal area and cervix. Then, the iodine application should be followed almost immediately by an injection of magnesium sulfate. Of course, you'll need a doctor's help with both of these steps (for a referral, contact the American College for Advancement in Medicine at 800-532-3688; www.acam.org).

Over the past 30 years, I've also used SSKI to treat at least 30 women—one of them my own daughter—for ovarian cysts. These cysts usually disappear within two to three months with the same quantity of SSKI mentioned above for breast cysts.

But please do not use this treatment for either of these conditions without monitoring your thyroid function (see "Using SSKI Safely" on page 454). Testing for fibrocystic breast disease and ovarian cysts and treatment of them using SSKI requires the help of a physician skilled and knowledgeable in nutritional and natural medicine, who can also help with monitoring thyroid function.

It's very likely that SSKI helps eliminate fibrocystic breast disease and ovarian cysts at least partly through its interaction with estrogens... which brings me to another important use for SSKI. Various forms of iodine, including SSKI, can help your body to metabolize estrone (a slightly carcinogenic human estrogen) and 16-alpha-hydroxyestrone (a much more dangerous metabolite of human estrogen) into estriol, an anti-carcinogenic—or, at worst, neutral—form of human estrogen. I've reviewed literally hundreds of hormone tests in over 26 years—all of which have proven this point.

Iodine's benefits may save you the pain and embarrassment of some sensitive conditions

"But what ever happened to the old way iodine was used?" you might wonder. "What about applying it to my skin? Does it have any benefits that way?" It's a good question with an even better answer—a resounding yes.

Iodine has just as many topical applications as internal, and the results are just as great. In fact, some of the topical applications might save you from the continued pain and embarrassment of some rather sensitive (and I mean that in every sense of the word) conditions.

Mainstream medicine has plenty of options for people with hemorrhoids—over-the-counter creams, pads, and ointments, those inflatable "donuts" to sit on, and, of course, surgery. Unfortunately, the less drastic ones aren't very effective, and the more drastic are just that—drastic. But my colleague Richard Kunin, M.D., (a world-class expert on the use of SSKI and other forms of iodine) has found that hemorrhoids will disappear—sometimes literally overnight—when a mixture of 20 drops of SSKI and 1 ounce of flaxseed oil is applied to them at bedtime. SSKI alone will do the same job, but Dr. Kunin's patients have reported that it "really stings" when applied by itself.

This loosening of thickened tissue also works for scars, especially keloids, which are abnormally thick (sometimes up to an inch) scars. Rubbing SSKI into a keloid at least twice daily will ultimately flatten it down to a normal scar. But patience really is a virtue here: It can take many months to a year for particularly bad ones. You can help the treatment go a bit faster if you mix SSKI "50-50" with a substance called dimethyl sulfoxide (DMSO), which is available in most natural food stores and even some pharmacies.

The pictures are worth a thousand words: SSKI fights cholesterol buildup and unclogs arteries

Over 30 years ago, two ophthalmologists observed that when they gave patients a combination tablet called "Iodo-niacin" (which contained 120 milligrams of iodide and 15 milligrams of niacin) and instructed them to take it for several months, the supplement actually reversed atherosclerotic clogging of arteries. And it's hard to argue with their proof: They took pictures of clogged arteries in the backs of the eyes before and after treatment. The published "after" photographs showed a significant lessening of the cholesterol-laden artery clogging.

Amazingly enough, no follow-up study has ever been published (probably because niacin and iodide aren't patentable). But the published pictures speak clearly for themselves.

I learned about iodine's power to help "dissolve" oils, fats, and waxes (cholesterol is actually a wax) way back as a pre-med student. The famous Harvard chemistry professor Louis Feiser made a point of demonstrating this to my classmates and me, and he urged us to remember it in our medical practices (he told us he was sure it wouldn't be taught in medical school—he was right).

I took Professor Feiser's advice to heart and still recommend 4 to 6 drops of SSKI and a niacin-containing B-complex vitamin as part of a daily supplement regimen for anyone with significant cholesterol-related clogged arteries.

From toenail fungus to pimples: Get rid of those nagging, bothersome problems once and for all

Now, let's move on to some bothersome conditions that just about all of us have experienced at one point or another—and I'll tell you how SSKI can help.

When my children were teenagers, they always knew where to find the SSKI bottle. Whenever one of them got a pimple, she or he knew to rub SSKI into it every hour or two. The offending "zit" disappeared in 24 to 48 hours or less (and let me tell you—this approach saved the day for more social events than I can count).

Then there's infected hangnails. Most people never even think to try to "cure" them, but they're very easy to clear up (as are nagging bacterial infections around the edges of the toenails) by applying the 50-50 SSKI/ DMSO mixture to them. Rub in the mixture several times daily, and the problem's usually gone in a few days. Cold sores (and other herpes outbreaks) can be stopped cold in the same way, but it often takes longer for the sore to heal itself over.

Toenail fungus is one of those annoyingly persistent conditions that just doesn't seem to respond well to many treatments. Even conventional antifungal drug treatment takes months to work, and using them means you need to have monthly liver function tests for safety reasons. The SSKI and DMSO mixture doesn't work any faster, but it's just as effective as antifungal drugs—and definitely safer. Rub it on, around, and under the affected toenails. And make sure to wear old socks, because SSKI and other forms of iodine leave an orange-brown stain. (If you really don't want to ruin your socks, you can also use oregano, geranium, or tea tree oils mixed with DMSO for toenail fungus.)

SSKI can also help clear up vaginal infections. Twenty to 30 drops in water, used in a small "douche" once daily for five to 10 days will usually do the job. (There's actually a prescription-only iodine preparation available for vaginal infections, too.) However, iodine preparations of any sort for vaginal infections aren't usually very popular because of the inevitable orange-brown stains they leave on clothing.

And last, but not least, there's also a gastronomic use for SSKI. I'm sure you know the little song (popular among most 10-year-olds): "Beans, beans, they're good for your heart. The more you eat, the more you…" well, you know the rest. It might be a silly and slightly crass song, but it does speak the truth! But, sure enough, SSKI can help reduce the gas we all get from eating beans. If you soak beans before cooking them, add 1 or 2 drops of SSKI, and let them soak for another hour or so. (Make sure to rinse them and use fresh water for the actual cooking process). You'll be surprised at how much less gas you feel later. (For those who want a technical explanation: There's a naturally occurring enzyme inhibitor in

Using SSKI safely:
Three important things you need to know

As you've read, SSKI has enormous potential benefits. But there are three hazards you need to know about when using it: Staining, allergy, and a very small possibility of thyroid suppression with long-term use.

Staining can be a big nuisance, but it's not a health hazard. When SSKI is applied to skin, it can leave a faint to moderate orange-brown color, which fades away once SSKI is no longer being applied.

Iodine allergy is possible, although, in nearly 30 years of medical practice, I've only seen it maybe a handful of times. Usually, it causes a red, bumpy skin rash, which is almost never a serious emergency. The rash generally goes away after SSKI or other iodine use is discontinued.

But if you're still worried or if there's any suspicion at all of iodine allergy, it's best not to use it without testing for the allergy.

The last precaution for you to be aware of is suppressed thyroid function. Many of the uses described for SSKI in this chapter are short term, from a few days to a week or two. If you stop using SSKI at that point, there's almost no chance of significant thyroid suppression. However, if SSKI is to be used for two to three weeks or longer, and especially if it's to be used continuously, monitoring thyroid function is very important. A physician can help you order and interpret thyroid function tests.

A final safety note: If you use SSKI or other iodine long term, make sure your diet contains plenty of essential fatty acids (both omega-3 and omega-6) as well as the amino acids methionine and cysteine. If you eat meat or other animal protein on a daily basis, you're probably getting enough of these two amino acids, but if you're vegetarian (or close) and using long-term SSKI, then be sure to take 300 to 500 milligrams of each daily.

beans that interferes with starch digestion—this is what produces gas. SSKI inactivates this enzyme inhibitor.)

Getting your hands on this all natural "cure-all"

By now you're probably wondering why—with all of its benefits—you haven't heard or read much about SSKI. Well, basically, it all boils down to the fact that the FDA forbids companies from making "claims"—even truthful ones—on product labels or advertisements. Unless, of course, they're paid an enormous amount of money (in the neighborhood of $250 million) for "approval." Since SSKI can't be patented, and no one can make back all that money they paid for approval...well, you know how it works.

SSKI can be obtained without prescription in some compounding pharmacies, some health food stores, from on-line sources, and through the Tahoma Clinic Dispensary (with which I am, of course, affiliated) in a convenient travel-size dropper bottle. To locate a compounding pharmacy near you, contact the International Academy of Compounding Pharmacists (800-927-4227; 281-933-8400; www.iacprx.org).

Chapter 12:

From tooth decay to sinus infections: Sugar cane miracles that pack a powerful punch

Medicine is filled with irony. Professional dentists, doctors, and many, many moms said for years that sugar rots teeth and is generally just plain bad for you. Well, it turns out that's only partially true. Refined sugar IS very harmful to your health. But there are other sugars—particular simple, natural sugars—that have shown some amazing health-promoting abilities. These sugars appear to protect us from tooth decay, ear infections, bladder infections, asthma, sinusitis, and a host of other health problems—even high cholesterol.

Boost your immune system with polysaccharide power

Simple sugars transmit information, particularly to immune system cells that defend us against infection. When these simple sugars combine in chains along with uronic acid, they're called "polysaccharides." Polysaccharides cause the immune cells to be much more active and vigilant against bacteria and other germs. They help in both the prevention and the treatment of infection. Echinacea, aloe vera, and many types of mushrooms are all rich sources of polysaccharides.

Beat bladder infections in 3 days or less, naturally

Approximately 90 percent of all bladder infections are caused by E. coli bacteria. (The E. coli I'm referring to here are normal inhabitants of all human and animal intestinal tracts. They are not the same as the food-contaminating, deadly, mutant E. coli O157:H7 bacteria.) And while most physicians will throw a prescription for antibiotics at you, you can eliminate this painful condition in just a few days—without putting your immune system at risk.

As I mentioned in the previous chapter, SSKI is a very effective treatment for bladder and urinary tract infections, but there's also another safe, natural option you might want to consider. The simple sugar D-mannose has the ability to detach E. coli from the walls of the bladder without upsetting the balance of the friendly bacteria necessary for good health. After being loosened from bladder walls, the bacteria are then rinsed away by normal urination. The E. coli aren't killed; they're simply relocated—"from the inside to the outside"—and the infection is gone.

People who treat their own bladder infections with cranberry juice are, in fact, using a form of D-mannose therapy. Cranberry juice, as well as pineapple juice, contains more D-mannose than other foods. However, the amounts are too low to be significantly effective against serious infections.

For adults, 1/2 to 1 teaspoonful of D-mannose, dissolved in water and taken every 2 to 3 hours, will eliminate almost any bladder infection caused by E. coli. It also has the great advantage of tasting very good!

Despite being classified as a "sugar," D-mannose is very safe. Very little of it is actually metabolized by the body. Large doses are washed away in the urine, and the amounts not excreted into the urine are so small that they do not affect blood sugar levels—even in diabetics.

D-mannose is available through compounding pharmacies, as well as many health food stores and alternative medicine practitioners. You can also order it from the Tahoma Clinic Dispensary (425-264-0059; www.tahomadispensary.com).

Never get stuck with another sinus infection

Another substance that has similar abilities is xylitol ("zye-lit-all"). Xylitol is a natural substance, but it actually looks and tastes like table sugar.

One study found that a solution containing 5 percent xylitol blocks the ability of more than half of all harmful bacteria to "stick" to the tissues inside the back of the nose. As with D-mannose, xylitol prevents the bacteria from infecting you without actually killing it.

Dr. Lon Jones, a physician in Texas, pioneered the use of intranasal xylitol in his medical practice. I've spoken to Dr. Jones, and he tells me that he has seen a 93 percent reduction in ear and sinus infections in his patients when they spray the inside of their noses regularly with the xylitol solution. Not only does the xylitol appear to "unstick" the bacteria that adhere to the cells lining the nose and sinuses but also stimulates the body's normal defensive drainage in the back of the nose (where the bacteria causing these conditions usually live).

Rinse away your allergies—maybe even throw away that inhaler

In addition to stimulating nasal drainage, xylitol spray also removes other pollutants that trigger allergic reactions and consequent asthma attacks. (Asthma can be triggered by infection in the back of the nose and sinuses, other upper respiratory infection, chronic sinus problems, and allergies.)

Dr. Jones' patients control their asthma simply by rinsing away pollutants from the back of the nose on a regular basis. Dr. Jones says that for many of his patients no other asthma medications are needed. This unique nasal spray is available as a product called Xlear (pronounced Klear). Xlear may be available at your own natural food store or compounding pharmacy. It is also available from the Tahoma Clinic Dispensary (425-264-0059; www.tahomadispensary.com).

Sink your teeth into this irony: A sugar reduces tooth decay by 80 percent

I've grown rather annoyed with dentistry. Along with everyone else, I've brushed, flossed, and used "water-pressure" devices for my teeth and gums. I haven't knowingly consumed any refined sugar or refined carbohydrates for nearly 30 years. Yet every so often the dentist has informed me it's time to have another filling or two. Furthermore, to this day, no dentist has informed me—or anyone else—of the existence of a simple, safe, good-tasting way to significantly reduce the incidence of dental cavities. Not only does this method exist, but it first appeared in dental and other journals in the 1970s—and there's now no question at all that it really works.

No, it's not that hazardous (but politically correct) toxic waste by-product, fluoride. So what is it? Believe it or not, it's xylitol—the same derivative of a natural, simple sugar that I mentioned above for sinus infection, allergy, and asthma relief.

You see, xylitol can prevent cavities because cavities are caused by the bacteria *Streptococcus mutans* (S. mutans).

Dr. John Peldyak, a dental researcher from the University of Michigan who has been involved in most of the dental research with xylitol in this country, has summed up the results of the past 25 years of clinical studies involving xylitol and tooth decay: Chewing xylitol gum once a day provides little protection. Twice a day reduces tooth decay by 40 percent. Three times a day, by 60 percent, and five times a day—80 percent.

Chewing gum containing xylitol is available through many natural food stores and compounding pharmacies, as well as through the Tahoma Clinic Dispensary or through Xlear Inc. (877-599-5327; www.xlear.com). If you have dental work that doesn't permit chewing gum, a variety of all-natural xylitol lozenges are also available.

Chapter 13:

Toss the Ritalin and eliminate the hidden culprit behind ADD

Jeremy, a second grader, began having sudden "anger spells" when he was in pre-school, at the age of four. His achievement levels in reading and other basic school subjects were also low, and his teachers were concerned about his attention span. When they recommended Ritalin, Jeremy's mother, Susannah, brought him to see me at the Tahoma Clinic in the hopes of an alternative. She'd noticed some strange symptoms on Jeremy—dark under eye circles and horizontal creases on his lower eyelids—and she wondered if he had allergies.

She was right. Nearly all children diagnosed as "hyperactive" have allergies and sensitivities, especially food allergies.

I learned about the link between allergy and sensitivity and attention deficit disorder back in 1979 when I read Dr. James C. Breneman's book *Basics of Food Allergy.*

There are many ways to identify food sensitivity. Physicians and other health care practitioners have found that elimination diets, certain types of skin tests, blood tests, muscle testing, electrodermal testing, and radionics are all helpful in the identification of food sensitivity. Not all techniques work for everyone, and food sensitivity testing and evaluation can be just as individual as the food sensitivities themselves. Treatments for these sensitivities are also very individualized and can include an array of techniques.

Dr. Breneman's technique involves following an elimination diet. During the first week, you'll eat only foods that are less likely to cause allergies (Dr. Breneman had his patients eat things like rice, spinach, and beef). Then you add back the foods you normally eat, one at a time to see if they cause your symptoms to return.

If you'd rather explore other testing options, contact the American Academy for Environmental Medicine (316-684-5500; www.aaem.com) for a list of physicians near you who are skilled in allergy screening and treatment.

It turned out that Jeremy was sensitive to milk and dairy products, wheat, soy, oranges, and 27 other foods. With the help of a nutritionist, Susannah put together a temporary diet plan for Jeremy while desensitization was done. It took seven months to complete Jeremy's desensitization. During this time, he also began taking a multiple-vitamin/mineral combination along with 50 milligrams of vitamin B6 and 100 milligrams of magnesium per day.

By the third grade, Jeremy's behavior was described by his teachers as "not hyperactive at all, just normal and bright." His "anger spells" were gone entirely. He caught up in all his subjects, and by the end of the year he had started to excel.

Chapter 14:

Soothing solutions for anxiety

For some people, caffeine can be a hidden source of anxiety. Caffeine-induced anxiety, or "caffeinism," occurs most often in individuals from families with blood sugar problems. Eliminating your intake of refined sugar is likely to reduce your anxiety, and, of course, eliminating caffeine will help too.

Vitamin and mineral supplements can also be sources of relief. Niacinamide, a form of vitamin B3, helps most people with anxiety and, to some degree, depression (especially for individuals whose family has a history of blood sugar problems). I usually recommend taking 500 to 1,000 milligrams a day along with a good B-complex vitamin supplement. The B-complex helps "back up" the niacinaminde, and it also helps settle anxiety on its own.

Herbal remedies like ginkgo (40 milligrams of a standardized extract, three times a day) and Siberian ginseng (100 to 200 milligrams, three times a day) can also be a big help.

Chapter 15:

The great-tasting way to beat bladder and urinary tract infections

Ninety percent or more of all urinary tract infections are caused by the common intestinal bacterium E. coli. D-mannose literally makes it impossible for this particular bacterium to "stick" to the bladder or the rest of the urinary tract, so infections are just "rinsed away" with normal urination. Even better, D-mannose is harmless and tastes good.

For adults, 1/2 to 1 teaspoon of D-mannose dissolved in a glass of water and taken every two to three hours will eliminate almost any bladder or urinary tract infection in about three days.

D-mannose is a simple sugar, but it isn't at all bad for you—not even for diabetics. See, very little of it is actually metabolized by the body. Large doses are washed away in your urine and the amounts left behind are so small they don't affect blood sugar levels.

You can get D-mannose from some natural food stores or from the Tahoma Clinic Dispensary (425-264-0059; www.tahomadispensary.com).

Chapter 16:

Stomp out chronic fatigue and get back your old get-up and go

When Kathy came to see me at the Tahoma Clinic, she'd already been diagnosed with chronic fatigue syndrome by her physician. The first thing I had Kathy do was undergo an adrenal-function test. This test measures how the adrenal glands respond to stress of any kind, physical or mental. Adrenal glands are stress-response glands and should make considerably more of each steroid hormone when stressed. It wouldn't be normal for our hearts to beat at the same rate or even a little slower after exercise than before, and it isn't normal for adrenal glands to make the same amount of hormone after stress as before. When they make less, weakness becomes a serious problem. They "go all out" just to keep you walking around. When they're called on to do more…exercise, working hard…they just can't do it.

If your adrenal glands are overstressed, stress reduction is a necessary part of recovery. But even though it's necessary, it can't usually do the job on its own. So Kathy began taking a number of supplements to combat her weak adrenal glands, beginning with cortisol, DHEA (15 milligrams per day), and salt. Extra salt is important in the production of a hormone called aldosterone. The main function of aldosterone is to regulate minerals like potassium and sodium, and it is a major factor in enabling our bodies to retain salt. You couldn't survive if your body didn't retain salt. If you're not eating much salt, your body has to make more aldosterone to make up for it. But if salt intake is high, it's actually normal for your adrenal glands not to make any aldosterone at all. So, if you eat enough salt, your adrenal glands don't need to make aldosterone, and that saves them some work.

Extra salt, cortisol, and DHEA help to rest the adrenal glands so they have more energy to repair themselves. But, you can help the repairs go even faster with the right diet, nutrients, herbs, and other supplements.

People with weak adrenal glands should never follow a low-carbohydrate diet. Weak adrenal glands are among the causes of low blood sugar levels, and a low-carbohydrate diet is meant to control blood sugar. Perhaps the most surprising nutritional recommendation given for strengthening adrenal gland functioning is incorporating six or more pieces of licorice (with no added artificial color or sugar) into your diet daily. Licorice contains substances that slow the liver's breakdown of steroid hormones.

In addition to these dietary modifications, vitamins A, E, and the entire B complex are thought to help the functioning of the adrenal glands. Usually, any good multivitamin and B-complex supplements from a natural food store will contain enough. Other supplements found to be helpful in treating weak adrenal glands are "Adren-Plus" and an "adrenal glandular." Adren-Plus is a combination of botanicals that have been shown to improve adrenal health. Adrenal glandulars are whole, dehydrated, animal adrenal cortex. Adren-Plus is available through the Tahoma Clinic Dispensary (425-264-0059; www.tahomadispensary.com).

Just two months after Kathy began treatment for her weak adrenal glands, she found that her old energy was back, and she was able to do things she hadn't been able to do for years.

Chapter 17:

The natural depression solution to try before St. John's wort

Aided mightily by the media, many people have the impression that St. John's wort is the only alternative treatment for depression. There's no doubt that St. John's wort is often effective, but it's actually one of the last natural treatments to try. One of the basic principles of nutritional and natural medicine is to always replace any "missing" essential nutrients first before turning to or adding other natural treatments.

In a large number of cases, depression is actually caused by a neurotransmitter deficiency, which can be treated by supplementing with relatively large quantities of the essential amino acids the depressed individual is missing, along with any supporting nutrients or metabolites.

Tryptophan, tyrosine, and phenylalanine are all especially common deficiencies, so have your levels of these checked and corrected before turning to or adding St. John's wort.

You'll need a doctor's help testing your levels of amino acids and determining how much of each to take to bring your levels back up to normal. Contact the American College for Advancement in Medicine (800)532-3688 or www.acam.org for a list of natural physicians near you.

Chapter 18:

The best varicose vein treatments around

Varicose veins are often considered an unavoidable part of getting older. Maybe they even run in your family. Most likely, they're due to the lack of sufficient dietary fiber intake over the years. Lack of fiber allows pressure to build up in the abdomen. This abdominal pressure, in turn, creates "back pressure" on the veins from the legs, dilating them. Foods containing bioflavonoids (like blueberries, blackberries, plums, and purple cabbage) can help alleviate this condition. Also try taking 200 to 600 milligrams of magnesium and 400 to 800 IU of vitamin E each day.

But the best varicose vein treatments are herbs. Check your local natural food store for butcher's broom supplements, which can increase the tone of blood vessel walls and help them function better. If you can find capsules containing 20 to 40 milligrams of a butcher's broom extract called ruscogenin, take them two times a day.

Horse chestnut is probably the best-known and most effective treatment for varicose veins. Take 600 milligrams of horse chestnut (containing 100 milligrams of an extract called escin) each day.

Sometimes combining butcher's broom and horse chestnut works even better—it's definitely worth a try.

Chapter 19:

Breathe easy with these safe, natural asthma remedies

Eighty percent of asthmatic children have low levels of stomach acid and pepsin. This hurts digestion and lowers nutrient absorption, gradually increasing food allergies. Stomach malfunction impairs vitamin B12 nutrition. In childhood asthma, a series of vitamin B12 injections often eliminates asthmatic wheezing entirely. When I'm working with an asthmatic child, I almost always ask a nurse to teach the parents how to give the injections at home. Depending on the child's size, I use between 1,000 and 3,000 micrograms of vitamin B12 daily, and taper off both the quantity and frequency according to the response. If you find the vitamin B12 hasn't reduced symptoms at all after 2 or 3 weeks, you should discontinue the daily injections.

For both childhood and adult asthma, magnesium and vitamin B6 intravenous injections given during acute attacks almost always eliminate them, although sometimes you need more than one injection to do the job. Both of these nutrients are also good to take orally, and can cut down on the frequency of asthma attacks. For adults, I usually recommend taking 50 to 100 milligrams of vitamin B6, along with 200 milligrams of magnesium three times a day.

As far as herbal treatments for asthma, Boswellia is the best bet. In one clinical study, 80 patients with chronic asthma were treated with 900 milligrams per day of Boswellia gum resin. Seventy percent of patients taking the Boswellia improved. Improvements were observed for shortness of breath, number of attacks, and respiratory capacity as well as indicators of inflammation.

These treatments are all good for reducing the symptoms of asthma, and sometimes they can even eliminate it altogether. But for adult asthma, allergy elimination or desensitization are usually necessary in the long run. For help with allergy screening and treatment, contact the American Academy for Environmental Medicine at (316)684-5500 or www.aaem.com.

Chapter 20:

Supplement solutions for emphysema

Erwin's story is a good example of how emphysema can be treated when nutritional deficiencies are taken into account, and when obvious symptoms are not ignored. When he came to the Tahoma Clinic, Erwin looked blue. Not bright blue, but a more dull, mottled blue with red tones, darker around the lips and cheeks, a little lighter on the rest of his face. The skin of his hands was more red with blue mottling; it was lighter on his fingers, where yellow-brown-orange cigarette stains also appeared. He was obviously working hard for each breath. He had been smoking for 54 years and was diagnosed with bronchial obstructive disease and emphysema.

The first step in treating Erwin was to have him tested for allergies. Allergies increase bronchial secretions and congestion and possibly constrict the bronchial tubes. He was also prescribed a number of vitamin and mineral supplements, beginning with 200 milligrams of magnesium citrate twice daily. Magnesium promotes healthy lung functioning in two ways. First, it acts as a bronchodilator, preventing the bronchial passages from going into spasm. Second, it plays a key role in the production of energy, which is needed by chest-wall muscles and the diaphragm to perform the work of breathing.

To help the function of breathing muscles, 250 milligrams of L-carnitine three times daily is also recommended. To thin and loosen bronchial secretions, 500 milligrams of N-acetylcysteine should be taken two times a day, as well as six drops, in liquid, of SSKI (a saturated solution of prescription potassium iodide). In addition to these recommendations (not prescription items), taking 50,000 units of vitamin A, 2,000 milligrams of vitamin C, and two 19-grain capsules of lecithin each day, as well as vitamin E, copper, and zinc is beneficial. These supplements improve the health of the cells lining the bronchial tubes and the rest of the lungs.

Ten weeks later, Erwin's condition was much improved. Although there was still a slight blue-red tinge to his skin, it was definitely less noticeable, and much less mottled. His breathing was much less labored.

After he'd improved to this point, I prescribed a new inhalant treatment to Erwin. It's called glutathione (which is a natural metabolite), and it should be inhaled two or three times a day. Glutathione plays a crucial role in the natural antioxidant-defense system, which helps prevent oxidation damage to lung tissue.

After two months using the glutathione, Erwin returned. "The lung doctor can hardly believe how well I'm doing," he said. "When I told him this glutathione thing was in regular medical journals, he didn't believe me, but then he looked it up and called me back. He says he's going to use it for all his other patients!"

The glutathione therapy is available by prescription only, and can be obtained through a compounding pharmacy. To locate a compounding pharmacy near you, contact the International Academy of Compounding Pharmacists (800)927-4227; www.iacprx.org).

Chapter 21:

Wipe out migraines in minutes for less than $10

I've seen so many people come to the Tahoma Clinic suffering from migraines who just aren't getting the relief they need from the expensive patent medicines their doctor has prescribed to them. Most of the time, these people are more than a little skeptical when I tell them there's an all-natural, safe, and cheap solution that can stop migraines in their tracks. Who can blame them for doubting it? After all, they've heard similar claims hundreds of times before. But it usually only takes a few minutes to convince them—because that's how long it takes for this treatment to work.

It involves a simple injection of magnesium and vitamin B6. Magnesium appears to do most of the "work" in relieving migraine pain. Vitamin B6 helps the magnesium do its job. In general, relatively rapid intravenous injection of magnesium quickly re-regulates and relieves acute muscle contraction/relaxation disorders. (These injections are also useful for recurrent back pain.)

Even better, the shot itself—needle, syringe, and contents—usually costs less than $10. And a nurse can teach you how to give these injections to yourself right at home.

Chapter 22:

Two amazing treatments for "incurable" multiple sclerosis (MS)

Imagine watching a woman who had been suffering from multiple sclerosis for many years—and who had previously needed a walker to help her get around—get up and walk several times around a room, without any help, at good speed and with no balance problems. Imagine listening to her say she's sleeping better, her energy is much improved, and that she's able to think more clearly. Imagine hearing another woman, even more severely afflicted, report that she's able to feed herself again and that her friends and relatives had all noticed her speech is easier to understand. It sounds amazing, I know—and it was even more amazing to watch firsthand. But I saw these things happen as a result of treatment with an amino-acid derivative called Procarin.

Procarin is actually a histamine that is combined with another natural amino acid. It's not known exactly how Procarin works. One theory is that it may reverse the blood vessel spasms associated with MS, restoring normal blood flow to the affected tissue.

In the research we've compiled at the Tahoma Clinic, 67 percent of patients being treated with Procarin report at least one significant improvement in symptoms, and some many more.

Procarin is available as a skin patch and can be obtained by prescription from any compounding pharmacy. To find a compounding pharmacy near you, contact the International Academy of Compounding Pharmacists at (800)927-4227. Physicians familiar with Procarin and able to prescribe it (if appropriate) can be found through the American College for Advancement in Medicine (ACAM) at (800)532-3688.

Another frequently helpful treatment for patients suffering from multiple sclerosis is called calcium aminoethylphosphate, or CaAEP. This treatment was introduced by Dr. Hans Nieper of Germany, a pioneer in natural medicine. Since then, CaAEP has become one of the few substances to cause clinical improvement in the majority of those patients who have taken it. CaAEP is an injectable supplement, available through "natural medicine" physicians. The chemical works by protecting the integrity of cell membranes, sealing them off from autoimmune complexes but still permitting nutrients to enter. Of the 293 individuals surveyed who tried the intravenous CaAEP, 235 noticed improvement on an average of 13 out of the 36 possible symptoms listed on the survey. The American College for Advancement in Medicine can also help you locate a physician in your area who can tell you more about CaAEP.

Procarin and CaAEP are innovations that offer victims of MS a ray of hope for what was previously believed to be an inevitably deteriorating condition. The use of these two treatments gives us not only a revival of hope, but a much improved chance of making very real improvements in the symptoms of individuals suffering from multiple sclerosis. Even better, the shot itself—needle, syringe, and contents—usually costs less than $10. And a nurse can teach you how to give these injections to yourself right at home.

Chapter 23:

A vitamin victory over psoriasis

If you're one of the 5 million people in the United States suffering from psoriasis, you know just how resistant to treatment it can be. Conventional medicine generally treats psoriasis with topical cortisone preparations. While these can alleviate the symptoms of psoriasis, there are a number of potential side effects including bruising, changes in skin color, and dilated blood vessels. In addition, it is common for a patient to become resistant to the cortisone preparation after several months of treatment, which means that dosages must be consistently increased.

Food allergies and sensitivities are common in most cases of psoriasis, so thorough testing and desensitization should be done under the supervision of a physician. Once allergies have been determined and treated, there are a number of vitamins, minerals, and herbs that can drastically improve—even eliminate—psoriasis.

1.25 dihydroxy vitamin D is a naturally occurring metabolite of vitamin D that can be very effective for most cases of psoriasis. However, it is available only by prescription through compounding pharmacists. To locate a compounding pharmacy in your area, contact the International Academy of Compounding Pharmacists at (800)927-4227 or www.iacprx.org.

Vitamin B12 and folic acid are also helpful in treating psoriasis. To achieve the highest level of relief, these nutrients should be taken over the same period of time. (Just keep in mind that it can take two to three months to experience results.) Because the dosages required are fairly large—1,000 to 3,000 micrograms of vitamin B12 daily and 50 milligrams of folic acid taken two or three times per day—you might need a prescription from a doctor skilled in nutritional medicine. For a referral to one in your area, contact the American College for Advancement in Medicine at (800)532-3688 or www.acam.org.

The rapid cell division that occurs in psoriasis is attributed to an abnormal ratio of two different cell growth-regulating factors. This ratio can often be normalized with an herbal remedy called Forskolin, which is often used in Ayurvedic medicine. Forskolin does not appear to have any toxic side effects and is available in many health food stores, as well as through the Tahoma Clinic Dispensary (425-264-0059; www.tahomadispensary.com). Most preparations offer 5 milligram tablets and capsules; take two or three of these daily, for a total dose of 10 to 15 milligrams per day.

In medicine, the element nickel is usually thought of as a "bad guy"—a frequent cause of skin reactions to jewelry (nickel dermatitis). But, as ironic as it sounds, relatively recent research has shown that nickel can be a very effective treatment for psoriasis when it's combined with another natural substance called bromide. Often, psoriasis disappears completely. Other times, it's substantially improved. It's worth trying—especially since the quantities of nickel and bromide required are quite low and adverse reactions are few.

For more information on some specific nickel-bromide preparations, contact Loma Lux Laboratories at (918)664-9882 or www.lomalux.com.

Chapter 24:

Heal cuts and bruises faster than ever

Digestive enzymes are one of the most useful tools I've used in my practice for accelerating the healing process and suppressing inflammation.

Pancreatin (usually from a beef, pork, or lamb source), bromelain (from pineapple), papain (from papaya), and other "plant source" digestive enzymes are all effective. Three or four tablets or capsules should be taken three or four times daily on an empty stomach. Try to avoid food for at least an hour (if possible) before and after. Taking the enzymes before unavoidable trauma (like surgery), as well as after, makes the treatment even more effective.

If the injury is an accident, you can start taking the enzymes as soon as reasonably possible, and you should continue until you're completely healed.

Enzymes are nontoxic and are safe for even small children, although they don't need as much to do the same job. For children too small to swallow capsules or tablets, chewable enzymes (which usually are pineapple- or papaya-flavored and taste good) are very useful.

If you've never tried this approach before, I think you'll be pleasantly surprised: Swelling goes down more rapidly, there's less pain, and injuries are "back to normal" much more quickly. Enzymes are available at any natural food store, as well as through online vitamin distributors.

In the case of people who bruise very easily, supplemental vitamin K is a good idea. Severe vitamin K deficiency causes uncontrollable bleeding, but mild to moderate degrees of such a deficiency don't ordinarily cause such obvious problems. Easy bruising is one physical sign of such mild to moderate deficiency. While easy bruising can also be due to a lack of flavonoids (which help keep small blood vessels strong), it's definitely safe and worth a try to use supplemental vitamin K (5 to 10 milligrams daily) to try to stop the problem. After six to eight weeks, it should be possible to tell whether it's helpful or not.

Alternative Health Resources

American Academy of Environmental Medicine (AAEM)
Phone: (316)684-5500; www.aaem.com

American Association of Naturopathic Physicians
Phone: (866)538-2267; www.naturopathic.org

American College for Advancement in Medicine (ACAM)
Phone: (888)439-6891; www.acam.org

International College Integrative Medicine
Phone: (866)464-5226; www.icimed.com

Meridian Valley Laboratory
Phone: (425)271-8689; www.meridianvalleylab.com

Nutrition & Healing
www.WrightNewsletter.com

Tahoma Clinic (for appointments only)
Phone: (425)264-0059; www.tahoma-clinic.com

Tahoma Dispensary (for supplement orders only)
Phone: (425)264-0051 or (888)893-6878; www.tahomadispensary.com

References

Part I: Cancer

Toss your sunscreen and step out of the shadows!
You can prevent skin cancer and still enjoy time the sun this summer

[1] Wang Z et al.. Ultraviolet irradiation of human skin causes functional vitamin A deficiency, preventable by all-trans retinoic acid pre-treatment. *Nature Medicine* 1999; 5(4): 418-422

The cancer-fighting mineral you can't afford to ignore

[1] Eskin BA, Shuman R, Krouse T, Merion JA. Rat mammary gland atypia produced by iodine blockade with perchlorate. *Cancer Res.* 1975 Sep;35(9):2332-9.

[2] Aceves C, Anguiano B, Delgado G. Is iodine a gatekeeper of the integrity of the mammary gland? *J Mammary Gland Biol Neoplasia* 2005 Apr;10(2):189-96.

[3] Shrivastava A, et al. Molecular iodine induces caspase-independent apoptosis in human breast carcinoma cells involving the mitochondria-mediated pathway. *J Biol Chem.* 2006 Jul 14;281(28):19762-71

[4] Arroyo-Helguera O, Anguiano B, Delgado G, Aceves C. Uptake and antiproliferative effect of molecular iodine in the MCF-7 breast cancer cell line. *Endocr Relat Cancer.* 2006 Dec;13(4):1147-58.

[5] Tretsch D, et al. Acute iodide intoxication with cardiac irritability. *Arch Int Med* 1074;134:760-762

The "unimportant" molecule curing cancer: Do-it-yourself tips for boosting your levels—without Big Pharma's help

[1] Tinley TL, Leal RM, Randall-Hlubek DA, et al. "Novel 2-methoxyestradiol analogues with antitumor activity." *Cancer Research* 2003; 63: 1,538-1,549

[2] Pribluda VS, Gubish ER Jr., Lavallee TM, et al. "2-methoxyestradiol: an endogenous antiangiogenic and antiproliferative drug candidate." *Cancer Metastasis Rev* 2000; 19(1-2): 173-179

[3] Golebiewska J, Rozwadowski P, Spodnik JH, et al. "Dual effect of 2-methoxyestradiol on cell cycle events in human osteosarcoma 143 B cells." *Acta Biochemica Polonica* 2002; 49(1): 59-65

[4] Drissa A, Bennani H, Giton F, et al. "Tocopherols and saponins derived from Argania spinosa exert an antiproliferative effect on human prostate

cancer." *Cancer Invest* 2006; 24(6): 588-592

[5] Mueck AO, Seeger H, Huober J. "Chemotherapy of breast cancer-additive anticancerogenic effects by 2-methoxyestradiol?" *Life Sci* 2004; 75(10): 1,205-1,210

[6] Gomez LA, de Las Pozas A, Reiner T, et al. "Increased expression of cyclin B1 sensitizes prostate cancer cells to apoptosis induced by chemotherapy." *Mol Cancer Ther* 2007;6(5): 1,534-1,543

[7] Schumacher G, Hoffmann J, Cramer T, et al. "Antineoplastic activity of 2-methoxyestradiol in human pancreatic and gastric cancer cells with different multidrug-resistant phenotypes." *J Gastroenterol Hepatol* 2007; 22(9): 1,469-1,473

[8] Mueck AO, Seeger H, Wallwiener D, Huober J. "Is the combination with 2-methoxyestradiol able to reduce the dosages of chemotherapeutics in the treatment of human ovarian cancer? Preliminary in vitro investigations." *Eur J Gynaecol Oncol* 2004; 25(6): 699-701

[9] Golebiewska J, Rozwadowski P, Spodnik JH, et al. "Dual effect of 2-methoxyestradiol on cell cycle events in human osteosarcoma 143 B cells." *Acta Biochemica Polonica* 2002; 49(1): 59-65

[10] Shogren KL, Turner RT, Yaszemski J, Maran A. "Double-stranded RNA-dependent protein kinase is involved in 2-methoxyestradiol-mediated cell death of osteosarcoma cells." *J Bone Miner Res* 2007: 22(1): 29-36

[11] She MR, Li JG, Guo KY, et al. "Requirement of reactive oxygen species generation in apoptosis of leukemia cells induced by 2-methoxyestradiol." *Acta Pharmacologica Sinica* 2007; 28(7): 1,037-1,044

[12] Fong YC, Yang WH, Hsu SF, et al. "2-methoxyestradiol induces apoptosis and cell cycle arrest in human chondrosarcoma cells." *J Orthop Res* 2007; 25(8): 1,106-1,114

[13] Miller KD, Haney LG, Pribluda VS, Sledge VW. "A phase I safety, pharmacokinetic and pharmacodynamic study of 2-methoxyestradiol (2ME2) in patients with refractory metastatic breast cancer." *Proceedings of the American Society of Clinical Oncology* 2001; 170: 20-43a

[14] Davoodpour P, Landstrom M, Welsh M. "Reduced tumor growth in vivo and increased c-Abl activity in PC3 prostate cancer cells overexpressing the Shb adapter protein." *BMC Cancer* 2007; 7: 161

[15] Ho A, Kim YE, Lee H, et al. "SAR studies of 2-methoxyestradiol and development of its analogs as probes of anti-tumor mechanisms." *Bioorg Med Chem Lett* 2006; 16(13): 3,383-3,387

[16] Tinley TL, Leal RM, Randall-Hlubek DA, et al. "Novel 2-methoxyestradiol analogues with antitumor activity." *Cancer Research* 2003; 63: 1,538-1,549

[17] "Drug found effective in treating, preventing breast cancer," Science Daily (www.sciencedaily.com), 11/4/07

[18] Cicek M, Iwaniec UT, Goblirsch MJ, et al. "2-methoxyestradiol suppresses osteolytic breast cancer tumor progression in vivo." *Cancer Res* 2007; 67(21): 10,106-10,111

[19] Miller KD, Haney LG, Pribluda VS, Sledge VW. "A phase I safety, pharmacokinetic and pharmacodynamic study of 2-methoxyestradiol (2ME2) in patients with refractory metastatic breast cancer." *Proceedings of the American Society of Clinical Oncology* 2001; 170: 20-43a

[20] Miller KD, Haney LG, Pribluda VS, et al. "A phase I study of 2-methoxyestradiol (2ME2) plus docetaxel in patients with metastatic breast cancer." *Proceedings of the American Society of Clinical Oncology* 2002; 21: 111a.

[21] Dahut W, Lakhani NJ, Gulley JL, et al. "Phase I clinical trial of oral 2-methoxyestradiol, an antiangiogenic and apoptotic agent, in patients with solid tumors." *Cancer Biology & Therapy* 2006; 5(1): 22-27

[22] Sweeney C, Liu G, Yiannoutsos C, et al. "A phase II multicenter, randomized, double-blind, safety trial assessing the pharmacokinetics, pharmacodynamics, and efficacy of oral 2-methoxyestradiol capsules in hormone-refractory prostate cancer." *Clinical Cancer Research* 2005; 11: 6,625-6,633

[23] Salama SA, et al. "Estrogen metabolite 2-Methoxyestradiol induces apoptosis and inhibits cell proliferation and collagen production in rat and human leiomyoma cells: a potential medicinal treatment for uterine fibroids." *J Soc Gynecol Invest* 2006; 13: 542-550

Part II: Heart

Could a stroke steal your future?

[1] Keli S et al. Dietary flavonoids, antioxidant vitamins, and incidence of stroke: the Zutphen Study. *Arch Int Med* 1996;156(6) 637-642

[2] Joshipura KJ et al. Fruit and vegetable intake in relation to risk of ischemic stroke. *JAMA* 1999;282(13):1233-1239

[3] Khaw KT, Barrett-Connor E. Dietary potassium and stroke-related mortality: a 12-year prospective population study. *NEJM* 1987;316(5):235-40

[4] Liu S et al. Whole grain consumption and risk of ischemic stroke in women: a prospective study. *JAMA* 2000;284;(12):1534-1540

[5] Bone K, Mills S. Hawthorn. In Principles and Practice of Phytotherapy. Churchill Livingstone, London, 2000. pp. 439-447

[6] ibid, pp. 404-417

[7] Murray M. Gotu Kola. in The Healing Power of Herbs, Prima Publishing, Rocklin, California, 1995. pp. 173-183

[8] Bone K, Mills S. Hawthorn. In Principles and Practice of Phytotherapy. Churchill Livingstone, London, 2000. pp. 439-447

[9] Sumi H et al. A novel fibrinolytic enzyme (nattokinase) in the vegetable cheese natto, a typicl and popular food in the Japanese diet. *Experientia* 1987;43:1110-1111

[10] Sumi H et al. Enhancement of the fibrinolytic activity in plasma by oral administration of nattokinase. *Acta Haematol* 1990;84:139-145

Part III: Pain

Two weeks to bursitis relief minus the aspirin, NSAIDs, and cortisone shots

[1] Klemes, Irving, M.D. Vitamin B12 in acute subdeltoid bursitis. *Industrial Medicine & Surgery* 1957; 26:290-292.

Part IV: Diabetes

Five steps to curing the common condition your doctor may be overlooking

[1] Laboratory Medicine 1975; 6(2): 10-20

Do-it-yourself pain relief for diabetic neuropathy: Even the "last resort" is natural and side-effect-free!

[1] Jamal GA, et al. "Gamma-linolenic acid in diabetic neuropathy," *Lancet* 1986; 1: 1098

[2] Ziegler D, et al. "Treatment of symptomatic diabetic neuropathy with the anti-oxidant alpha-lipoic acid," *Diabetologica* 1995; 38: 1,425-1,433

[3] Ruhnau KJ, et al. "Effects of 3-week oral treatment with the antioxidant thioctic acid (alpha-lipoic acid) in symptomatic diabetic polyneuropathy," *Diabet Med* 1999; 16: 1,040-1,043

[4] Hixson JR. "Hot stuff for diabetic neuropathy:capsaicin," *Med Tribune*, 9/14/89, pages 12-13

[5] Lee P, Chen R. "Vitamin D as an analgesic for patients with Type 2 diabetes and neuropathic pain," *Arch Intern Med* 2008; 168(7): 771-772.

Get your type 2 diabetes under control... without a single drug

[1] Yin, J., H. Xing, et al. (2008). Efficacy of berberine in patients with type 2 diabetes mellitus. *Metabolism* 57(5): 712-7.

[2] Zhang, Y., X. Li, et al. (2008). Treatment of type 2 diabetes and dyslipidemia with the natural plant alkaloid berberine. *J Clin Endocrinol Metab* 93(7): 2559-65.

[3] Turner, N., J. Y. Li, et al. (2008). Berberine and its more biologically available derivative, dihydroberberine, inhibit mitochondrial respiratory complex I: a mechanism for the action of berberine to activate AMP-activated protein kinase and improve insulin action. *Diabetes* 57(5): 1414-8.

[4] Lee, Y. S., W. S. Kim, et al. (2006). Berberine, a natural plant product, activates AMP-activated protein kinase with beneficial metabolic effects in diabetic and insulin-resistant states. *Diabetes* 55(8): 2256-64.

[5] Ma, X., T. Egawa, et al. (2010). Berberine-induced activation of 5'-adenosine monophosphate-activated protein kinase and glucose transport in rat skeletal muscles. *Metabolism.*

[6] Hwang, J. T., D. Y. Kwon, et al. (2009). AMP-activated protein kinase: a potential target for the diseases prevention by natural occurring polyphenols. *N Biotechnol* 26(1-2): 17-22.

[7] Zhang, H., J. Wei, et al. (2009). Berberine lowers blood glucose in type 2 diabetes mellitus patients through increasing insulin receptor expression. *Metabolism* 59(2): 285-92.

[8] Kong, W. J., H. Zhang, et al. (2009). Berberine reduces insulin resistance through protein kinase C-dependent up-regulation of insulin receptor expression. *Metabolism* 58(1): 109-19.

[9] Chen, C., Y. Zhang, et al. (2010). Berberine inhibits PTP1B activity and mimics insulin action. *Biochem Biophys Res Commun* 397(3): 543-7.

[10] Yu, Y., L. Liu, et al. (2009). Modulation of glucagon-like peptide-1 release by berberine: in vivo and in vitro studies. *Biochem Pharmacol* 79(7): 1000-6.

[11] Al-masri, I. M., M. K. Mohammad, et al. (2009). Inhibition of dipeptidyl peptidase IV (DPP IV) is one of the mechanisms explaining the hypoglycemic effect of berberine. *J Enzyme Inhib Med Chem* 24(5): 1061-6.

[12] Ni YX (1988) Therapeutic effect of berberine on 60 patients with type II diabetes mellitus andexperimental research [article in Chinese]. *Zhong*

Xi Yi Jie He Za Zhi 8:711–713.

[13] Wei J, Wu J, Jiang J, Wang S, Wang Z (2004). Clinical study on improvement of type 2 diabetesmellitus complicated with fatty liver treatment by berberine [article in Chinese]. *Zhong Xi Yi JieHe Ganbing Za Zhi* 14:334–336.

[14] Xie P, Zhou H, Gao Y 2005 The clinical efficacy of berberine in treatment of type 2 diabetes mellitus [article in Chinese]. *Chin J Clin Healthcare* 8:402–403.

Part V: Digestion

Age and antacids—a double whammy against your body's optimal health

[1] Reference cited in Wright JV and Lenard L, Why Stomach Acid Is Good for You, Natural Relief From Heartburn, Indigestion, and GERD, Chapter 5.. M. Evans and Company, New York City, 2001

[2] Dial S, Delaney JA, Barkun AN, Suissa S. Use of gastric acid-suppressive agents and the risk of community-acquired Clostridium difficile-associated disease. *JAMA* 2005 Dec 21;294(23):2989-95.

[3] Yang YX, Lewis JD, Epstein S, Metz DC. Long-term proton pump inhibitor therapy and risk of hip fracture. *JAMA* 2006 Dec 27;296(24):2947-53.

[4] Laheij RJ, et al. Risk of community-acquired pneumonia and use of gastric acid-suppressive drugs. *JAMA* 2004 Oct 27;292(16):1955-60.

[5] Clemons TE, Milton RC, Klein R, Seddon JM, Ferris FL 3rd; Age-Related Eye Disease Study Research Group. Risk factors for the incidence of Advanced Age-Related Macular Degeneration in the Age-Related Eye Disease Study (AREDS) AREDS report no. 19. *Ophthalmology* 2005 Apr;112(4):533-9.

[6] Age-related Eye Disease Study Group (AREDS). Risk factors associated with Age-related macular degeneration, *Ophthalmology* 2000:107:2224-2232.

[7] Henry EB, Carswell A, Wirz A, Fyffe V, McColl KE. Proton pump inhibitors reduce the bioavailability of dietary vitamin C. *Aliment Pharmacol Ther*. 2005 Sep 15;22(6):539-45.

[8] All references cited in Wright JV and Lenard L, Why Stomach Acid Is Good for You, Natural Relief From Heartburn, Indigestion, and GERD, Chapter 5. M. Evans and Company, New York City, 2001

The 99.9 percent effective technique for eliminating gallbladder attacks forever

[1] Breneman, James C. Basics of Food Allergy. Springfield (IL): CC Thomas (pub), 1978.

[2] Breneman JC Allergy Elimination as the Most Effective Gallbladder Diet. *Annals of Allergy* 1968; 26; 83-89

Part VI: Immune System

Dangerous grains linked to serious disease!

[1] H gene theory of inherited autoimmune disease. *Lancet* 1980; 1(8165): 396-8

[2] Braly, James and Ron Hoggan. Dangerous Grains: Why Gluten Cereal Grains May Be Hazardous to Your Health. New York: Avery Penguin Putnam, July 2002.

5 ways to make sure you've had your last bout with the common cold: And 3 cures you never knew could work so well

[1] "Listing of the ISTERH/NTES/HTES '07 Scientific Program," International Society for Trace Element Research in Humans website (http://www.angelfire.com/nd/isterh/2007conference/glimpse.html), accessed July 28, 2007

[2] Prasad AS, Fitzgerald JT, Bao B, Beck FW, Chandrasekar PH. "Duration of symptoms and plasma cytokine levels in patients with the common cold treated with zinc acetate. A randomized, double-blind, placebo-controlled trial," *Ann Intern Med*;133(4): 245-252

[3] Eby GA, Davis DR, Halcomb WW. "Reduction in duration of common colds by zinc gluconate lozenges in a double-blind study." *Antimicrob Agents Chemother* 1984;25(1): 20-24

[4] "History of Zinc Lozenges in Treating and Curing Common Colds" George Eby Research website (http://george-eby-research.com/html/history.html), accessed July 28, 2007

Part VII: Women's Health

Forget your annual mammogram! New tool offers better, earlier breast cancer detection (and it's pain-free, too!)

Kuhl CK. "The 'Coming of age' of non-mammography screening for breast cancer." *JAMA* 2008; 299(18): 2,203-2,205

Miller AB, Baines CJ, To T, Wall C. "Canadian National Breast Screening Study: 1. Breast cancer detection and death rates among women aged 40 to 49 years." *CMAJ* 1992; 147(10): 1,459-1,476

Miller AB, To T, Baines CJ, Wall C. "The Canadian National Breast Screening Study-1: breast cancer mortality after 11 to 16 years of follow-up. A randomized screening trial of mammography in women age 40 to 49 years." *Ann Intern Med* 2002; 137(5 Part 1): 305-312

Miller AB, Baines CJ, To T, Wall C. "Canadian National Breast Screening Study: 2. Breast cancer detection and death rates among women aged 50 to 59 years." *CMAJ* 1992;147(10):1477-88

Warner E, Plewes DB, Hill KA, et al. "Surveillance of BRCA1 and BRCA2 mutation carriers with magnetic resonance imaging, ultrasound, mammography, and clinical breast examination." *JAMA* 2004; 292(11): 1,317-1,325

Leach MO, Boggins CR, Dixon AK, et al; MARIBS study group. "Screening with magnetic resonance imaging and mammography of a UK population at high familial risk of breast cancer: a prospective multicenter cohort study (MARIBS)." *Lancet* 2005; 365(9,473): 1,769-1,778

Tilanus-Linthorst M, Verhoog L, Obdeijn IM, et al. "A BRCA1/2 mutation, highbreast density and prominent pushing margins of a tumor independently contribute to a frequent false-negative mammography." *Int J Cancer* 2002; 102(1): 91-95

Lehman CD, Isaacs C, Schnall MD, et al. "Cancer yield of mammography, MR and US in high-risk women: prospective multi-institutional breast cancer screening study." *Radiology* 2007; 244(2): 381-388

Sardinelli F, Podo F, D'Agnolo G, et al. "Multicenter comparative multi-modality surveillance of women at genetic-familial high risk for breast cancer (HIBCRIT study): interim results." *Radiology* 2007; 244(2): 698-715

Part VIII: Men's Health

Drop the finasteride!

[1] Hart JP, Cooper WL. Vitamin F in the treatment of prostatic hypertrophy. Report Number 1, Lee Foundation for Nutritional Research, Milwaukee, Wisconsin, 1941.

[2] Bush IM, et al. Zinc and the prostate. Presented at the annual meeting of the American Medical Association, Chicago, 1974

[3] Fahim MS, Fahim Z, et al. Zinc treatment for reduction or hyperplasia

of the prostate. *Fed Proc* 1976;35:361

[4] Thompson IM, Goodman PJ, Tangen CM, Lucia MS, Miller GJ, Ford LG, Lieber MM, Cespedes RD, Atkins JN, Lippman SM, Carlin SM, Ryan A, Szczepanek CM, Crowley JJ, Coltman CA. The influence of finasteride on the development of prostate cancer. *N. Engl. J. Med.* 2003 Jul 17;349(3):215-24

[5] De Stefani E, Deneo-Pellegrini H, Boffetta P, et al. Alpha-linolenic acid and risk of prostate cancer: a case-control study in Uruguay. *Cancer Epidemiol Biomarkers Prev* 2000;9:335-8.

[6] Ramon JM, Bou R, Romea S, et al. Dietary fat intake and prostate cancer risk: a case-control study in Spain. *Cancer Causes Control* 2000;11:679-85.

[7] Pandalai PK, Pilat MJ, Yamazaki K, et al. The effects of omega-3 and omega-6 fatty acids on in vitro prostate cancer growth. *Anticancer Res* 1996;16:815-20.

[8] De Toit PJ, van Aswegen CH, du Plessis DJ. The effect of essential fatty acids on growth and urokinase-type plasminogen activator production in human prostate DU-145 cells. *Prostaglandins Leukot Essent Fatty Acids* 1996;55:173-7.

[9] Leitzmann MF, Stampfer MJ, Wu K, Colditz GA, Willett WC, Giovannucci EL. Zinc supplement use and risk of prostate cancer. *J Natl Cancer Inst.* 2003 Jul 2;95(13):1004-7.

[10] Imamov O, Lopatkin NA, Gustafsson JA. Estrogen receptor beta in prostate cancer. *N. Engl. J. Med.* 2004 Dec 23;351(26):2773-4.

Part IX: Anti-Aging, Memory, Hearing, and Vision

Five ways to avoid that hearing aid

[1] Ochi K, Kinoshita H, Kenmochi M, Nishino H, Ohashi T. Zinc deficiency and tinnitus. *Auris Nasus Larynx.* 2003 Feb;30 Suppl:S25-8.

[2] Arda HN, Tuncel U, Akdogan O, Ozluoglu LN. The role of zinc in the treatment of tinnitus. *Otol Neurotol.* 2003 Jan;24(1):86-9.

The mineral breakthrough helping terminal patients defy death: And why you should be taking a little of it, too

[1] Moore G J, et al. "Lithium-induced increase in human brain grey matter." *Lancet* 2000; 356: 1,241-1,242

[2] Chuang DM, Hashimoto R, Kanai H., et al. "Lithium stimulates

progenitor proliferation in cultured brain neurons." *Neuroscience* 2003; 117(1): 55-61

[3] Nonaka S, Chuang DM. "Neuroprotective effects of chronic lithium on focal cererbral ischemia in rats." *Neuroreport* 1998; 9(9): 2,081-2,084

[4] Manji HK, Chen G, Moore GJ. "Lithium at 50: Have the neuroprotective effects of this unique cation been overlooked?" *Biological Psychiatry* 1999; 46(7): 929-940

[5] Chuang DM. "Lithium exerts robust neuroprotective effects in vitro and in the CNS in viv Therapeutic implications." *Neuropsychopharmacology* 2000; 23(S2): S39

[6] Takashima A, Murayama M, Murayama O, et al. "Lithium inhibits amyloid secretion in COS7 cells transfected with amyloid precursor protein C100." *Neuroscience Letters* 2002; 321(1-2): 61-64

[7] Diaz-Nido J, Alvarez G, Avila J, et al. "Lithium protects cultured neurons against beta-amyloid-induced neurodegeneration." *FEBS Letters* 1999; 453(3): 260-264

[8] Zhong J, Lee WH. "Lithium: a novel treatment for Alzheimer's disease?" *Expert Opin Drug Saf* 2007; 6(4): 375-383

[9] Schrauzer GN, Shreshta KP. "Lithium in drinking water and the incidence of crimes, suicides, and arrests related to drug addiction." *Biological Trace Elements Research* 1990; 25: 105-113

[10] McMillan TM. "Lithium and the treatment of alcoholism: a critical review." *British Journal of Addiction* 1981; 76: 245-258

[11] Fornai F, Longone P, et al. "Lithium delays progression of amyotrophic lateral sclerosis." *Proc Natl Acad Sci* USA 2008; 105(6): 2,052-2,057

Forget those needles—erase your wrinkles with a powdered drink mix: Plus 2 other all-natural age-fighters your skin will thank you for

[1] Kantor I, Donikyan LA, Simon R, Wollschlaeger B. "Results of a study evaluating the use of a dietary supplement formula in the management of age-related skin changes in women with moderate to severe wrinkling of the peri-orbital area." Stephen Kemp & Associates (www.how-to-reverse-skin-joint-aging.info), accessed 11/12/07

[2] Punnonen R, Vaajalahti P, Teisala K. "Local oestriol treatment improves the structure of elastic fibers in the skin of postmenopausal women." *Ann Chir Gynaecol Suppl* 1987; 202: 39-41

[3] Schmidt JB, Binder M, Demschik G, et al. "Treatment of skin aging

with topical estrogens." *Int J Dermatol* 1996; 35(9): 669-674

[4] Purba MB, Kouris-Blazos A, Wattanapenpaiboon N, et al. "Skin wrinkling: can food make a difference?" *Journal of the American College of Nutrition* 2001; 20(1): 71-80

Part X: Essential Health Secrets

Vitamin K: What's it good for?

[1] *J Dent Res* 1948;27:235-241

[2] *J Canad Dent Assoc* 1943;9(8):359-356

[3] Merkel RL. The use of menadione bisulfite and ascorbic acid in the treatment of nausea and vomiting of pregnancy. *Am J Ob Gyn* 1952;64(2):416-418

[4] Kubovic M et al. Analgesic effect of vitamin K. *Proc Soc Exp Biol Med* 1955;90:660-662

[5] Hart JP et al. Circulating vitamin K levels in fractured neck of femur. *Lancet* 1984;2:283

[6] Hart JP et al. Electrochemical detection of depressed circulating levels of vitamin K1 in osteoporosis. *J Clin Endocrinol Metab* 1985;60:1268-1269

[7] Tomita A. Post-menopausal osteoporosis: 47Ca study with vitamin K2. *Clin Endocrinol* (Japan) 1971;19:731-736.

[8] Knapen MHJ et al. The effect of vitamin K supplementation on circulating osteocalcin (bone Gla protein) and urinary calcium excretion. *Ann Intern Med* 1989;111:1001-1005

[9] Bouckaert JH Said AH. Fracture healing by vitamin K. *Nature* 1960;185:849

[10] Seyuma Y et al. Comparative effects of vitamin K2 and vitamin E on experimental arteriosclerosis. *J Vit Nutr Res* 1999;69(1):23-26

[11] Jie K-SG et al. Vitamin K status and bone mass in women with and without aortic atheroclerosis. *Calcif Tiisue Int* 1996;59:352-356

[12] Mitchell T. Vitamin K. Life Extension (magazine) 2000;6(2):32-38

1 program, 2 months, lasting relief from almost any symptoms—And the older you are, the better it works

[1] James Breneman, James, M.D., Basics of Food Allergy, Springfield (IL): Charles C. Thomas Publisher, 1978

Send even the most stubborn infections—cold sores, toenail fungus, and more—into hiding for good

[1] Buck DS, Nidorf DM, Addino JG. "Comparison of two topical preparations for the treatment of onychomycosis: Melaleuca alternifolia (Tea Tree) oil and clotrimazole." *J Family Practice* 1994; 38(6): 601-605

[2] Bassett IB, Pannowitz DL, Barnetson RS. "A comparative study of tea-tree oil versus benzoyl peroxide in the treatment of acne. Medical Journal of Australia." *Med J Australia* 1990; 153(8): 455-458

[3] Satchell AC, Saurajen A, Bell C, et al. "Treatment of interdigital tinea pedis with 25% and 50% tea tree oil solution: a randomized, placebo-controlled, blinded study," *Australas J Dermatol* 2002; 43(3): 175-178

[4] Belaiche P. "Treatment of vaginal infections of Candida albicans with the essential oil of Melaleuca alternifolia." *Phytotherapy* 1985; 15: 13-15

[5] Pena EF. "Melaleuca alternifolia oil. Its use for trichomonal vaginitis and other vaginal infections," *Obstet Gynecol* 1962; 19: 793-795

[6] Wölbling RH, Rapprich K: *Der Deutsche Dermatologe* 1983; 10(31): 1,318-1,328

[7] Wölbling RH, Milbradt R. *Therapiewoche* 1984; 34: 1,193-1,200

[8] Koytchev R, Alken RG, Dundarov S. "Balm mint extract (Lo-701) for topical treatment of recurring herpes labialis," *Phytomedicine* 1999; 6(4): 225-230

[9] Saller R, Buechi S, Meyrat R et al. "Combined herbal preparation for topical treatment of Herpes labialis," *Forsch Komplementarmed Klass Naturheilkd* 2001; 8(6): 373-382

Harnessing the healing power of light
Part 1: What you need to know about UV rays—beyond sunburn

[1] Miner AL, Losina E, Katz JN, et al. "Infection control practices to reduce airborne bacteria during total knee replacement: a hospital survey in four states." *Infect Control Hosp Epidemiol* 2005; 26(12): 910-915

[2] Kujundzic E, Matalkah F, Howard CJ, et al. "UV air cleaners and upper-room air ultraviolet germicidal irradiation for controlling airborne bacteria and fungal spores." *J Occup Environ Hyg* 2006; 3(10): 536-546

[3] Ritter MA, Olberding EM, Malinzak RA. "Ultraviolet lighting during orthopaedic surgery and the rate of infection." *J Bone Joint Surg Am* 2007; 89(9): 1,935-1,940

[4] Miner AL, Losina E, Katz JN, et al. "Infection control practices to reduce airborne bacteria during total knee replacement: a hospital survey in four states." *Infect Control Hosp Epidemiol* 2005; 26(12): 910-915

[5] Kujundzic E, Matalkah F, Howard CJ, et al. "UV air cleaners and upper-room air ultraviolet germicidal irradiation for controlling airborne bacteria and fungal spores." *J Occup Environ Hyg* 2006; 3(10): 536-546

[6] Ritter MA, Olberding EM, Malinzak RA. "Ultraviolet lighting during orthopaedic surgery and the rate of infection." *J Bone Joint Surg Am* 2007; 89(9): 1,935-1,940

[7] Koek M, Buskens E, Steegmans P, et al. "UVB phototherapy in an outpatient setting or at home: a pragmatic randomized single-blind trial designed to settle the dispute. The Pluto study." *BMC Med Res Methodol* 2006; 6: 39

[8] Silva SH, Guedes ACM, Gontijo B, et al. "Influence of narrow-band UVB phototherapy on cutaneous microbiota of children with atopic dermatitis." *Journal of the European Academy of Dermatology and Venereology* 2006; 20(9): 1,114-1,120

[9] Marshall S. "Technology insight: ECP for the treatment of GvHD – can we offer selective immune control without generalized immunosuppression?" *Nature Clinical Practice Oncology* 2006; 3: 302-314

[10] Edelson R, Berger C, Gasparro F, et al. "Treatment of cutaneous T-cell lymphoma by extracorporeal photochemotherapy. Preliminary results." *NEJM* 1987; 316: 297-303

[11] Kumar V, Lockerbie O, Keil SD, et al. "Riboflavin and UV-light based pathogen reduction: extent and consequence of DNA damage at the molecular level." *Photochem Photobiol* 2004; 80: 15-21

[12] Edelson R, Berger C, Gasparro F, et al. "Treatment of cutaneous T-cell lymphoma by extracorporeal photochemotherapy. Preliminary results." *NEJM* 1987; 316: 297-303

[13] Vowels BR, Cassin M, Boufal MH, et al. "Extracorporeal photochemotherapy induces the production of tumor necrosis factor-? by monocytes: implications for the treatment of cutaneous T-cell lymphoma and systemic sclerosis." *Journal of Investigative Dermatology* 1992; 98: 686-692.

[14] Potashov LV, Cheminava RV. "Reinfusion of the patient's own irradiated blood in surgical patients." *Vestn Khir Im II Grek* 1980; 125(10): 144-146

[15] Boudurov N, Filipov ZH. "Effect of ultraviolet ray-irradiated autogenous blood on hematological indices in horses." *Vet Med Nauki* 1976;

13(10):11-19.

[16] Ivanov EM, Shakirova OV, Zhurayskaia NS. "Use of auto-transfusion of UV-irradiated blood in chronic bronchitis." *Klin Med* (Mosk) 2002; 80(6): 21-25

[17] Paleev NR, Vetchinnikov ON, Plaksina GV, Brucheeva IS. "The efficacy of the extracorporeal ultraviolet irradiation of autologous blood in the treatment of chronic nonspecific lung diseases." *Vestn Ross Akad Med Nauk* 1993; 3: 3-6

[18] Kuvshinchikova VN, Shmelev EI, Mishin VI. "Effectiveness of extracorporeal ultraviolet blood irradiation in treatment of chronic obstructive bronchitis in pulmonary tuberculosis." *Probl Tuberk* 1998; 3: 48-50

[19] Isaev IuV, Dzhangirova GM, Padenko AV, Lipikin AA. "Use of UV autologous blood irradiation for preventing the occurrence of tracheobronchitis during tracheostomy." *Vestn Khir Im II Grek* 1987; 138(4):116-118

[20] Alizade IG, Karaeva NT. "Experience in the use of auto-transfusions of laser-irradiated blood in treating hypertension patients." *Lik Sprava* 1994; May-Jun(5-6): 29-32

[21] McGlade JP, Gorman S, Zosky GR, et al. "Suppression of the asthmatic phenotype by ultraviolet B-induced, antigen-specific regulatory cells." *Clinical & Experimental Allergy* 2007; 37(9): 1,267–1,276

[22] Bernstein JA, Bobbitt RC, Levin L, et al. "Health effects of ultraviolet irradiation in asthmatic children's homes." *Journal of Asthma* 2006; 43: 255-262

[23] Paleev NR, Cherniakov VL, Vetchinnikova ON. "Ultraviolet irradiation of the blood in the treatment of pyo-inflammatory complications in patients with terminal renal failure." *Vestn Akad Med Nauk* SSSR 1991; 3: 15-20

[24] Gaiseniuk LA. "Use of re-infusions of isolated irradiated auto-blood for the correction of hematopoietic disorders." *Med Radiol* (Mosk) 1987; 32(11): 15-18

[25] Hansen E, Knuechel E, Altmeppen J, Taeger K. "Blood irradiation for intraoperative auto-transfusion in cancer surgery: demonstration of efficient elimination of contaminating tumor cells." *Transfusion* 1999; 39(6): 608-615

[26] Hansen E, Bechmann V, Altmeppen J. "Intraoperative blood salvage in cancer surgery: safe and effective?" *Transfus Apher Sci* 2002; 27(2): 153-157

[27] Sawyer L, Hanson D, Castro G, et al. "Inactivation of parvovirus B19 in human platelet concentrates by treatment with amotosalen and ultra-

violet A illumination." *Transfusion* 2007; 47(6): 1,062-1,070.

[28] Thai TP, Houghton PE, Campbell KE, Woodbury MG. "Ultraviolet light C in the treatment of chronic wounds with MRSA: a case study." *Ostomy Wound Manage* 2002; 48(11): 52-60

[29] Thai TP, Keast DH, Campbell KE, et al. "Effect of ultraviolet light C on bacterial colonization in chronic wounds." *Ostomy Wound Manage* 2005; 51(10): 32-45.

[30] Conner-Kerr TA, Sullivan PK, Gaillard J, et al. "The effects of ultraviolet radiation on antibiotic-resistant bacteria in vitro." *Ostomy Wound Manage* 1998; 44(10): 50-6.

[31] Phoenix DA, Harris F. "Light activated compounds as antimicrobial agents—patently obvious?" *Recent Patents Anti-Infect Drug Disc* 2006; 1(2): 181-99.

Harnessing the healing power of light
Part 2: Time-tested strategies for beating superbugs and more of today's deadliest health threats

[1] Douglass WC. Into the Light: Tomorrow's Medicine Today. Second Opinion Publishing, Inc, Dunwoody, GA 1995.

[2] www.Nobelprize.org

[3] Ude WH. *Journal of Surgery* 1943; 61(1)

[4] Knott EK. "Development of Ultraviolet blood irradiation," *American Journal of Surgery* 1948; 76: 165-171

[5] Hancock VK, Knott EK. "Irradiated blood transfusion in treatment of infections," *Northwest Medicine* 1934; 33: 200

[6] Miley G. *Archives of Physical Therapy* 1943; 23: 536

[7] Douglass WC. Into the Light: Tomorrow's Medicine Today. Second Opinion Publishing, Inc, Dunwoody, GA 1995.

[8] Rebbeck EW. "Ultraviolet irradiation of blood in the treatment of Escherichia coli septicemia," *Archives of Physical Therapy* 1943; 24: 158-167

[9] Rebbeck EW. "Ultraviolet irradiation of auto-transfused blood in the treatment of postabortional sepsis," *American Journal of Surgery* 1942; 55:476-486

[10] Miley GP. "Ultraviolet blood irradiation therapy in acute poliomyelitis," *Archives of Physical Therapy* 1946; 25: 651-656

[11] Miley G. *American Journal of Bacteriology* 1943; 45:303

[12] Edelson RL. "Photopheresis: a clinically relevant immunobiologic response modifier," *Annals of the New York Academy of Sciences* 1991; 636(1): 154-164

[13] Barr ML, Meiser BM, Eisen HJ, et al. "Photopheresis for the prevention of rejection in cardiac transplantation," *The New England Journal of Medicine* 1998; 339(24): 1,744-1,751

[14] Malawista S, Trock DH, Edelson R. "Treatment of rheumatoid arthritis by extracorporeal photochemotherapy: a pilot study," *Arthritis Rheum* 1991; 34: 646-654

[15] Ludvigsson J, Samuelsson U, Ernerudh J, et al. "Photopheresis at onset of type 1 diabetes: a randomized, double blind, placebo controlled trial," *Arch Dis Child* 2001; 85: 149-154

[16] Rostami AM, Sater RA, Bird SJ, et al. "A double-blind placebo-controlled trial of extracorporeal photopheresis in chronic progressive multiple sclerosism," *Neurology* 1990; 40(Suppl 1): 393-394

[17] Miley GP, Seidel RE, Christensen JA. "Preliminary report of results observed in 80 cases of intractable bronchial asthma," *Archives of Physical Therapy* 1943; 24: 533

[18] Miley GP, Seidel RE, Christensen JA. "Ultraviolet blood irradiation in apparently intractable bronchial asthma," Archives of Physical Medicine 1946; 27:24

[19] Douglass WC. Into the Light: Tomorrow's Medicine Today. Second Opinion Publishing, Inc, Dunwoody, GA 1995.

[20] Miley GP, Seidel RE, Christensen JA. "Ultraviolet blood irradiation in apparently intractable bronchial asthma," *Archives of Physical Medicine* 1946; 27:24

[21] Miley GP. "Efficacy of ultraviolet blood irradiation therapy in the control of Staphylococcemias," *American Journal of Surgery* 1944; 64: 313-322

[22] Miley GP, Christensen JA. "Ultraviolet blood irradiation therapy: Further studies in acute infections," *American Journal of Surgery* 1947; 73: 486-493

[23] Miley GP. "Present status ultraviolet blood irradiation (Knott technic)," *Archives of Physical Therapy* 1944; 25: 368-372.

[24] Miley GP, Rebbeck EW. "The Knott technic of ultraviolet blood irradiation as a control of infection in peritonitis," *Review of Gastroenterology* 1943; 10: 1

[25] Miley GP. "The Knott Technic of ultraviolet blood irradiation in acute pyogenic infections. A study of 103 cases with clinical observations on the effects of a new therapeutic agent," *New York State Journal of Medicine* 1942, 42(1): 38-46

[26] Miley GP, Christensen JA. "Ultraviolet blood irradiation therapy: Further studies in acute infections," *American Journal of Surgery* 1947; 73: 486-493

[27] ibid

[28] ibid

[29] Edelson R, Berger C, Gasparro F, et al. "Treatment of cutaneous T-cell lymphoma by extracorporeal photochemotherapy. Preliminary results," *New England Journal of Medicine* 1987; 316: 297-303

[30] Gollnick K. "Chemical aspects of photodynamic action in the presence of molecular oxygen." In Nygaard OF (ed): Radiation Research: Biomedical, Chemical, and Physical Perspectives. New York: Academic Press, 1975, pp. 590-611.

[31] Olney RC. "Treatment of viral hepatitis with Knott technic of blood irradiation," *American Journal of Surgery* 1955; 90: 402-409

[32] Dougherty TJ, Kaufman JE, Goldfarb A, et al. "Photoradiation therapy for the treatment of malignant tumors," *Cancer Research* 1978; 39: 2,628-2,635

[33] McCaughton JS. "Overview of experiences with photodynamic therapy for malignancy in 192 patients," *Photochemistry and Photobiology* 1987; 46: 903-909

[34] McCaughton JS, Doughtery TJ. "Summary of clinical reports of photodynamic therapy," *Postgrad Gen Surg* 1989

[35] Miley GP. "The Knott Technic of ultraviolet blood irradiation in acute pyogenic infections. A study of 103 cases with clinical observations on the effects of a new therapeutic agent," *New York State Journal of Medicine* 1942, 42(1): 38-46

[36] Miley GP, Rebbeck EW. "The Knott technic of ultraviolet blood irradiation as a control of infection in peritonitis," *Review of Gastroenterology* 1943; 10: 1

[37] Miley GP, Christensen JA. "Ultraviolet blood irradiation therapy: Further studies in acute infections," *American Journal of Surgery* 1947; 73: 486-493

[38] Miley G, Christensen JA. "Ultraviolet blood irradiation therapy in

acute virus-like infections," *Review of Gastroenterology* 1948; 15: 271-277

[39] Miley GP. "Ultraviolet blood irradiation," *Archives of Physical Therapy* 1942; 23: 536

[40] Miley GP. "Ultraviolet blood irradiation: Therapy in acute pyogenic infection at Hanhemann Hospital," *Hahnemannian Monthly* 1940

The two vitamins that could save your life in the ICU—and why many hospitals won't give them to you

[1] Powell-Tuck J. "Nutritional interventions in critical illness." *Proc Nutr Soc* 2007; 66(1): 16-24

[2] Goodyear-Bruch C, Pierce JD. "Oxidative stress in critically ill patients." *Am J Crit Care* 2002;11(6): 543-551.

[3] Bulger EM, Maier RV. "Antioxidants in critical illness." *Arch. Surg* 2001; 136: 1,201-1,207

[4] Lemineur T,Deby-Dupont G, Preiser JC. "Biomarkers of oxidative stress in critically ill patients: what should be measured, when and how?" *Curr Opin Clin Nutr Metab Care* 2006; 9(6) 704-10

[5] Abiles J, de la Cruz A, Castano J, et al. "Oxidative stress is increased in critically ill patients according to antioxidant vitamins intake, independent of severity: a cohort study." *Crit Care* 2006; 10(5): R146

[6] Crimi E, Sica V, Slutsky AS, et al. "Role of oxidative stress in experimental sepsis and multisystem organ dysfunction." *Free Radic Res* 2006; 40(7) 665-672

[7] Gutteridge JM, Mitchell J. "Redox imbalance in the critically ill." *Br Med Bull* 1999; 55: 49-75.

[8] Nathens AB, Maier RV, et al. "Randomized, Prospective Trial of Antioxidant Supplementation in Critically Ill Surgical Patients," *Annals of Surgery* 2002; 236(6): 814-822

[9] Preiser JC, Van Gossum A, Berre J, Vinvent JL, Carpentier Y. "Enteral feeding with a solution enriched with antioxidant vitamins A, C, and E enhances the resistance to oxidative stress." *Crit Care Med* 2000; 28(12): 3,828-3,832

[10] Berger MM. "Antioxidant functions of micronutriments in the general population and critically ill patients." *Nutrition Clinique et Metabolisme* 2004; 11(2): 125-132

[11] McGregor GP, Biesalski HK. "Rationale and impact of vitamin C in clinical nutrition." *Curr Opin Clin Nutr Metab Care* 2006; 9(6): 697-703

[12] Berger MM, Shenkin A. "Role of trace elements and other antioxidants in the critically ill." *Crit Car Ill* 2004; 19(4): 120-125

[13] Crimi E, Liguori A, Condorelli M, et al. "The beneficial effects of antioxidant supplementation in enteral feeding in critically ill patients: a prospective, randomized, double-blind, placebo controlled trial." *Anesth. Analg* 2004; 99: 857-863

[14] Friedl HP, Till GO, Ward PA. "Roles of histamine, complement and xanthine oxidase in thermal injury of skin." *American Journal of Pathology* 1989; 135: 203-217

[15] Horton JW. "Free radicals and lipid peroxidation mediated injury in burn trauma: the role of antioxidant therapy." *Toxicology* 2003; 189 (1-2): 75-88

[16] Tanaka H, Matsuda T, Miyagantani Y, et al. "Reduction of resuscitative fluid volumes in severely burned patients using ascorbic acid administration: a randomized, prospective study." *Arch Surg* 2000; 135: 326-331

[17] Matsuda T, Tanaka H, Yuasa H. "The effects of high-dose vitamin C therapy on postburn lipid peroxidation." *J Burn Care Rehabil* 1993; 14: 624-629

[18] Berger MM. "Antioxidant micronutrients in major trauma and burns: evidence and practice." *Nutr Clin Pract* 2006; 21(5): 438-449

[19] Sakr Y, Reinhart K, Bloos F, et al. "Time course and relationship between plasma selenium concentrations, systemic inflammatory response, sepsis, and multiorgan failure." *Br J Anaesth* 2007; 98 (6): 775-784

[20] Geoghegan M, McAuley D, Eaton S, Powell-Tuck J. "Selenium in critical illness." *Curr Opin Crit Care* 2006; 12(2): 136-141

Killer appliances? 9 ways to protect yourself from the new pollution more deadly than lead poisoning

[1] Milham S, Morgan L. "New electromagnetic exposure metric: high frequency voltage transients associated with increased cancer incidence in teachers in a California school," *American Journal of Industrial Medicine* 2008; 51(8):579-586

[2] Havas M, Stetzer D. "Dirty electricity and electrical hypersensitivity: five case studies," World Health Organization Workshop on Electrical Hypersensitivity, October 25-26, Prague, Czech Republic. (Accessed at www.stetzerelectric.com)

[3] Wertheimer N, Leeper E. "Electrical wiring configurations and childhood cancer." *Am J Epidemiol* 1979; 109: 273-284

[4] Milham S, Morgan L. "New electromagnetic exposure metric: high frequency voltage transients associated with increased cancer incidence in teachers in a California school," *American Journal of Industrial Medicine* 2008; 51(8):579-586

[5] Ahlbom A, Cardis E, Green A, et al. "Review of the epidemiologic literature on EMF and health." *Environmental Health Perspectives* 2001; 109 (Suppl 6): 911-933

[6] Green LM, Miller AB, Villeneuve PJ, et al. "A case-control study of childhood leukemia in southern Ontario Canada and exposure to magnetic fields in residences." *Int J Cancer* 1999; 82: 161-170

[7] Greenland S, Sheppard AR, Kaune WT, et al. "A pooled analysis of magnetic fields, wire codes, and childhood leukemia." *Epidemiology* 2000; 11: 624-634

[8] Kheifets LI, Afifi AA, Buffler PA, Zhang ZW. "Occupational electric and magnetic field exposure and brain cancer: a metaanalysis." *J Occup Environ Med* 1995; 37: 1,327-1,341

[9] Kheifets LI, Gilbert ES, Sussman SS, et al. "Comparative analyses of the studies of magnetic fields and cancer in electric utility workers: studies from France, Canada, and the United States." *Occup Environ Med* 1999; 56: 567-574

[10] Blackman C, Blank M, Kundi M, Sage C. "BioInitiative report: A rationale for a biologically-based public exposure standard for electromagnetic fields (ELF and RF)." The BioInitiative, 8/31/07. (Accessed at www.bioinitiative.org)

[11] "The Health Consequences of Involuntary Exposure to Tobacco Smoke: A Report of the Surgeon General." US Department of Health and Human Services (US DHHS), 2006. (Accessed at www.surgeongeneral.gov/library/secondhandsmoke)

[12] Hardell L, Carlberg M, Söderqvist F, et al. "Long-term use of cellular phones and brain tumours: increased risk associated with use for > or =10 years." *Occup Environ Med* 2007; 64(9): 626-632

[13] Lahkola A Tokola K, Auvinen A. "Meta-analysis of mobile phone use and intracranial tumors." *Scand J Work Environ Health* 2006; 32(3):171-177

[14] Kan P, Simonsen SE, Lyon JL, Kestle JRW. "Cellular phone use and brain tumor: a meta-analysis." *J Neurooncol* 2008; 86(1): 71-78

[15] Lowenthal RM, Tuck DM, Bray IC. "Residential exposure to electric power transmission lines and risk of lymphoproliferative and myeloproliferative disorders: a case controlled study." *Int Med J* 2007; 37(9): 614-619

[16] Stevens RG. "Electric power use and breast cancer: a hypothesis." *Am J Epidemiol* 1987; 125: 556-561

[17] Stevens RG, Davis S, Thomas DB, et al. "Electric power, pineal function, and the risk of breast cancer." *FASEB J* 1992; 6: 853-860

[18] Erren T. "A meta-analysis of epidemiologic studies of electric and magnetic fields and breast cancer in women and men." 2001. *Bioelectromagnetics* 2001; Suppl 5: S105-S119

[19] Havas M. "Dirty electricity elevates blood sugar among electrically sensitive diabetics and may explain brittle diabetes." *Electromagnetic Biology and Medicine* 2008; 27(2): 135-146

[20] Havas M, Stetzer D. "Dirty electricity and electrical hypersensitivity: five case studies," World Health Organization Workshop on Electrical Hypersensitivity, October 25-26, Prague, Czech Republic. (Accessed at www.stetzerelectric.com)

[21] Hakansson N, Gustavsson P, Johansen C, Floderus B. "Neurodegenerative diseases in welders and other workers exposed to high levels of magnetic fields." *Epidemiology* 2003; 14: 420-426

[22] Savitz DA, Checkoway H, Loomis DP. "Magnetic field exposure and neurodegenerative disease mortality among electric utility workers." *Epidemiology* 1998; 9: 398-404

[23] Blackman C, Blank M, Kundi M, Sage C. "BioInitiative report: A rationale for a biologically-based public exposure standard for electromagnetic fields (ELF and RF)." The BioInitiative, 8/31/07. (Accessed at www.bioinitiative.org)

[24] ibid

[25] www.electricalpollution.com

[26] ibid

[27] ibid

[28] Havas M, Stetzer D. "Graham/Stetzer Filters Improve Power Quality in Homes and Schools, Reduce Blood Sugar Levels in Diabetics, Multiple Sclerosis Symptoms, and Headaches." Presented at the International Scientific Conference on Childhood Leukemias, 9/6/04. (Accessed at www.electricalpollution.com)

[29] "The health effects of electrical pollution." National Foundation for Alternative Medicine. (Accessed at www.stetzerelectric.com)

[30] Havas M, Stetzer D. "Graham/Stetzer Filters Improve Power Quality in Homes and Schools, Reduce Blood Sugar Levels in Diabetics, Multiple

Sclerosis Symptoms, and Headaches." Presented at the International Scientific Conference on Childhood Leukemias, 9/6/04. (Accessed at www.electricalpollution.com)

[31] ibid

[32] "The health effects of electrical pollution." National Foundation for Alternative Medicine. (Accessed at www.stetzerelectric.com)

[33] Havas M, Illiatovitch M, Proctor C. "Teacher and student response to the removal of dirty electricity by the Graham/Stetzer Filter at Willow Wood School in Toronto, Canada." Presented at the 3rd International Workshop on the Biological Effects of Electromagnetic Fields, 10/4/04. (Accessed at www.emrpolicy.org)

[34] Havas M. "Electromagnetic hypersensitivity: Biological effects of dirty electricity with emphasis on diabetes and multiple sclerosis." *Electromagnetic Biology and Medicine* 2006; 25: 259-268

[35] www.electricalpollution.com

[36] Boyd EB. "Can you hear me now?" Conscious Choice, 9/08, p. 22

Nature's equal opportunity libido booster

[1] Vakina TN, et al. "Dehydroepiandosterone and sexual function in men with chronic prostatitis." *Urologia* 2003; Jan-Feb(1): 49-52